Praise for **HEALING WITHOUT HURTING**

"Pure excellence! I tell all my patients to read *Healing Without Hurting*. If you are a family with a special needs child, this book will give you the answers you've been looking for."

—Dr. Jared M. Skowron, Defeat Autism Now (DAN) doctor, vice president of the Pediatric Association of Naturopathic Physicians, and Amazon bestselling author of *100 Natural Remedies for Your Child*

"Jennifer Giustra-Kozek has used her experience as a therapist and mother to write a comprehensive guide book to inspire others. Her book is truly an invaluable resource for parents whose first priority is to 'do no harm'."

—Kelly Dorfman, MS, clinical nutritionist and award-winning author of *Cure Your Child with Food*

"*Healing Without Hurting* should be a bible for parents and physicians alike. If your child or patient is suffering from any of these biological disorders that negatively affect behavior and mental function, your solution is bound to be in here."

—William Kelley Eidem, natural health expert and author of *The Doctor Who Cures Cancer*

"I highly recommend this educational book, which offers a very useful guideline for all those who are seeking a way to improve their health and quality of lives aside from the mainstream of deceptive doctrines pushed by the profit-driven economy."

—Dr. Nick Moskalev, PhD in organic chemistry, www.Dyediet.com, and creator of Dye Diet Calculator of Health Risk and Nutritional Values of Any Packed Food

"The epidemics of autism, ADD/ADHD, and other neurobehavioral disorders have hit this country so rapidly that the medical community is struggling to provide answers for affected families. While it is possible to reverse these conditions in many children, the process for finding the right resources and healing strategies can be overwhelming. Jennifer Giustra-Kozek makes this process much more manageable for parents and healthcare providers alike. In *Healing Without Hurting*, Giustra-Kozek shares her encyclopedic knowledge of the many healing supports that can get a child onto the road of recovery. Whether you are just starting your healing journey or are a parent or caregiver who has 'tried everything' for your child, *Healing Without Hurting* is a fantastic resource."

—Beth Lambert, founder of Epidemic Answers and author of *A Compromised Generation: The Epidemic of Chronic Illness in America's Children*

"Truly inspirational! *Healing Without Hurting* should be mandatory reading for every parent, caregiver, and extended family member affected by autism, ADHD, apraxia, and even many mental health conditions challenging our families, educators, medical, and government services systems. Jennifer has incredible fortitude. *Healing Without Hurting* provides a list of comprehensive avenues to explore to improve the lives of affected children/adults. Her inspirational story paves the way for families to find a natural solution for their child, so they can have a better quality of life, a greater set of capabilities, more normal behavior and social integration, and in some cases, functional recovery."

—Douglas Baker, father of an autistic son, national speaker, special needs advisor, writer, educator, and advocate with over 20 years' experience assisting families in navigating the "special needs" community

"Jennifer has written an exceptional resource guide for any family that has a child with special needs. This is not only a must-read, but also a book you should tell all of your friends about because it will change their life. You will want to read *Healing Without Hurting* over and over again."

—Gary James, A4CWSN.com (Apps for Children with Special Needs)

"*Healing Without Hurting* is a much-needed breath of fresh air, given the fact that the author came from a western medical paradigm for treating mental issues that typically promotes the use of pharmaceuticals to manage symptoms. Jennifer shows us, step by step, how she used nutrition and other 'alternative' health practices to heal ADHD, autism, and neurodevelopmental issues. She makes clear that these disorders are not just mental issues, but medical issues of toxicity, gut dysbiosis, and nutritional deficiencies as well. It is my belief that as more and more mainstream practitioners, like Jennifer, discover how to recover their own children, they will be able to teach mainstream parents that there are natural solutions to healing their children."

—Maria Rickert Hong, certified holistic health counselor at AADP; owner of Maria Rickert Hong Nutritional Healing; mother of two sons recovered from sensory processing disorder, asthma, and acid reflux; board member and media director of Epidemic Answers, a 501(c)3 Non-Profit; media director of Canary Kids Film Project

HEALING WITHOUT HURTING

Treating ADHD, Apraxia, and Autism Spectrum Disorders Naturally and Effectively Without Harmful Medication

JENNIFER GIUSTRA-KOZEK, LPC, NCC

CHANGING LIVES PRESS

The information provided in this book is designed to provide helpful information on the subjects discussed. This book is not meant to be used, nor should it be used, to diagnose or treat any medical condition. For the diagnosis or treatment of any medical problem, consult your own physician or practitioner. The publisher and author are not responsible for any specific health or allergy needs that may require medical attention or supervision and are not liable for any damages or negative consequences from any treatment, action, application, or preparation given to any person reading or following the information in this book. References are provided for informational purposes only and do not constitute endorsement of any websites or other sources. Readers should be aware that the websites listed in this book may change.

Changing Lives Press
P.O Box 140189
Howard Beach NY
www.changinglivespress.com

Library of Congress Cataloging-in-Publication Data is available through the Library of Congress.

ISBN: 978-0-98945-298-4

Cover and interior design: Gary A. Rosenberg • www.thebookcouple.com

Printed in the United States of America

10   9   8   7   6   5   4   3   2   1

*In loving memory of the 26 beautiful lives
lost on December 14, 2012, at Sandy Hook Elementary,
and for all those who need love and healing!*

Contents

Contents

Acknowledgments

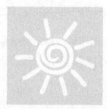

First, I would like to thank Evan, my spirited, angelic, loving boy who brings so much light and joy into our lives. His struggles and his determination to overcome them led to the writing of this book.

I would also like to thank my loving husband, Steve, for his unwavering support through our journey to help our son. Steve is the best dad a child could ask for. At times, cautious and skeptical, it was difficult for him to accept treatments that were far outside mainstream approaches. Thankfully, he showed faith, and it paid off big time for our family.

I would also like to thank my lovely daughter, Elaina, who has patiently waited through Evan's numerous medical appointments. She has been a wonderful and affectionate little sister.

In addition, I would like to thank all of the members of our family for their support and love. I thank my mom, Nancy, for sitting me on the counter as a young child to teach me how to cook nutritious meals. My dad, for giving me cod liver oil throughout my childhood and insisting that I do not eat too much fast food. I take inspiration from my grandparents. "Gran'ma" taught me how to garden and raid the beehives, always believing that healthy eating came from nature. And Grandpa passed down all of his baking recipes, believing that store-bought cookies were not as healthy as homemade. I want to thank Evan's great-aunt Joan, whose strong and consistent championing of alternative medicine, despite our initial resistance, put us on the right path, and Evan's grandmother, Carol, who was invaluable in finding creative, and delicious, ways to execute Evan's alternative treatments.

I must acknowledge Randy Peyser at Author One Stop who contributed to the success of this book by providing guidance and direction, along with my editors Hy Bender, Melanie Votaw, and pediatrician Allison Bloom, MD, who provided her medical expertise and polishing of my manuscript. Words cannot express my gratitude to Francesca Minerva at Changing Lives Press for believing in my project and understanding the importance of this book.

Foreword

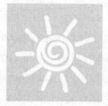

How does a family find the courage and strength to carry on when their child displays many behaviors that cause them alarm? How do they move past the day their child is diagnosed with a debilitating condition? What prevents them from becoming paralyzed in fear?

The answer is love. The love for a child can be so infinite that we as parents will do anything for them.

We enter parenthood with the naivety that childhood can be perfect, a wonderful time of life with no responsibilities or worries. We see our children smile at us. We hear them say, "Mama" and "Dada," and we watch them as they look at us to fix their boo-boos and change their dirty diapers. As they start to walk, they explore and find jubilation in simple things, like seeing a bird flying or listening to a dog barking.

Then, for some, that child is stolen away. The light doesn't shine in their eyes anymore. The innocent laughter is gone. The "Mama," "Dada," and "I love you" are not heard. Everything becomes a struggle. Screaming replaces laughter. Anger replaces joy. Sleep deprivation can be true torture.

We reach out to our families, we reach out to our pediatrician, and we reach out to the Internet. Many times we are told, "It's a phase" or "He'll grow out of it." But in reality, those are lies. This doesn't change. He doesn't grow out of it; it gets worse. Your friends and family members have similar age children who are growing up and learning the alphabet, but not your child. You wait, and wait, and wait, and wait . . . for nothing.

While you're waiting, every day can be worse than the last. Is this the joy of parenting you were hoping for? The struggles, the arguments, the depression? Eventually someone mentions the word "Autism" or "PDD-NOS," along with "There's no hope," or "He won't get any better," or "Put him in a home and forget about him." Those words sink like a lead weight into the soul. But you're a parent with infinite love for your child. You won't accept that for an answer. That's why you're reading this book. That's why you're reading this Foreword (which most people skip). It's because you have the conviction that there is an answer. You will not rest until you have wrestled your child back from whomever has stolen him. You will look under every rock and on every webpage until you find your solution. Trust me. You've found it.

I've been working with special needs children (autism, PDD-NOS, sensory, developmentally delayed, etc.) for over ten years of private practice. I have seen miracles. I have seen children talk when they couldn't talk before. I have seen children smile when they couldn't smile before. I have heard, "I love you, Mommy" in my office, and I have cried with the mothers sitting next to me, overjoyed that their child is coming back. I have heard pediatricians say, "This child's not autistic. They must have been misdiagnosed."

I have seen recovery, and it is possible. Please, please, please understand that there is hope. There is an answer. There is a solution to every problem. It's just that in the beginning of the twenty-first century, we're still trying to figure it out.

When Jenn Kozek walked into my office with her son, I was immediately impressed. She knew what she was talking about. She outpaced the knowledge of most of my colleagues. Jenn had the passion to fight for her child. She has accumulated the information to help your child, too, and most important, she describes it in the language of a mother. She shares with you her story—a story of hope, a story of recovery, a story that should be shouted from the mountains that you can have your child back!

Many of us look for someone to blame. The years taken from our child and from ourselves can never be regained. Even if you find the thief, they can't give you anything back. The answer lies elsewhere. The future is unwritten. Tomorrow can have a smile, a hug, a kiss, and even laughter. Believe.

Dr. Jared M. Skowron
Defeat Autism Now (DAN) Doctor
Vice President of the Pediatric Association of Naturopathic Physicians
Amazon bestselling author of *100 Natural Remedies for Your Child*

*"It takes a village to raise a child.
It takes a child with autism to raise
the consciousness of the village."*

COACH/SPEAKER ELAINE HALL

Introduction

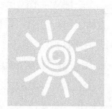

I'm a working psychotherapist who has over thirteen years of experience treating patients with attention deficit disorder (ADD), attention deficit hyperactivity disorder (ADHD), Asperger's syndrome, Tourette's syndrome, obsessive-compulsive disorder, and a myriad of other ailments.

All of the scores of psychiatrists and general practitioners I've encountered on the job have focused on medication as the primary treatment option. Yet, I always aimed at working with the more enlightened doctors who recognized the importance of therapy alongside their pharmaceutical treatments. This is because I've frequently seen medications change sweet and agreeable children into angry, depressed, and/or foggy kids their parents didn't recognize.

For a long time, I wondered about the cavalier prescribing of drugs but bit my tongue. Who was I to question physicians with the benefit of many more years of medical training?

This changed in 2006 after I gave birth to a sweet, funny, beautiful boy named Evan. After several years, my son was diagnosed as having ADHD, pervasive developmental disorder, obsessive-compulsive disorder, and apraxia. I was told he was on the mild to moderate end of the autism spectrum.

At first, I was in denial, but I also recognized the many signs that Evan had special challenges.

I knew doctors would eventually recommend medication. I also knew that I didn't want my son to go down that road for fear it would severely damage his lively, wonderful spirit.

As my husband, Steve, and I tried to make do with physical and behavioral therapies, I received a medical journal article from my aunt Joan about a link between malabsorption and malnutrition issues and apraxia. This led me to wonder whether Evan's disorders could be a medical illness treatable with natural remedies that didn't involve intrusive, personality-altering medication.

I started reading numerous medical journal articles and posts on the Internet from mothers who found alternative and natural treatments genuinely helpful. While I was skeptical at first, the potential rewards were so high that these methods outside the mainstream seemed well worth trying.

I'm now so grateful that my husband and I did try. It has made all the difference in Evan's health and well-being.

If you, your child, your relative, or your friend is struggling with ADHD or with one or more autism-related disorders, and you are looking for natural, effective treatments, this book is for you.

If you're a doctor, nurse, therapist, or other professional who deals with patients and craves something better than the hammer-like approach of mainstream medicine, this book is for you, too.

Everyone is different and requires individual care. So, rather than provide just one solution, I'll cover a full menu of natural treatment options that I discovered in my quest to help my son. You can pick and choose the ones that are the best fit for you or the person you're caring for, designing a personal treatment plan.

Conventional medicine is incredibly powerful for dealing with a variety of ailments, ranging from a broken leg to a heart attack. When it comes to more nuanced disorders, however, Western doctors are trained to virtually ignore holistic approaches and natural remedies—even when the latter aren't only cheaper and more effective, but sometimes the *only* good option.

This book is by someone who's been working for over a decade in the world of mainstream medicine and has a strong understanding of both its strengths and weaknesses. But I'm also a mom who fiercely loves her son, and for his sake, I explored all available options, eventually finding better solutions than any conventional specialist had ever offered.

If you feel frustrated or hopeless about the progress of your child, I've "walked in your shoes." I've been there and may well have the answers you've been seeking. At minimum, this book may provide you with a new way of evaluating your options and give you the tools you need to look beyond traditional treatments.

As you follow me on my journey, you may recognize, identify with, and relate to some of my stories. I recognize your stressors and your fears, and I support you on your own journey to treat and care for your child.

CHAPTER 1

Our Journey Begins

At thirty-two weeks pregnant, I found myself up in bed at 4:00 a.m. counting my contractions. Could I be going into labor eight weeks prematurely? By coincidence, my next gynecologist appointment was for that morning at 10:00 a.m. When I told the doctor my suspicions, she replied, "Oh, no, you're much too early. These must be Braxton Hicks contractions." But my body and instincts told me differently.

After twenty minutes in her office, my doctor wanted to send me home without completing an internal exam. I refused to leave. It was the first of a number of decisions contrary to doctor's orders that would save Evan's life.

After completing an internal exam, my doctor confirmed that I really was in labor. She told me to go across the street to the hospital. While the contractions intensified, I drove my car to the hospital's parking garage. As I waited by the hospital elevator, I pulled out my cell phone to reach my husband, Steve. Then I noticed a sign saying the elevator was out of order. In a panic, I began walking five long flights of stairs to the maternity floor.

I could feel that something wasn't right. The nurses hooked me up to a monitor and gave me an ultrasound immediately. It was bad news—little Evan was positioned with his butt down and his legs over his head like a jackknife. Luckily, the nurses told me his heartbeat was going strong, and they'd try to stop the contractions.

Steve arrived but couldn't do much other than comfort me. Still, that counted for a lot.

At 8:00 p.m., Steve left to get a bite to eat at a local Mexican restaurant. I hadn't eaten anything all morning, and since I might end up needing surgery, no one would feed me. I was starving.

As I waited for Steve, a doctor came in and told me they needed to keep me overnight because the contractions weren't slowing down as quickly as they had hoped. I began to worry that my instincts were right. I remembered how many times I had gone for fetal movement tests, concerned something was wrong with my son. I had never felt butterflies fluttering or those reassuring kicks everyone always talked about.

Steve returned within an hour and helped me get to the bathroom, despite the fact that I was hooked up to a bunch of IVs and monitor leads. When I returned to bed, I heard alarms, and hospital personnel scrambled into my room. I felt like my body was no longer my own. An oxygen mask was strapped around my mouth and nose. As tears ran down my face, I saw Steve being escorted out. An anesthesiologist asked me to roll onto my side, and he jammed an epidural into my spine. Within minutes, I couldn't feel my legs, and the doctors were performing an emergency Caesarean section.

My tiny baby boy was delivered within minutes, weighing four pounds, two ounces. I had one quick look at him before he was taken away by the neonatal intensive care unit (NICU) team. He had a full head of dark hair and a slightly flattened little nose.

I was told later that the team had needed to act quickly because his umbilical cord had been wrapped so tightly around his little body that it had caused his oxygen levels to drop. The medical team needed to work on him for quite a while.

How did this happen?

I was thirty-two when Steve and I tried to start a family. I considered myself relatively healthy. I had been on birth control pills for fifteen years and expected that, after being on them for so long, pregnancy would happen rather quickly. It actually took eight months to get the good news. I scheduled a GYN appointment to discuss infertility treatment options, and it was during that appointment that the nurse informed me I was approximately six weeks pregnant. A blood test confirmed the findings. Steve and I were elated.

I ate relatively well and exercised regularly during my pregnancy. I took my natural, whole-food prenatal vitamins after hearing that they were more bioavailable and contained more B "brain" vitamins than many of the prescribed counterparts. I also took omega-3 fish oil for over a year, and I followed all of the prenatal guidelines. I attended every scheduled appointment, drank plenty of water, and avoided raw eggs, tuna, and other big fish that could contain mercury. I avoided over-the-counter medications and alcohol, and I refused to get my hair dyed.

I had terrible heartburn, however, so my doctor insisted that taking an antacid was absolutely acceptable. I popped them like candy on some days without realizing how much aluminum they contain. (It wasn't until recently that I learned that too much aluminum can affect a baby's developing brain. Nor did I know that antacids, especially ones that contain aluminum, can interfere with iron, calcium, zinc, and magnesium absorption and function.) I had little nausea throughout my pregnancy, but perhaps some afternoon queasiness if I hadn't eaten. My blood pressure was always on the low to normal side.

With every ultrasound, I was reassured that my little baby was growing normally. I was at the doctor's office often so that they could perform a stress test or an additional ultrasound to monitor fetal movement. Each time, they told me that the baby's heartbeat was strong and that everything was all right. At twenty weeks, it was confirmed that I was having a little boy, and I started preparing his nursery. Most of my pregnancy was uneventful until the unforeseen happened.

Neonatal Intensive Care Unit (NICU)

Evan spent five and a half weeks in the NICU, mostly in an incubator. As a premature baby, his lungs were underdeveloped, and he lacked coordination for sucking, swallowing, and breathing. He had an underdeveloped digestive system; he couldn't even digest my breast milk.

Nevertheless, he was an attractive baby who enjoyed the comfort of familiar faces and daily routine. From birth, he benefited from lots of cuddles and love. One NICU nurse commented, "Evan is such a sweet baby and a definite snuggle bug—he nuzzles right up on my shoulder."

The doctors supplemented Evan's nutrition with an IV for weeks until he could finally metabolize my milk, and he was tube-fed until he was coordinated enough to breastfeed successfully.

After a few weeks in the NICU and only thirty-five weeks gestation, Evan started putting on some weight. The doctors wanted to give him his first of a series of three hepatitis B vaccines. I was concerned because he wasn't even a full-term baby yet, but I had always been a rule follower.

A soft-spoken and even-tempered neonatal physician reassured me that the benefits of vaccinating greatly outweighed the associated risks. Up to that point, I saw the doctors as angels on earth, and I was a very trusting person. After all, it was their quick decision to take Evan out of me by emergency C-section that saved his life, and it was their miraculous work that was giving him optimal health. So, when the neonatal doctor informed me that Evan needed his first shot before he left the hospital, I consented.

Evan continued drinking breast milk, breathing on his own, and gaining weight. When he weighed 5.5 pounds, the hospital decided to discharge him and let him come home with me.

Baby Days

I was so in love with my little boy as he gazed up at me with a look that said, "I love you, Mommy." I quickly learned within only a few days that Evan loved regular breastfeeding times, nap times, and bath times.

He loved his comfortable, cozy blankets and was a sensory-seeking baby. Like most infants, he liked to suck on a pacifier or his upper lip and seemed to need a soothing touch. However, he appeared sensitive to certain textures, tags or seams on his clothing, certain mushy foods, and loud noises. He became startled very easily. He had an aversion to bare feet on the grass and seemed to have many other sensory issues.

As a preemie, Evan started physical therapy almost immediately. The NICU sent us straight to a physiatrist at a pediatric rehabilitation center. He needed a prescription so that the insurance company would cover vigorous physical therapy. Well, that was a joke, considering it covered twenty visits per calendar year, and we needed to pay for the rest. I was thankful that Steve and I had some savings.

Evan was diagnosed with hip dysplasia due to his breech position and hypotonia (decreased muscle tone). Hip dysplasia in pediatrics/neonatal orthopedics is used to describe unstable/dislocated hips and poorly developed hipbone sockets. In addition, he had acute torticollis, a condition sometimes called "wry neck," and a flat head. A corrective helmet was recommended by the pediatric neurologist in the NICU.

A friend recommended a local craniosacral therapist, however, who was wonderful. It was my first taste of alternative treatment that proved successful. In weeks, she was able to correct Evan's flat head, and she resolved the torticollis within a few months.

As we started the long trek of treatment, it was recommended that Evan attend therapy sessions at least four days a week. This was the beginning of feeling that my life was no longer my own. I immediately went straight into Mommy Mode. I was lucky to be able to take five months off from my psychotherapy practice, because I felt it was my obligation to do everything I could to help my son. My own life took a backseat to his treatment, and I remember feeling increasingly alone as contact with my friends and colleagues dwindled.

As a first-time mother and the mother of a preemie, I listened to the advice of doctors and therapists who said that Evan was within the normal range for a premature baby and that he would catch up by age three. I was told that I needed to correct for his true gestational age, and that he was just a laid back and happy little fellow who enjoyed hours in his bouncy chair or baby swing. I realize now that being a "good" baby isn't always the best thing. He wasn't interested in exploring the world around him. He sat on my lap without a wiggle.

In the first year of therapy, we made very little progress. The inexperienced physical therapist told me that Evan was either extremely laid back or stubborn because, at almost a year old, he was still not rolling over. He was right-side dominant and didn't cross midline. Evan would protest with gut-wrenching screams when the therapist or I tried to put him on his belly or in the confines of a swaddling therapy swing.

Everyone told me that he probably had a slight developmental delay, but eventually he would really want something and would find a way to get it. A part of me believed them because I was a late walker myself, but I think a deeper part of me knew there was more going on.

CHAPTER 2

A Chronically Sick Child Is a Warning That Something Isn't Right

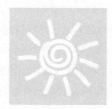

Even though Evan was a relatively easy baby who was content in his baby swing and could stay there for hours without a fuss, he was often sick. He had colds, viral-induced asthma, bronchiolitis, and respiratory illnesses such as pneumonia, sinus infections, RSV (respiratory syncytial virus), and GERD (gastroesophageal reflux disease). "He was a preemie. You should expect Evan to have a less than perfect immune system," the doctors assured us.

So, we gave Evan every recommended flu shot and immunization. We asked the pediatrician to spread out the vaccine schedule so that Evan did not receive more than two on any given visit.

We visited the pediatrician and ENT nearly twenty times that first year. Often, in the cold winter months, Evan developed croup, and I would need to wrap him in a blanket and take him for long car rides with the windows rolled down. Sometimes, I would have to give him a steroid and call for an ambulance in the middle of the night because he struggled to breathe.

Within days after the croup, Evan often developed bronchitis and a double ear infection. He would be up nights coughing for up to three weeks, for which he was treated with various antibiotics for serious sinus infections. These infections were followed by many more courses of antibiotics, which were necessary to prevent an even worse infection. What I didn't realize at the time was that, with every round of the meds, his immune system was damaged further.

He chronically and frequently excreted mucus from his eyes and got bad eye infections such as conjunctivitis or uveitis. Evan further suffered from chronic constipation. Not one doctor linked these sicknesses to a more serious digestive issue or suggested that he could be suffering from a systemic illness that needed to be researched further. The doctors almost always responded by treating Evan with more antibiotics and steroids to save him from infection and respiratory distress. For his constipation, they prescribed MiraLAX, which I know now was compounding the problem.

Evan's long parade of doctor visits was exhausting. Beyond his pediatrician, we saw many specialists. He needed to see an ear, nose, and throat specialist (ENT), a pediatric ophthalmologist, and an allergist. Each physician treated Evan's symptoms in isolation without considering how his different conditions might relate to each other and without taking into account that he was a severely sensitive child whose gut was reacting badly to the medications they prescribed. When Evan took an antibiotic, a bad yeast infection would typically follow.

He was very prone to thrush, athlete's foot, and other fungal infections. Doctors responded by treating him with heavy-duty antifungal medications that have the potential to cause liver damage.

Between the ages of ten months and three and one-half years, Evan had multiple surgeries. (I will discuss the potential damaging effects of anesthesia later on.) There were operations for ear tubes and adenoids, an eye stint to unblock his tear ducts, and a four-hour operation under anesthesia for hernia and testicle repair. Evan also had a tonsillectomy. During this surgery, the ENT discovered a large amount of scar tissue in his esophagus due to silent acid reflux. Prevacid was prescribed immediately.

Starting from age one-and-a-half, Evan developed trouble sleeping soundly, waking up many times during the night. I thought getting his tonsils removed would help, but it didn't. I brought him back to the ENT to check on whether his adenoids had grown back. They hadn't.

The doctor recommended Evan start on a small dose of melatonin, which is often recommended by both alternative and conventional physicians. Many parents told me melatonin really helped their child's sleep issues, but I was afraid to give it to Evan longterm after reading about the possible side effects. These include increased seizure activity, testicular atrophy (reduced testicle size and/or loss of function), and increased risk of type 2 diabetes, agitation, nightmares, constipation, and other behavioral changes. Also, I had read that melatonin supplementation could signal the body to stop making it naturally.

The tonsillectomy reduced the frequency of Evan's colds. However, when he did get sick, his "bad immune system" led to his taking a nebulizer with albuterol three to four times a day—and even so, his eyes got very congested. Within a couple of weeks, he was inevitably on another round of antibiotics for eye and sinus infections.

Evan was diagnosed by his pediatrician as having viral-induced asthma. She recommended we take him to an allergist and continue him on the necessary steroids. The allergist did a 150-common allergen test, during which Evan's skin didn't react to anything except dust mites. The allergist agreed with the pediatrician and recommended a slightly different steroid for bronchial flare-ups. At that time, I accepted that Evan wasn't "allergic" to anything. This was all before I realized the difference between a classic allergic reaction and a sensitivity or intolerance that inflames the gut and affects the immune system.

I also often wondered about sugar and the effects it could be having on Evan. If he didn't eat every two to three hours, he became irritable, emotional, anxious, frustrated, and cranky with a low attention span likely from the drop in blood sugar. Every doctor I consulted said, "It's normal for children to need to eat every few hours," or "Every child reacts negatively to sugar." So, I never thought anything else. Retrospectively, it seemed the hypoglycemia Evan was suffering from was causing some of his symptoms.

Hypoglycemia is a condition that occurs when a person's blood sugar (glucose) is too low. Some of the other symptoms of hypoglycemia include headaches, aggression, blurred vision, antisocial behavior, sugar addiction, faintness, and depression.

I later discovered while reading literature from the Hypo-glycemic Health Association, that allergies, including food allergies, as well as food intolerances/sensitivities, can be closely related to hypoglycemia due intestinal inflammation and the effect they can have on blood sugar (that is, from adrenaline surges after eating) and vitamin and mineral levels.[1]

Our friends and family told us that it was normal for young children to be sick frequently and that Evan was just building his immune system. But they were not living my life. Evan was sick for weeks at a time. Could everyone be wrong? Were we doing enough to keep him healthy? Was daycare the wrong environment for him?

No, that wasn't it. We did everything that was humanly possible. Yet, my son was still suffering. I felt guilty and confused.

CHAPTER 3
Developmental and Behavioral Concerns

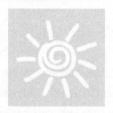

O n Evan's first birthday, I can remember clearly how he entertained people with his infectious smile and animated personality. He wore a light blue felt hat with a large candle sticking out of the top. He squealed with delight when surrounded by our friends and family and seemed to be acting for the video camera.

It was around this time, however, that it became increasingly clear that Evan wasn't developing normally. I had read numerous books about normal child development, so I became very concerned. When I asked for advice, people would say things like "Stop reading those books" or "He's a boy; they're all a little behind."

He wasn't pointing to things or using any gestures to communicate, and his language wasn't progressing past minor grunts.

He had great difficulty retaining information and would often "forget" what he was doing. He daydreamed and exhibited extremely low energy for a one-year-old boy.

Evan's speech started to emerge at age two and one-half. Most of the time, we couldn't understand one word he said. He sounded more like a little alien than a small child with his own high-pitched babbling language. He couldn't imitate sounds. He often groped for words, lost complete thoughts, and omitted or distorted consonants in a way that made his speech unintelligible.

There were instances that petrified me. One morning during

breakfast, I continuously had to prompt Evan to eat. He would take one bite, then sit at the table with a blank look on his face. When I asked him why he wasn't eating, he replied, "me a—ga ha." Surprisingly, I knew what he was saying. I sternly said, "Evan, you are home, honey. You are at our kitchen table eating your breakfast." He just looked at me with a puzzled stare.

I Was Uncoordinated as a Child, but This Was Ridiculous

It was clear that Evan was missing many of his important milestones. He didn't start rolling, standing, or crawling at the normal age. He enjoyed the outdoors and could spend hours in a sandpit, but he was unable to put objects into a container or take them out.

It wasn't until Evan was eighteen months old that he was finally sitting up without assistance, and he enjoyed watching the world around him. He played on a blanket with his favorite spinning toy, which lit up. He was only able to play with infant toys at this point, though, because he wasn't coordinated enough to operate anything too complicated.

When he fell, he would not catch himself with his hands, so he'd fall straight on his face, often scraping his face on a toy.

While Evan loved company, I became extremely discouraged on playdates with my girlfriends and their conventionally developing children. It pained me to watch the other children behaving so normally. I would also worry that Evan would get hurt, because he couldn't physically or verbally protect himself from other active boys his age.

Again, when I questioned this, his pediatrician and numerous therapists told me that he wasn't autistic because he was affectionate, smiled, and looked for praise. My gut feeling, even at that point, was that so many of his issues and behaviors mimicked that of an autistic child, so perhaps he was somewhere on the spectrum. But I didn't want to believe it. I choked on the "A" word many times, becoming very defensive and even angry when my mother-in-law, Carol, or my aunt, Joan, suggested that my son had autistic features.

I contacted Connecticut's early intervention sponsored services to have Evan evaluated. Fortunately, he qualified for its services, which eased financial pressures. When I asked for a definitive diagnosis from the Birth to Three team, however, they couldn't give me one.

By the time Evan reached age two, my heart was breaking. He struggled so much. All of the occupational, physical, and play therapy he was receiving was helpful, but he still couldn't walk. He felt frustrated and anxious with virtually every movement he made. I wanted so desperately to help him get better, but I often felt powerless to do so.

As time went on, it became more and more obvious that my little boy wasn't typical. At eighteen months old, he still struggled to roll. He wasn't crawling normally; instead, he scooted on his butt. He could stand but needed maximum assistance to do so. He could only sit on his own for short periods, and the fine motor pinch of his thumb and forefinger was slow to progress. He still didn't fully grasp time and space, showing little awareness of his surroundings.

Evan didn't start walking until he was twenty-six months old. It was Memorial Day weekend when he took his first wobbly steps unassisted. We were all elated, dancing around the kitchen. Evan looked up at us with glee in his eyes because he was as proud of himself as we were of him. It seemed like a "forever" journey, so the holiday barbeque turned into a "walking party" in his honor. It was perfect timing because the whole family had come over.

The progress continued from that day, but it was very slow. Despite Evan's many hours of therapy, he was very accident-prone. There were numerous falls, trips to the emergency room, and plastic surgery for stitches on his mouth and lips. He continued to fall straight on his face without any scrapes on his hands, arms, or elbows. There was still no defensive reaction that caused him to put his hands out to break his fall.

As a result, Evan became increasingly afraid of walking down a flight of stairs. He clung to the handrail and often forgot his footing. I would need to prompt him step by step on how to bend his knees and look carefully for the next step. Consequently, riding the Batman Big Wheel he got for his birthday was nearly impossible.

For your reference, I have included "Childhood Developmental Guidelines" in Appendix B to help you determine if your child is meeting all of the recommended milestones.

Beyond the Terrible Two's—My Poor Baby

I had a beautiful and seemingly happy two-year-old, except when he had terrible tantrums and fits of rage. I knew what the terrible two's looked like, and this was worse. His temper was so extreme that it frightened us at times.

Evan frequently hit himself and threw things. The simplest task could create a lot of frustration for him and send him into an episode of crying and screaming.

On one particular Christmas, he struggled desperately to use a little tow truck he had gotten from his grandfather. He needed to pull a small lever on the right side of the truck to work it, and even after numerous attempts to teach him, he couldn't figure it out. As the entire family watched, he sat there beating himself up, emotionally as well as physically. This type of scene was repeated often. As a psychotherapist and a mom, this concerned me most. I wanted my son to be a happy, well-adjusted kid with a good sense of self-esteem.

Yet, there was clearly a deeper part of him that knew something was wrong. It reminded me of when my grandmother started developing dementia. She would look in the mirror and ask out loud, "What's happening to me?"

At this point, my poor little boy still couldn't blow a bubble or stick out his tongue. Naturally, these inabilities escalated his anxieties, and he began showing signs of rigidity. He was rigid in his eating routines and also displayed rigid thinking patterns. He needed things in a certain way or order, and he would become very upset if we needed to change the original "plan."

He hoarded his toys, and he became extremely upset if his hands got dirty or sticky, so he wanted to wash his hands often. He displayed tic-like behaviors when he was anxious or tired, and he pulled at his face and eyelashes or sucked on his bottom lip. When one behavior seemed to wane, another one would pop up. Evan also exhibited pressure-seeking behavior, pushing his body against objects and people. He had difficulties with time and space—e.g., distinguishing where he ended and a table began. This led to such accidents as smacking his head numerous times against the table.

Additionally, Evan exhibited ritualistic behavior to soothe his fears and bring him a sense of control. He often retreated into his own silent world, focusing on one particular thing. He spent so much time in his head that it prevented him from engaging socially.

Evan's Sensory Issues

Evan's sensory issues seemed to also get worse during his toddler years. When he was about three, he was very excited to go to the *Max & Ruby* play at a community theater because it was his favorite cartoon. When we arrived, he jumped right in Steve's lap and became impatient because the show didn't start quickly enough for him. As soon as it began, though, Evan covered his ears and displayed some flapping gestures. He buried his head in his dad's shoulders. I vividly remember the disappointed look on Steve's face. We felt so heartbroken that Evan was going to miss the whole experience when he had looked forward to it so much.

Steve immediately covered Evan's ears with his hands to muffle some of the loud noises, and we were able to get through the rest of the performance.

Evan also craved undesirable objects and foods for sensation's sake. He would try to eat sand, pebbles, and rocks, especially on spring and summer days at the park when he would seek out the sandbox. We needed to watch him like a hawk. I had to do the Heimlich maneuver a handful of times because he shoved food into his mouth to the point that he made himself choke. Steve and I often felt on edge with the responsibility of keeping Evan alive.

One day, Grandpa came over with his homemade spicy chili. To my surprise, Evan dug right in. He actually couldn't get enough. Evan had always been a fairly good eater, but I thought it was strange for such a small child to appreciate a hot bowl of spicy chili. I later learned that children with low muscle tone often enjoy spicier foods.

A friend suggested books on sensory issues, so I read *The Out-Of-Sync Child* by Carol Stock Kranowitz, *The Sensory Processing Disorder Answer Book* by Tara Delaney, and *Raising a Sensory Smart Child* by Lindsey Biel and Nancy Peske. I also referred to the Sensory Processing Disorder Foundation website from time to time for the latest research.

Evan exhibited all of the signs of a sensory processing disorder. These resources were eye-opening and helped me greatly, giving me lots of hints and tricks for helping my son. I just had to be careful to not overanalyze every single thing.

For example, one fall afternoon when Evan was about three and one-half years old, we were walking in a park with my girlfriend Nicole and her two sons. Evan started stomping in the leaves and seemed amused by the rustling noise that he could make with his feet. I looked up at my girlfriend and said, "Oh, look at Evan; he's such a sensory kid."

She smiled and said, "Jenn, every three-year-old loves running through crunchy leaves." I had to laugh because I could easily forget that he was at times simply exhibiting normal childlike behavior.

Troubling School Days

Evan started a special education preschool program at age three. He loved being at school and enjoyed his highly structured school environment. Teachers reported that he was a pleasure to have in the class.

Nevertheless, Evan's obsessive behaviors were a problem, and he had a meltdown if his "plan" got disrupted in any way. He seemed off in his own world at times and became easily distracted by background noise.

He had a difficult time retaining the information that he was taught. His receptive language (the ability to receive information and understand instruction), for example, was better than his expressive language, so he couldn't always effectively demonstrate or communicate what he had learned.

Evan repeatedly ran out of the classroom and had trouble waiting his turn. When I asked him why he ran out, his answer was always, "Me no do. Me t—red." When asked a question, he frequently acted silly and guessed at answers. It was my belief that when things got tough, he bolted for the door; when he needed a break from sensory overload, he asked to go to the nurse or the bathroom; and when he became frustrated, he would joke around to distract the teachers.

Steve and I were afraid that as Evan advanced in school and didn't have the same level of hand-holding, he would encounter serious problems. His behaviors and attention issues could become a real roadblock to success, and we feared that he could quickly become discouraged and lose his enthusiasm for school altogether.

CHAPTER 4

My Search for
an Official Diagnosis

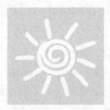

Much of the time, Evan was an absolute joy. He was a charming, warm, and loving child to whom everyone gravitated. He was a "pleaser," never wanting anyone to be mad at him.

I would look into my beautiful son's eyes, and I saw his gifts and spiritual nature. Evan was a single-minded little guy, inspired and focused in some areas and scattered in others. He was funny, quirky, and creative, a child who thought outside the box. He was helpful and cooperative. He was a visual learner who was imaginative, intuitive, eager, and friendly. I wanted to keep all of his wonderful attributes intact, and I was afraid if we ever needed to medicate him for his inattention and anxiety-related issues that he would be changed forever.

In our quest for a proper diagnosis, we visited a neurologist to get the appropriate tests and rule out worst-case scenarios. We needed to find out: Was Evan suffering from a brain tumor? Did he have a seizure disorder? Did he suffer from lack of oxygen at birth and have mild cerebral palsy?

An MRI and EEG were performed—and all the tests came back negative. The neurologist couldn't come up with any reason for Evan's behavior. Wasn't this the most informed person in the field of brain/neurological disorders? It was obvious Evan had something wrong neurologically, but this doctor was as puzzled as Evan's therapists. The neurologist told me that children develop at different paces. He said that I could take Evan to a physical therapist, but my son would probably be fine by age seven.

He also told us that we could go for genetic testing if we wanted, but those tests are often inconclusive and wouldn't change the treatment plan. As it turned out, this was terrible advice. Much later, I learned that genetic testing can prove immensely helpful in understanding root causes. It would help us identify nutritional deficiencies and neurotransmitter imbalances (more on that later).

Steve and I decided against the genetic testing because no one pointed us in the direction of low-cost and noninvasive genetic urine and saliva tests. We were already spending so much money on specialists that the thought of spending more and putting Evan through yet more testing didn't sit well with us.

As a psychotherapist, I just chalked Evan's symptoms up to a mental issue that was potentially genetic because my entire family has some form of learning disabilities, ADD, social awkwardness, anger, and anxiety-related issues. In addition, both my dad and I were late walkers. At the time, I had no idea my whole family was suffering from food sensitivities, gut issues, and gene mutations that affected the metabolism of essential nutrients, nor did I realize that these issues could have been remedied with appropriate nutritional therapies and complementary treatments and therapies.

The Therapies That Seemed to Work

We did take Evan to a behavioral optometrist and hearing specialist to rule out vision problems and hearing loss, however. The hearing test proved that Evan's hearing was within normal limits. The behavioral optometrist found that he had some issues with his ability to track and focus, so he suggested some practice at home and supplied us with eye exercises. Getting tested and treated by a qualified behavioral optometrist is often very helpful, especially with children who have issues with clumsiness, spatial awareness, dyslexia, and learning.

Meanwhile, we continued with specialized speech and occupational therapy and saw some good progress. Therapy was helping to harness the brain to heal itself. Using specific stimulation, brain balancing, and behavioral therapies, Evan's brain was being altered, and new pathways were being created. But in my heart, I felt there was more we could do to help our son. We were just at a loss as to what.

Evan had been in private therapies since birth, but he continued having a very difficult time with fine and gross motor skills. Tasks that required the utilization of his small muscles created a tremendous challenge for him. Brushing his teeth, getting dressed, and grasping a spoon, pencil, or crayon between his thumb and finger were difficult for him.

He also continued to struggle with coordinating his larger muscles to run, hop, and join in the regular activities of the other boys his age. He showed little to no potty-training readiness at age four. He didn't seem to know when he had an urge to go, never mind the physical ability to carry out the task.

His speech was still unintelligible. When he made sounds, they were distorted, repeated, or left out. People around him would lose the entire meaning of the words he spoke. He had many impaired social skills and lacked the ability to play imaginatively.

I felt his school was doing everything its budget allowed for, and I remained grateful for their attention, especially after talking with parents in other school districts who received considerably less for their children. Many of them needed to hire advocates and attorneys to force their school system to act. I felt extremely blessed that the teachers and therapists at Evan's school were working so hard on his behalf.

His school psychologist was hesitant to diagnose him with ADD or autism, however, since she wasn't a trained medical professional. School psychologists may sometimes use rating scales as a diagnostic tool to identify symptoms for their own knowledge but will often encourage parents to seek testing with a professional outside of the school setting.

As I noticed more and more that Evan exhibited many of the same traits as children on the autism spectrum, I grew impatient. I wanted more answers and an official diagnosis.

Was Apraxia Part of the Picture?

Interestingly, while I was attending an apraxia walk for my friend Michele's son, she observed Evan and pulled me aside to encourage me to make an appointment with Baron Therapy Services, LLC. She thought Evan might have apraxia (a specialized motor planning disorder) or what is sometimes called developmental dyspraxia, a neurological disorder beginning in early childhood. It can affect the motor planning of movements and coordination because brain messages are not correctly transmitted to the body.

My friend explained apraxia in more detail and told me that more than eighty-five percent of children with speech apraxia also have some gross motor and fine motor problems.

Michele also told me that going to her therapy practice would ensure that Evan got a thorough evaluation. She reassured me that if he needed treatment, he would be in the right place with professionals who understood how to treat apraxia and related disorders. She said, "Lisa, the director of Baron Therapy, has a gift that I have not encountered before. She understands apraxia and exactly how to treat it. She knows how to deal with behavioral challenges of children that often shut down in their therapy sessions when the work gets too difficult. She is a very talented therapist and, in my opinion, a true expert."

During this conversation, I learned that the therapeutic techniques used to treat apraxia are quite different from treatments provided by traditional speech and occupational therapists. Apparently, Michele had been to a few therapists who achieved nothing notable with her nonverbal son. It wasn't until she found her current therapists, who specialized in apraxia, that real progress was made. I was grateful for the information and happy that we could avoid the trials she had experienced. As a result of this meeting, I learned that a parent recommendation is one of the most valuable tools for finding a qualified diagnostician to evaluate your child.

I also discovered that it's essential to find speech therapists and occupational therapists who specializes in apraxia and autism spectrum disorders. It is important to find therapists who can conduct a thorough motor speech and motor skills evaluations. I was lucky to have a friend who was able to point me in the direction of a group of practitioners who are experts at evaluating and treating such disorders.

Finally, Some Understanding

I was very nervous walking into the specialist's office that Evan would be diagnosed with autism. However, I recognized that a proper diagnosis would help the therapists and teachers create a more specialized therapeutic treatment plan. Up to this point, I had never heard of any effective medical treatments for apraxia or autism, so I felt somewhat hopeless.

I sat there as the therapists played with him and completed their very thorough assessment. This experience was unnerving, but I felt in my heart that we were in the right place.

After the evaluation, the therapists brought me into their office to talk to me about what the tests had revealed. Lisa started by saying, "Evan has moderate to severe apraxia." Evan fell in the disordered range in almost all areas of physical and speech development.

Lisa went on to explain why Evan couldn't get himself out of a wicker laundry basket and why he couldn't fall "correctly" with arms down. It was because his body was never able to develop a "motor plan" to carry out the simplest of tasks. It finally all started to make sense.

It was also brought to my attention that although Evan babbled as a baby by saying "da, da, da, da," a more appropriate babble would have sounded like "da, ba, la, do, ba." A baby without apraxia starts to produce many variegated syllables while babbling.

Apraxia/Dyspraxia

Just what is apraxia? It's a disorder that can stand alone, or more often than not, it coexists with other conditions. It is a neurological-based motor planning disorder that impacts speech and often affects gross motor (crawling, walking, and jumping) and fine motor sequencing (writing, dressing, and brushing teeth). Confusion around this condition is reflected by the number of terms used to define it, including childhood apraxia of speech, developmental apraxia, developmental dyspraxia, and speech dyspraxia. Evan especially has trouble with motor planning. He was diagnosed with limb apraxia, oral motor apraxia, and speech apraxia.

A typical child is able to learn an action after performing it once or a few times. In contrast, Evan couldn't carry out even the simplest of tasks without significant repetition. He would need to move one foot in front of the other hundreds of times before mastering how to walk up stairs. This is an example of issues related to limb apraxia.

Evan also lacked proper muscle tone around his mouth, lips, and tongue, and he had extreme difficulty as a baby coordinating normal eating movements. These problems were most likely linked to oral motor apraxia.

He needed to create a memory for each and every movement of his lips, tongue, and mouth to create each and every consonant or vowel sound. This is symptomatic of speech apraxia.

The American Speech-Language-Hearing Association (ASHA) defines Childhood Apraxia of Speech (CAS) as "a neurological childhood (pediatric) speech sound disorder in which the precision and consistency of movements underlying speech are impaired in the absence of neuromuscular deficits (e.g., abnormal reflexes, abnormal tone). CAS may occur as a result of known neurological impairment, in association with complex neurobehavioral disorders of known or unknown origin, or as an idiopathic neurogenic speech sound disorder. The core impairment in planning and/or programming spatiotemporal parameters of movement sequences results in errors in speech sound production and prosody."[1]

Apraxia often causes many problems with general activities of daily living such as toileting. Besides his difficulties with toilet training, Evan had trouble dressing, putting on his socks and shoes, and imitating and repeating movements that come so naturally to other children. I took for granted the ability to dance and sing a song at the same time without thinking about it. Evan had to be taught in very small steps to do virtually everything, and he had to think about every movement to coordinate the simplest task. He would need to spend countless hours with an occupational therapist who knew how to treat apraxia and its motor planning challenges.

Evan was also diagnosed with pervasive developmental disorder, suggesting he wasn't severely autistic but exhibited some autistic features. He had a multifaceted neurobiological condition affecting his development of language, social interaction, and behavior. He also had some hyperactivity and attention-focusing issues that categorized him as ADHD, even though at times he would exhibit extremely low energy.

The speech and language pathologist (SLP) went on to discuss that her test pointed to some learning issues and a "sensory processing disorder," including sensory integration and self-regulatory issues. Evan experienced abnormal pain sensations, for example. He had balancing issues and a difficult time positioning himself in relation to the other neighboring parts of his body.

I felt less overwhelmed after the diagnosis was more clearly explained, and I was extremely comforted by the therapists' words, "These labels don't change who Evan is, but they help us understand how to treat him."

I also found so much support in the therapists' waiting rooms with parents who had patience and understanding. I talked to and learned quite a lot from other parents. For example, I learned that apraxia and autism are frequently accompanied by ADD/ADHD, anxiety, Tourette's syndrome, obsessive-compulsive disorder, and oppositional defiant disorder.

To learn more about speech apraxia, to locate a local chapter near you, or to find a SLP specializing in apraxia, please visit the Childhood Apraxia of Speech Association of North America (CASANA) at www.apraxia-kids.org.

CHAPTER 5

Outlining the Most Common Labels and Behaviors

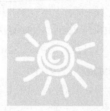

It's important to remember that many of the behaviors I am about to explain are common in "normal" or "healthy" children, and it has been my experience that some children are given psychiatric labels too prematurely. So we need to be careful that we are not over-diagnosing bright and creative children who are simply "marching to the beat of their own drum." However, in the cases of children like Evan, these behaviors are out of normal range for his age and chronic with a particular intensity and persistence. There is a significant overlap of many of these conditions, and there is a familial relationship among them.

I discussed apraxia in the last chapter, but let's look at some of the other common diagnoses.

ADD and ADHD

It's normal for all children to forget their homework or occasionally daydream in class. Children and adults with attention deficit disorder (ADD) and attention deficit hyperactivity disorder (ADHD), however, exhibit symptoms that become more and more prevalent.

Signs and Symptoms of ADD

• Seems spacey and off in his/her own world

- Appears unmotivated and lazy at times
- Inability to focus
- Easily distracted
- Under performs
- Guesses at answers and acts silly when asked a question
- Forgetful and has problems retaining information

Signs and Symptoms of Hyperactivity

- Interrupts others
- Runs out of the classroom
- Acts impulsively
- Has trouble waiting his/her turn
- Exhibits squirmy and fidgety behavior

Autistic Spectrum Disorders (ASD)

On March 20, 2013, the Centers for Disease Control (CDC) released a *National Health Statistics Report* indicating that approximately 1 in 50 of American school-aged children are on the autism spectrum. This study was released after the government surveyed 100,000 parents across the country. This number is significantly higher than the official government estimate of 1 in 88 American children in 2007. It supports the belief that many affected children are being missed by the surveillance methods the CDC uses to produce its official estimate. It also suggests that the rates are increasing. This study also revealed that school-aged boys were more than 4 times as likely as school-aged girls to have ASD.[1]

Children with ASD have mild to severe marked impairments in social interaction and communication, along with restricted, repetitive, and stereotyped patterns of behaviors, interests, and activities. These children often have difficulties regulating their emotions, and their thoughts can become rigid. This leads some children to obsessive thoughts and compulsive behavior. Some children with ASD exhibit ritualistic behavior called "stimming," which is short for self-stimulating behavior like hand-flapping or rocking.

Note that, for the purpose of this book, I will continue to recognize Asperger's syndrome and pervasive developmental disorders (PDD) as subtypes of autism, although there are significant changes in the definition of autism in the new edition of the *Diagnostic and Statistical Manual of Mental Disorders* (DSM-5). In the revised "bible" of psychiatry, any child exhibiting symptoms of autism will now be classified as having an autism spectrum disorder (ASD) and will no longer be broken down into subtypes. This manual is used by mental health professionals, insurance companies, schools, and other agencies responsible for covering or creating special provisions for individuals with developmental or mental disorders.

Many agree that this change will ensure that more children will get more therapy and more assistance. For example, some insurance companies were not covering services for Asperger's but were covering autism. This change will effectively alter that. On the other hand, some people are upset with the change because they believe that PDD and Asperger's must be recognized as separate disorders due to their less severe and unique features.

Pervasive Developmental Disorder

Pervasive developmental disorder (PDD) is a condition that falls on the autism spectrum and refers to a group of conditions that involve delays in development of many basic skills including talking, walking, communicating, socializing, using imagination, and understanding the world.

These kids typically fall behind their peer groups in many areas of development. Evan exhibited a delay in all of these areas and also shared many of the same behaviors of other more severely autistic children, including sensory processing issues and the desire to adhere to routines. He didn't have the same level of social impairment and was able to pick up on social cues easier than some children on the autism spectrum.

Evan did show some signs of impaired social interaction, such as poor eye contact. He often lived in his "head" in a daydreaming state instead of relating to the environment around him. Also, his verbal motor delays created many socially awkward moments for him. While everyone else was social, Evan couldn't complete a thought or verbalize it, never mind interact appropriately with peers his age.

He also displayed some of the same symptoms of autism like sleep issues, hyperactivity, temper tantrums, attention and focusing problems, apraxia, a learning disability, communication disorder, sensory issues, rigidity, finicky eating patterns, anger issues, and gastrointestinal problems. Still, Evan's problems were less extreme and fewer than for some children with severe autism.

Asperger's Syndrome—Impaired Social Skills

Children with Asperger's often have delays in the development of many basic skills; most notably, they lack nonverbal communication skills. They have problems interacting with peers and in groups. They often have poor eye contact and a difficult time picking up social cues —e.g., a friend stands in front of Michael, looking directly at him, his hands on his hips and his face taut, but Michael does not pick on the cues that indicate that his friend is upset with him.

Often these children show no sign of a cognitive or speech delay. However, they have problems socializing with others, using their imagination, and in some cases may also have problems feeling empathy for others. They have trouble making friends because of their dysfunctional social skills and have many problems maintaining reciprocal relationships. Children with Asperger's syndrome do not learn social skills the same way as typical children and need to be taught through social skills groups and other therapies.

At times, these children may not respond to their names when called and may act as if others around them do not exist. They may engage with adults long enough to get their needs met, but may ignore that same adult afterward. Adults are often more tolerant of the nonverbal skills deficits, so some Asperger's children often prefer to have relationships with adults over their peers.

Characteristically, these children appear awkward, exhibit eccentric repetitive movements, and often have limited interests. Often, they get stuck in a particular thought.

Childhood Disintegrative Disorder (CDD)

Disintegrative disorder (Heller's syndrome) is considered another subtype of autism. This rare disorder is normally diagnosed between the ages of two and ten years. Children with CDD have a marked regression in at least two areas of development, including language, self-help skills, social skills, and/or motor skills. The child begins losing important developmental milestones.

Landau-Kleffner Syndrome

Landau-Kleffner syndrome is manifested as a loss of language. A typically developing child starts to regress suddenly or gradually and loses the ability to comprehend and express themselves. It usually develops between ages three and seven, and it appears more common in males than females. Diagnosis of this syndrome is usually obtained by conducting an EEG and examining brain patterns during sleep. Individuals with this syndrome often also develop epilepsy (with or without convulsions). This syndrome is often diagnosed in conjunction with autism and may accompany symptoms of aggression, poor eye contact, rigidity, and sleep problems. According to Stephen M. Edelson, Ph.D., of the Autism Research Center in San Diego, California, the cause of Landau-Kleffner syndrome is not known. However, some suggested causes have been a dysfunctional immune system, exposure to a virus, toxins, and/or brain trauma.

Sensory Integration Disorders

Sensory integration disorder is not recognized in the DSM-5; however, many children with ASD appear to exhibit symptoms of this disorder. It is neurologically based and causes difficulties with taking in, processing, and responding to environmental stimuli. It occurs when sensory signals are not received through the senses in an organized way. This can cause inappropriate responses, behavioral problems, anxiety, and challenges in performing everyday tasks.

Learning Disabilities and Difficulties

Children with apraxia and ADHD often have special needs in the form of learning disabilities, as well as language and communication problems. I learned from experts in the field at apraxia and autism conferences that a multisensory approach to teaching is often best so that a child can participate more meaningfully in the classroom. It incorporates input that's visual, auditory, and tactile, which assists by doubling up on cues and giving the child more tools to remember and retain information.

For reading assistance to be the most successful, phonemic awareness and the structure of language must be taught in a structured and multisensory way. Many educators and experts in the field believe that the Wilson Reading System (WRS) is one of the most useful programs available.

Insomnia and Sleep Disorders

According to the May, 2004 edition of the *Journal of Sleep Research*, it is estimated that forty-three to eighty-three percent of children with autism have difficulty sleeping. The most frequent sleep problems quoted are difficulty falling asleep, restless sleep, not falling asleep in their own bed, and frequent waking. Among the least recorded are sleep walking, sleep apnea, and nightmares.[2] Evan had very inconsistent sleep routines, restlessness, and frequent and early waking.

Tourette's Syndrome

Tourette's syndrome is a neurological disorder characterized by multiple motor tics and at least one vocal tic—for example, motor tics may include continuous blinking of eyes, and vocal tics may include snorting or sniffing noises.

There seems to be comorbidity between tic disorders and other childhood disorders such as ADHD, OCD, and other specific learning disabilities. Although Evan was never officially diagnosed with Tourette's syndrome, I was concerned that Evan may have it. He would pull at his lips and eyelids, and suck on his bottom lip. He would also make sudden jerking movements. These behaviors intensified when he was anxious or tired, but would disappear while he slept. As he was a young child, I didn't believe Evan knew what he was doing or why.

As children get older, they often become more aware of their tic behavior and their inability to control it. Tourette's can affect their self-esteem and have many social impacts. As a psychotherapist, I was constantly thinking ahead. I knew medication is often used to control the OCD and tics—behavioral manifestations of an underlying anxiety disorder—but I also knew, from reading neuropsychology journals, that the use of stimulants and SSRIs intensifies tics for some children as well as adults.[3]

Seizures

Evan had frequent staring spells, so I, along with the therapists, worried that he might also have a seizure disorder. It's estimated that up to fifty percent of children on the autism spectrum suffer from seizures. These are caused by abnormal electrical activity in the brain and can produce a temporary loss of consciousness, body convulsions, unusual movements, and/or staring spells. Again, the thought of putting Evan on SSRIs and/or stimulants scared me. It has been widely publicized that these medications can contribute to the development of seizures.[4]

An EEG was performed on Evan, and the neurologist ruled out a seizure disorder. However, after recently reading *Silently Seizing* by Caren Haines, RN, I wonder if the testing failed to pick up a damaging seizure disorder.

Obsessive-Compulsive Disorder (OCD)

OCD is an anxiety disorder characterized by unreasonable thoughts and fears (obsessions) that lead a person to do repetitive behaviors (compulsions) to help relieve or manage anxious, fearful, or worrying feelings. Consciously, these individuals often realize that their thoughts are unreasonable and try to stop them. This usually increases the distress, and the individual is driven to perform even more compulsive acts.

Younger children with ADHD and/or autism are not generally diagnosed with OCD, yet they may display extremely rigid thoughts and repetitive behavior. As they become older, OCD may become one of their diagnoses.

Anger, Aggression, and Oppositional Defiant Disorder (ODD)

According to an article in *ADDitude*, "40% of children with ADHD will develop an Oppositional Defiant Disorder (ODD)."[5] This is characterized by temper tantrums and a pattern of uncooperative, angry, defiant, and sometimes hostile behavior. Symptoms must be perpetuated for longer than six months and must be considered beyond normal child behavior for a diagnosis to be given.

Signs and Symptoms of ODD

- Actively refuses to comply with rules
- Has a disregard for authority
- Deliberately annoys others
- Argues
- Blames others for own mistakes
- Often loses temper
- Is spiteful or seeks revenge
- Is touchy or easily annoyed

These behaviors often interfere significantly with academic and social functioning and can interrupt the family dynamic. Some experts suggest that ODD is tied to ADHD-related impulsivity or could be caused by the child's inability to cope with upsetting or painful emotions. ODD can also be accompanied by substance abuse and/or depressive disorders.

Depressive Disorders

The National Autistic Society published a guide geared toward understanding the mind and special challenges of a person with autism. It reminded me that children like Evan are vulnerable to depression and mood swing disorders (such as bipolar disorder) especially in late adolescence and in early adult life.[6] I was worried for my loving and happy son's future. I was concerned that if Evan did not resolve some of his issues and make significant gains that he might become depressed. I wanted him to be able to communicate his feelings and fit in with a peer group. I never wanted him to be bullied at school for being "different." I was concerned that others may take advantage of his sweet nature.

I wanted him to succeed in school to the best of his ability, and I didn't want him to start developing self-defeating thoughts. I was afraid that if he developed depression and a low self-esteem it could possibly lead to substance abuse, a dependence on pharmaceutical medication, and/or aggressive and violent behavior.

Most children with ADHD and autism are extremely loving and have the sweetest dispositions. Most of our children would never become angry or violent. However, we must not ignore the fact that some children with ADHD and autism do become socially withdrawn, anxious, angry, and depressed, and begin displaying impulsive behaviors. We must also recognize that the medication aimed to reduce these symptoms can actually make some children worse. Medications can potentially cause dangerous side effects, including paranoia, increased obsessive/compulsive thoughts and behaviors, and even psychosis. I fear that the wrong response to certain emotionally disturbed children can lead to more devastating tragedies, as witnessed on December 14, 2012, in Sandy Hook, Connecticut.

Given the options offered by both complementary and mainstream medicine, there is much to be said for "first do no harm" where natural therapies are undertaken to address underlying cause(s) of ADHD prior to falling back on more powerful but side effect–causing medications.

CHAPTER 6

Let's Talk About Medications

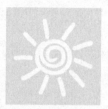

I was born and raised in the medical model. My mother was a nurse, and I went to graduate school to become a psychotherapist. I was trained by doctors in hospitals and by the pharmaceutical company reps who talked to me about the efficacy of certain medications to treat ADHD, anxiety, depression, panic attacks, obsessive thoughts and behaviors, and Tourette's.

As a psychotherapist for thirteen years, I spent years working with clients on stimulant drugs, and I knew that these drugs often came with the high price of negative side effects. I also knew that kids on the autism spectrum often react even more negatively to psychostimulants such as Ritalin because it prevents the natural breakdown of dopamine and can cause the levels to increase in a system with too much dopamine to begin with.[1] (Dopamine is a pleasure-producing neurotransmitter in the brain.)

Psychiatrists and doctors prescribe medication to help the person feel happier, more focused, and more cognitively stable. Medication blocks the reuptake of dopamine so that it circulates longer in the brain and so that it doesn't break down as quickly. It also works on another neurotransmitter called norepinephrine, which generally enhances a child's ability to concentrate and control impulsive behaviors. It works on the attention, motivation, and pleasure/reward centers in the brain.

When Evan was first diagnosed, I remember feeling very conflicted. Not medicating him went against everything I had learned from my psychiatrist mentors, graduate courses, and educational seminars on pharmaceuticals. Pharmaceutical reps told me repeatedly that "non-medicated" ADD/ADHD children were at a higher risk for alcohol and substance abuse because they would often look for ways to self-medicate their symptoms. I repeated those exact words to parents in my office who struggled with the decision to medicate their own children. I didn't know at that time that there may be safer or more natural ways to treat these symptoms or that many of these kids were suffering from a metabolic imbalance. And I certainly didn't want Evan to resort to addictive behaviors. After all, he comes from a family where substance abuse and alcoholism is rampant.

Still, I knew in my heart that medicating him was the last thing I ever wanted to do. I wanted to follow my motherly instincts even though I was afraid medication might be the only answer down the road despite the potential side effects.

Certainly, there are times that medication can be lifesaving—for example, in type 1 diabetes. If an individual has type 2 diabetes, they may need to take insulin to regulate blood sugar while they work on diet, exercise, and incorporate other healing practices. I also recognize that there are times when psychiatric medication may be necessary to prevent destabilization. We may need to use medication for a time as a "rescue remedy" while we address the many contributing factors and spend the time to heal and treat underlying conditions.

If your child is not in an acute state, you may be battling with the decision to medicate or not, and I realize it is not always an easy choice. You may have many questions and may feel very confused. The school may be telling you one thing, and your doctor may be telling you something completely different. Your child might be on medication already, and you don't want that. You may have already taken your child off a particular medication because it had more side effects than your child had symptoms, leaving you unsure where to turn next.

I am here to simply educate you about the types of drugs that are often prescribed to our kids and the benefits of each. In addition, I will provide a list of the potential side effects so that you can make a more informed decision. I am also here to balance the debate and speak of the ways these disorders can be treated naturally and effectively.

Most Frequently Prescribed Drugs for ADHD, Depression, and OCD

Medications are not prescribed for autism spectrum disorders, but for the symptoms and comorbid disorders associated with them.

Psychostimulants: Methylphenidate (Ritalin) and Similar Drugs

Psychostimulants are the primary drugs used to treat ADHD. These drugs increase circulating dopamine and stimulate the central nervous system; they can have a calming effect on a person with ADHD. These include Concerta, Ritalin, Metadate, Focalin, Dexedrine, Vyvanse, Adderall, Daytrana, and Methylin.

They work by blocking the reabsorption of the brain chemicals dopamine and norepinephrine. They increase blood flow to the prefrontal cortex of the brain that tends to be underactive in ADHD kids.

DID YOU KNOW?
Medications aimed at reducing ADHD symptoms contain some "inactive" ingredients that may actually cause neurotoxicity, digestive issues, and ADHD symptoms.

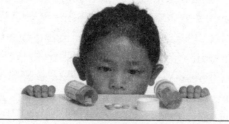

Nonstimulant: Atomoxetine (Strattera)

Strattera was the first FDA approved nonstimulant ADHD medication put on the market and the first one approved for the treatment of adult ADHD. The drug works by increasing the circulation of dopamine and norepinephrine, which are often lower than normal in individuals with ADHD.

Antidepressant: Bupropion (Wellbutrin)

Wellbutrin is commonly used in the treatment of ADHD, although it hasn't officially been approved by the FDA. It affects the reuptake of serotonin, norepinephrine, and dopamine neurotransmitters.

Antidepressants: Fluoxetine (Prozac), Paroxetine (Paxil), Sertraline (Zoloft), and Fluvoxamine (Luvox)

Prozac, Paxil, Zoloft, and Luvox belong in a class of drugs called selective serotonin reuptake inhibitors (SSRIs) and are used to treat a variety of conditions, including depression and other mental/mood disorders such as obsessive/compulsive disorder (OCD), post-traumatic stress disorder (PTSD), Tourette's syndrome (tics), social anxiety, panic disorders, and generalized anxiety disorders. These medications can help prevent suicidal thoughts/attempts and provide other important benefits.

Often, these drugs are combined with atypical antipsychotics such as aripiprazole (Abilify), most commonly used for aggression, and quetiapine (Seroquel) for manic depression, psychosis, and sleep disorders. These drugs are often added to SSRIs to enhance the effects by helping to adjust dopamine and serotonin.

Alpha-2 Agonists: Guanfacine and Clonidine

These include catapres (Clonidine) and guanfacine (Intuniv/Tenex). Intuniv was approved in 2009 for the treatment of ADHD in children as young as age six. These drugs are typically used in conjunction with a stimulant medication to enhance the treatment of impulsivity and hyperactivity. These medications regulate behaviors, attention, and emotion through acting on the alpha receptors in the prefrontal cortex of the brain.

So, What's the Harm?

In our quick-fix society, there are thousands of children each day marching to the nurse's office to take ADHD medication, Ritalin (methylphenidate), or another psychostimulant drug to help them focus and attend. They are also often prescribed psychoactive drugs such as Prozac, Paxil, and Zoloft for anxiety and depression. These drugs are designed to reduce symptoms quickly. However, it could be a dangerous solution if all factors aren't taken into consideration.

Evan was a good kid, and I knew it was only a matter of time before teachers and doctors would recommend medication to help him pay attention and focus more easily. In my heart, though, I knew that there wasn't a single pertinent drug out there without side effects. I imagined what a mess those effects could have on my son's developing brain.

Ongoing research suggests that early-life use of Ritalin (methylphenidate) affects brain development. A study published in *Biological Psychiatry* suggests that exposure of Ritalin in youth may later disrupt development of brain cells in the hippocampus, the region of the brain critical to memory, spatial navigation, and behavioral inhibition. Damage can lead to memory problems, disorientation, and depression in adulthood.[2]

In my practice, I had treated many older children diagnosed with ADHD, OCD, and depression—some of whom were also on the spectrum. I never really questioned the effects of the medications on their bodies. I did notice the stimulants often made my clients anxious or jittery, and sometimes more depressed and angry as well.

Often the doctors would reevaluate the medications and recommend a medication change or prescribe an atypical psychotropic mediction to the cocktail. In addition, they often recommended more intensive psychotherapy.

One of my private therapy clients, a younger man in his twenties, had been on psychotropic medication, from a young age. He was diagnosed by a psychiatrist as having bipolar disorder and ADHD. He also had many ASD features. He would come in and out of longer-term treatment facilities. The facilities would switch or increase his medications in an effort to stabilize him. The vicious cycle would continue; within six months, the police were called and he was back in a facility for violent and/or suicidal thoughts and behavior. Shortly after his last hospitalization, he started seeing me for individual psychotherapy. I spoke with his parents and encouraged him to see my naturopath. Lo and behold, his testing revealed that he had numerous food sensitivities and nutritional deficiencies. After approximately two months of treatment he was displaying remarkable progress. His eczema cleared up on his legs, his eye circles lessened, and he was gaining some weight. He stated that he felt better and his mood improved.

As published in *Child: Health Care and Development Journal*, "children with autism and ADHD can respond as well to stimulants as children with ADHD alone, with a reduction of many symptoms."[3] Yet we must not forget that many children on the autistic spectrum with ADHD symptoms do not respond as well to stimulant therapy. These medications can be ineffective and/or produce adverse effects such as increased anxiety, tics, mania, sleep disturbances, agitation, irritability, and worsening in behavior. As published in the *Journal of Developmental and Behavioral Pediatrics*, one particular study suggested that up to sixty-six percent of autistic children on stimulant medication may experience at least one negative side effect.[4]

We must also not forget, stimulant medication simply puts a Band-Aid on the problem, without addressing underlying causes. In addition, these medications mimic similar properties as "drugs on the street" and have some of the same side effects, including withdrawal and dependency, among many others.

Although some recent studies set out to refute the theory that stimulant medication can be addicting—especially among adolescents—I can personally attest to the countless times my drug-dependent clients told me that their drug addiction began when then started abusing their Adderall or Ritalin, and how they eventually graduated to bigger things. The U.S. Drug Enforcement Administration also stands strong in its beliefs. "Methylphenidate (Ritalin), a Schedule II substance, has a high potential for abuse and produces many of the same effects as cocaine or the amphetamines."[5]

Another interesting fact: according to Kenneth Bock, MD, author of *Healing the New Childhood Epidemics,* many autism spectrum kids already have too much circulating dopamine in their brains.[6] These drugs are so often doled out by conventional doctors and psychiatrists at the first sign of ADHD, but again, they can be ineffective or even harmful to a child on the spectrum. Rarely, if ever, do these doctors look deeper for possible medical causes and order specific metabolic, immunologic, and digestive testing before prescribing medications.

This can be a dangerous practice. If a child has too much circulating dopamine, he or she can become more impulsive, pleasure-seeking, aggressive, anxious, paranoid, compulsive, and filled with rage. One such compulsion could be to collect thousands of baseball cards. A more dangerous obsession could be to become infatuated with violent video games, guns, and mass shootings. Reading this was a lightbulb moment for me that explained why our medication practices may be pushing some kids toward rage and violent behavior.

While guns have been a common denominator in mass slayings at schools by teens, and there needs to be tighter laws on semiautomatic rifles, and stricter background checks to avoid loopholes, there's another familiar element that seems to be completely minimized, and that is the illness of the person pulling the trigger, planting a bomb, or bringing a knife to school.

There have been a numerous articles that have pointed to psychotropic medication as being linked to school shootings. One such article was featured on The Citizen's Commission on Human Rights website. "At least 31 school shootings and/or school-related acts of violence have been committed by those taking or withdrawing from psychiatric drugs resulting in 162 wounded and 72 killed. In other school shootings, information about their drug use was never made public."[7]

According to the Methylphenidate drug fact sheet, published by the National Institutes of Health–Medline Plus, Ritalin and similar drugs can also lead to other side effects such as seizures, tics, hallucinations, headaches, insomnia, growth issues, decreased appetite, addiction, malnutrition, heart valve weakness, kidney and liver problems, blood sugar destabilization, and/or severe fatigue.[8]

As the *Journal of Clinical Pharmacokinetics* points out, although a safety profile of short-term Ritalin use has been established, the specific effects of long-term use of methylphenidate, even at therapeutic doses, remain largely unknown.[9] However, it has been established that, although rare, psychostimulants like Ritalin can cause some children to become psychotic.

As stated by the *American Journal of Psychiatry*, "The potential for stimulants to induce psychosis-like or manic-like symptoms in children has been known for at least 35 years."[10] Psychotic symptoms from Ritalin can include hearing voices, visual hallucinations, urges to harm oneself, urges to harm someone else, suicide, severe anxiety, euphoria, grandiosity, paranoid delusions, confusion, increased aggression, and irritability.[11]

Knowledge of the effects of chronic use of Ritalin is poorly understood with regard to persisting behavioral and neuro-adaptational effects, and there are currently no sure methods for predicting who will be struck by methylphenidate psychosis. However, one study featured in *American Journal of Psychiatry* concluded that individuals with a diagnosis of bipolar or schizophrenia who were prescribed stimulants during childhood typically have a significantly earlier onset of the psychotic disorder and suffer a more severe clinical course of the disorder.[12]

"We can't blame medication alone. Aren't people who commit mass murder mentally ill?"

Understandably, we need to acknowledge that people committing murder are "mentally ill" for numerous reasons, and we must also recognize that not every child/teen on medication will commit such violence. However, my point is that we need to take better care of those that are diagnosed. We need to start asking why individuals are mentally ill. Why are their eyes so dull, almost dead, and seeming to draw light in instead of reflecting it out? Could school shooters like Adam Lanza, Elliot Rodgers, and so many others have food sensitivities triggering violent behavior? Could they have genetic mutations, nutritional deficiencies, heavy metal toxicity, leaky gut syndrome, PANDAS, Lyme disease causing Lyme rage, or amino acid deficiencies causing neurotransmitter imbalances?

There needs to more intense testing to determine if any of the above could be contributing to or at the root of their mental illness. Then we need to treat these underlying conditions. We need more long-term treatment facilities and more access to intensive outpatient programs. We need to address the breakdown of the American family, and we need more due diligence in our healthcare system. Simply handing out medications to address symptoms and hoping the client follows through with recommended weekly individual psychotherapy appointments is simply not enough.

MedWatch

MedWatch was created by the FDA to alert consumers of the potential risks associated with different medications across the board. In addition, it was established so that consumers could report all side effects. I encourage all parents to review and report possible side effects to this website, including minor effects. Since not enough parents know about it, the tool is underutilized. Visit www.fda.gov/Safety/MedWatch/default.htm. To access the reporting form, visit https://www.accessdata.fda.gov/scripts/medwatch/medwatch-online.htm.

I was first introduced to the MedWatch program through a Connecticut-based nonprofit organization called AbleChild, which was established to raise public awareness regarding the psychiatric labeling and the over-prescribing of psychiatric drugs to children, as well as the risks of mandatory mental health screening. This group is not affiliated with any religious or political organization, but acts as an independent advocate on behalf of parents whose children have been subjected to mental health screening, psychiatric labeling, and prescribed psychotropic drugs without receiving informed consent.

AbleChild works steadily to influence critical national policy debates and legislation by serving as a voice for caregivers and children. Its aim is to ensure that no law is passed that infringes on the rights of anyone to full informed consent and choice related to mental health screening, psychiatric labeling, and the use of psychotropic drugs in treatment of children. To learn more about their mission or gain more information, please refer to www.ablechild.org.

Another watchdog group is the Citizen's Commission of Human Rights International (CCHR). It was formed in California in 1969 as a global nonprofit watchdog committed to investigating and exposing human rights violations in the field of mental health. They are strong advocates against the arbitrary use of psychiatric drugs by children. The group is responsible for helping to enact more than 150 laws protecting children and individuals from abusive or coercive practices worldwide. CCHR has long fought to restore basic inalienable human rights to the field of mental health, including, but not limited to, full informed consent regarding the medical legitimacy of psychiatric diagnosis, the risks of psychiatric treatments, the right to all available medical alternatives, and the right to refuse any treatment considered harmful.

CCHR launched a free educational tool tool that is a definitive guide to documented psychiatric drug side effects. The Psychotropic Drugs Side Effects Search Engine can be located at www.cchrint .org/psychdrugdangers.

To learn more about CCHR, visit www.cchr.org.

To learn more about the effects of stimulants and other drugs, please refer to these other references as well:

"Long-term safety of stimulant medications used to treat children with ADHD" in the January 2008 issue of *Pediatric Annals*.[13]

"Methylphenidate-induced psychosis in adult attention-deficit/ hyperactivity disorder: report of 3 new cases and review of the literature" in volume 33 of *Clinical Neuropharmacology*.[14]

"Psychotic and manic-like symptoms during stimulant treatment of attention deficit hyperactivity disorder" in volume 163 of *The American Journal of Psychiatry*.[15]

CHAPTER 7

Our Movement Toward Alternative Treatments

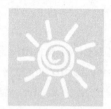

Until we found the path of alternative medicines and treatments, we had no idea that there were natural remedies available that could help Evan to heal from the conditions mentioned in Chapter 5. We also didn't realize that the underlying conditions plaguing children can mimic other classified autoimmune disorders.

Not one conventional doctor pointed us in that direction. It wasn't until I received correspondence from an unlikely source that we started our journey. It meant I needed to move away from everything I knew and everything that I had been taught about the treatment of these disorders.

My aunt, Joan, who lives in New York, had always leaned toward holistic health to address illness. From the time Evan was a baby, she insisted that something was medically wrong with him and that he had silent food sensitivities contributing to his illnesses and developmental delays. I didn't see it at first, or at least I didn't want to see it. I put her off time and time again and just told her what others were telling me: "Joan, don't worry; he was a preemie. Every child develops at his/her own pace."

Joan continued to send me articles about naturopathic and holistic treatments. She left me a barrage of emails and voice messages about treatments she thought might help Evan. She never had her own children, so I took her advice lightly.

In my mind, she was a "health nut" who had proclaimed for twenty years that she needed to avoid more than thirty foods. This seemed ridiculous to me. I thought it was in her head and that she was giving herself these "allergies" by avoiding the foods.

She often refused conventional medical advice and treatments. She even went as far as treating her own breast tumors using homeopathic doctors and dietary changes. My family thought she was "crazy."

I listened with one ear, while knowing in my heart that she made some sense. But I was a busy mom raising two babies, one an infant baby girl with terrible colic who screamed incessantly and the other with special needs who, at two years old, wasn't even walking. I was working as a psychotherapist in private practice and listening to everyone else's problems. I was shuffling around to countless doctor and therapy appointments. I was overwhelmed.

My aunt Joan is a persistent person, though, and when Evan was around five years old, she sent me the 2009 study about apraxia and malabsorption. It took me two months to finally get around to reading it. When I did, however, it opened up a whole new world of hope.

The article by Dr. Claudia R. Morris and Dr. Marilyn C. Agin was titled "Syndrome of Allergy, Apraxia, and Malabsorption."[1] It blew my mind and motivated me to read and learn as much as possible. So began our journey.

I started with Dr. Kenneth Bock's book called *Healing the New Childhood Epidemics: Autism, ADHD, Asthma, and Allergies—The Groundbreaking Program for the 4-A Disorders,*[2] cowritten with Cameron Stauth. The more I read, the more I was convinced that there is a direct connection between the intestinal tract and the brain. I learned that some sensitive kids are more prone to allergies, anxiety, apraxia, ADHD, and autism. I started to believe that Evan's issues could be directly affected by his diet and that nutritional interventions and supplementation could improve his health. I recognized that this wasn't mainstream thinking, but "alternative" doctors agreed there was help for such patients.

Sadly, many conventional doctors have little to no experience in

the area of nutritional deficiencies or in the underlying genetic mutations that may influence proper metabolic functioning.

Genes are segments of a person's DNA located on chromosomes.
A genetic mutation is a change or alteration in the DNA sequence.
Mutations cause changes in the genetic code that can lead to disease.
These mutations occur in two ways: (1) they can be inherited by a
parent, or (2) they can be acquired during a person's lifetime when
cells are exposed to environmental triggers, such as ultraviolet radiation, pollution, and toxic chemicals. Specific mutations can prevent
necessary chemical reactions in the body and can inhibit the body's
ability to digest foods, transport substances between cells, and utilize
nutrients appropriately.

Doctors often jump to treating symptoms with medications
instead of treating the root causes with immune system strengthening, gut rehabilitation, diet, and nutritional supplements. Before opt-
ing to pour more chemicals into the already inflamed systems of our
children, doctors might want to learn more about nutrition and
metabolic processes.

Traditionally, ADHD and autism spectrum disorders are diagnosed by therapists such as myself, psychologists, and psychiatrists,
who recommend traditional therapy and medications to address
neurological symptoms. Parents are told that their child's diagnosis
is complex and multifactorial in nature, a result of genetic, psychological, and others factors widely unknown. Most doctors are taught
to treat the emotional and mental component of these disorders with
medication. Yet, the physical or medical issues these children often
share are rarely noted or discussed. Some of those include eczema,
asthma, chronic illness, gastrointestinal distress, food sensitivities,
yeast overgrowth, leaky gut syndrome (a detailed explanation of this
syndrome is in Chapter 12), malnutrition, hypoglycemia, adrenal
fatigue, hormone imbalances, and sleep disturbances.

Typically, proper testing also reveals high levels of heavy metal
and environmental toxins relative to neurotypical children.[3]

As one article in the *Journal of Clinical Nutrition* points out, "Most
graduating medical students continue to rate their nutrition preparation as inadequate."[4] I had to find an integrative or functional

medicine physician, naturopath, homeopath, Medical Academy of Pediatric Special Needs (MAPS) physician, Defeat Autism Now (DAN) doctor, nutritionist, NAET practitioner, osteopath, chiropractor, and other complementary therapists.

I started collecting lots of data, studies, and articles on these subjects. The more I researched, the more I realized how much information was out there. Unfortunately, the mainstream medical community wasn't on board. Like many of you, I'm sure, I was programmed from a very young age to listen to and trust my doctor. After discovering so much, though, I was ready for a fight.

I remember feeling so hopeful that Evan could have a real medical condition that was preventing him from absorbing, utilizing, and metabolizing vitamins, minerals, and other important nutrients. For the first time, I felt like we could heal Evan of his ASD, ADHD, apraxia, and other issues by cleaning up his diet, removing environmental toxins as much as possible, addressing gastrointestinal issues, providing nutritional support, and boosting his immune system. I started to realize that I wasn't alone and that there was more help out there if I was willing to move away from the path of traditional medicine.

Coincidentally, shortly after reading the articles and making a connection, Evan had a bowel movement that presented itself with a lot of dark red blood. We immediately ran to the pediatrician. She sent Evan's stool to a lab to test for vitamin deficiency, as well as Crohn's disease and Celiac disease. Then, she referred us to a Pediatric Gastro Specialist at the Children's Medical Center in the Digestive Disease Department. The tests came back negative for both diseases.

Many of his vitamin levels were extremely low, however, and he presented with all of the symptoms of a sensitive child, including constipation, diarrhea, fatigue, abdominal bloating, gas, skin rashes, motor delays, and focus problems.

With all of my studies and articles in my hands and hope in my heart, I asked the doctor about "leaky gut" and the possibility that Evan might be suffering from gluten intolerance or other such sensitivities. I explained that both my aunt and father were diagnosed with food sensitivities and with a leaky gut. I told him that they also suffered from learning disabilities and many psychiatric symptoms. He raised his eyebrows and said, "You must be reading too much." It became obvious at that moment that this doctor wasn't reading enough.

He claimed that there was no evidence that leaky gut exists and that Evan didn't have a problem with gluten. He also mentioned that I could go to an allergist if I was concerned about allergies. I explained to him that we had already gone down that road. Obviously, he knew nothing about the difference between a histamine reaction in the skin and an internal "allergy" causing inflammation in the gut. Did he know anything about the brain/gut connection? He was a gastroenterologist! Why did I feel like I knew more about this than he did? When I asked why my little boy, who eats relatively well and takes many vitamins on a daily basis, came back vitamin deficient, his answer was, "If I tested all the children in Connecticut, they would all come back low in vitamin levels."

Steve looked at me with disbelief at what the doctor said to us. This man didn't know our child like we did. Evan wasn't eating fast food every day. We fed our son a well-balanced diet and supplemented it with vitamins. Unfortunately, this wasn't enough if Evan had a problem with his gut that was preventing the proper absorption and utilization of these nutrients. It wasn't enough if he had an underlying genetic mutation that was inhibiting vital metabolic processes from occurring.

It was obvious that I had challenged this doctor beyond his understanding—or his willingness to understand. I walked out of his office with more determination than ever to get someone to listen to me. I immediately crossed that doctor off the list and started reading more.

The "Syndrome of Allergy, Apraxia, and Malabsorption" article spoke volumes to me, by describing a new disease paradigm in which a problem with metabolism causes neurological dysfunction.[5] A total of 187 children with verbal apraxia, autism, sensory issues, low muscle tone, coordination difficulties, food allergies, and GI symptoms were treated with safe nutritional intervention in conjunction with additional speech and occupational therapy. In all, 181 families (97%) reported dramatic improvements in a number of areas, including speech, imitation, coordination, eye contact, behavior, sensory issues, and development of pain sensation. The article suggested to me that Evan deserved a more comprehensive metabolic workup and food sensitivity test.

About a week later, Steve came home with a business card from a colleague at his office whose wife had just started a naturopathic practice located only ten miles from our home. Steve wanted to help his friend's wife start her practice and thought I could refer some of my psychotherapy clients to her. I knew many of my clients hated being dependent on their medication for attention, focus, hyperactivity, anxiety, and depression issues, so they might want to pursue a more natural route.

Then it occurred to me that maybe this was a solution for Evan as well. We contacted Sharmilee Jayachandran, ND. We were hopeful, yet guarded, so we proceeded with caution.

We continued with all of the traditional therapies and simultaneously started treating Evan biomedically. This biomedical treatment is a systemic evaluation and treatment of the entire child. It is the combination of mainstream and alternative modalities working in harmony to heal the root causes of the symptoms. The protocol includes a close examination of the gastrointestinal, immune, and metabolic systems, and underlying conditions along with nutrient therapy.

Although biomedical treatment is considered alternative by the American Academy of Pediatrics, there is no denying that it was this treatment that dramatically enhanced the other, more traditional occupational and physical therapy and accelerated Evan's recovery. Within a few months, we saw minor improvements; and after a year, Evan showed notable improvements in all areas of development, both physically and emotionally. Thanks to Dr. Jayachandran, we were finally on our way!

CHAPTER 8

Genetic Vulnerability

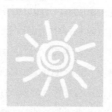

The doctors never determined why I went into spontaneous preterm labor with Evan, even after the hospital's lab biopsied the umbilical cord. I wasn't a drinker or a smoker, and I never suffered from high blood pressure or diabetes.

Coincidentally, researchers at the March of Dimes are studying a link between preterm labor and the mother's immune system response to infections. Labor can be triggered by inflammation caused by infections, so this could be one of the contributing factors in my situation.

The immune system requires optimal balance to counteract inflammation in the body. In autistic individuals, the immune system fails at this balancing act. Inflammatory signals dominate, and a state of chronic activation prevails. As explained by Moises Velasquez-Manoff in his bestselling book, *An Epidemic of Absence: A New Way of Understanding Allergies and Autoimmune Diseases*, "Nowhere are the consequences of this dysregulation more evident than in the autistic brain. Spidery cells that help maintain neurons—called astroglia and microglia—are enlarged from chronic activation. Pro-inflammatory signaling molecules abound. Genes involved in inflammation are switched on."

In the August 25, 2012 edition of *The New York Times*, Velasquez-Manoff added, "At least a subset of autism—perhaps one-third, and very likely more—looks like a type of inflammatory disease. And it begins in the womb."[1]

MTHFR Gene Mutations

An estimated forty percent of the population has a genetic defect called a MTHFR gene mutation that inhibits the body's ability to regenerate folate with help of vitamin B12. This genetic mutation can be problematic for developing babies. As we know, folic acid (the synthetic form of folate) is recommended to pregnant moms for proper brain development of their unborn child. Unfortunately, if a pregnant mother carries the mutated gene(s) and the correct dose and the correct form of this essential nutrient is not supplemented, many problems can arise. Doctors may recommended that a pregnant mother take methyl-B12 and folate instead of folic acid, at a much higher dose than what's normally prescribed.

Essentially, if the vitamin processing pathways are not functioning properly and your cells are trying to use defective enzymes, it can cause your body to malfunction and display a variety of symptoms and diseases. One such symptom is the malfunction of the central nervous system, affecting the making of serotonin, dopamine, and norepinephrine.

In addition, a study featured in the *British Medical Journal* showed that developing embryos may be adversely affected by toxic levels of homocysteine that result from such mutations, leading to tube defects, cleft palate, and miscarriages.[2] In addition, the June 18, 2012 edition of *Holistic Primary Care* states that a variation of MTHFR called C677T is associated with vascular, neurological, and other chronic disease states, and is suspected of increasing the risk of ADHD and autism.[3]

The remedy during pregnancy is taking about four times the normal dose of folate and substantially larger amounts of vitamins B6 and B12. Alternatively, if you already have a child on the autism spectrum or with ADHD or OCD who tests positive for these gene mutations, you may find that methyl-B12 supplements produce amazing positive results.[4]

I carry this gene mutation but was never checked for it during my pregnancy. Had my doctor performed a simple blood test, I could have taken more folate, B6, and B12 to help safeguard against problems.

My father and Evan also carry one MTHFR mutated gene, which means that all three of us are only able to metabolize vitamin B12 fifty to seventy percent of the time. Like many others, we can't rely on adequate food choices. We need to supplement our diets with a form of methyl-B12. It comes in the form of sprays and sublingually.

Studies, such as the one conducted on the effects of dietary folate on the gene expression of rats, concluded that those who carry both variations of C677T gene mutations are able to metabolize vitamin B12 only thirty percent of the time and are, therefore, at risk for substantially worse autistic symptoms, seizures, Celiac disease, Crohn's disease, and inflammatory bowel disease.[5] For these people, a high dose of methyl-B12 may need to be delivered via injections.

COMT Gene Mutations

COMT (catechol-O-methyltransferase) helps break down and regulate certain neurotransmitters. These include dopamine, epinephrine, and norepinephrine. Those that carry COMT (+/+) can have impaired enzyme function, which inhibits the body's ability to breakdown the neurotransmitters effectively. This can cause higher dopamine levels or fluctuations in the dopamine levels, which can lead to many neurological problems in the prefrontal cortex of the brain. This area of the brain is involved with personality, inhibition of behaviors, short-term memory, planning, abstract thinking, and emotion. COMT is also involved with metabolizing estrogens, so a mutation of the gene may be partially responsible for PMS.

As one can imagine, if the COMT is not functioning properly, it can cause a variety of problems, including irritability, hyperactivity, mood swings, anxiety, sleep issues, and lower frustration and pain tolerance. Lower executive function and a lower IQ has also been noted for some.

Individuals with COMT mutations can be supported nutritionally, and it is important to speak to your doctor or practitioner about an individualized treatment plan. Taking a B-complex supplement is often suggested. However, individuals with COMT often also have problems with methylation, so a morning B-complex containing methylcobalamin, L-5MTHF, and pyridoxine-5-phosphate is usually recommended. Often, part of the protocol also includes magnesium and amino acid (GABA) supplementation, detoxification practices, as well as botanical liver support. For PMS, modulating estrogen can also be helpful.

MAO-A Gene Mutations: "The Warrior Gene"

The MAO-A (monoamine oxidase A) is one of the two genes that encode mitochondrial enzymes, which catalyze the oxidative deamination of amines, such as serotonin, norepinephrine, dopamine, and adrenaline. Mutation of this gene results in Brunner syndrome. According to *BMC Psychiatry*, MAO dysfunction (too much or too little MAO enzyme activity) is thought to be responsible for a number of psychiatric and neurological disorders, including depression, mood swings, OCD, schizophrenia, substance abuse, migraines, irregular sexual maturation, as well as the behaviors associated with attention deficit disorder (ADD)[6] and autism. It is believed that too little enzyme activity can lead to aggressive, anti-social, and sometimes violent behavior, hence the name "Warrior gene."

This homozygous (+/+) mutation is thought to be quite common, especially among males. As I learned from an article published by the Public Library of Science, "prolonged periods of stress, violence, or trauma can lead to epigenetic changes that further decrease enzyme activity."[7]

Balancing and regulating serotonin levels becomes the important factor in managing people with this genetic mutation. In autism, serotonin levels seem to be greatly affected, which results in issues such as poor mood regulation, tantrums, and anxiety. Also, fine and gross motor skills, self-regulation problems, and sensory system imbalances such as touch, sound, etc. are prevalent, too.

There are nutritional and other more natural supports available to increase the activity of this important enzyme.

Some more common treatments include holistic remedies and 5HTP to help balance serotonin as well as addressing some factors that may be negatively impacting serotonin levels, such as the MTHFR mutation, BH4 deficiency often caused by aluminum toxicity, ammonia levels in the body, and others. There is also a product called Respen-A developed for autism with the intention of increasing MAO-A activity. Respen-A can only be obtained from compounding pharmacies and requires a prescription.

Respen-A is a topical homeopathic treatment for the symptoms of impaired social interaction, impaired communication, and repetitive behaviors. A small disc (about the size of a nickel) is applied to the skin once daily for 12 hours. In the disc is an ingredient called reserpine, a drug derived from the roots of certain species of the tropical plant *Rauwolfia*. The powdered whole root of the Indian shrub *Rauvolfia serpentina* historically had been used to treat snakebites, insomnia, hypertension, and emotional instability. In this case, a small dose that helps to promote MAO-A activity, and in doing so helps to turn serotonin over into what's called its "active aldehyde form." This aldehyde form called 5-hydroxyindoleacetaldehyde (5-HIAL) complexes with the postsynaptic serotonin receptor to influence the physiological effects of serotonin. Respen-A could reduce blood calcium greatly, apparently shifting it into bones and urine. Respen-A consequently requires 2g/day of supplemental calcium to compensate.

Reserpine is the active ingredient in Respen-A and has been used by physicians and naturopaths to also treat high blood pressure and relief of psychotic symptoms. One must realize, however, that reserpine can potentially cause dangerous side effects. Some parents report nasal congestion, loose stools, hyperactivity, and irritability (especially when used with antidepressants). This side effect has been remedied by either discontinuing or decreasing the antidepressants or decreasing Respen-A. Other possible side effects include increased asthma, depression, dizziness, hypotension, and stomach cramping.

Again, getting appropriate testing and talking with your doctor to determine your unique treatment plan is important.

VDR Mutations

The vitamin D receptor (VDR) gene encodes the nuclear hormone receptor for vitamin D3 and mediates most of the physiological actions of the vitamin. VDR is expressed in the intestine, thyroid, and kidneys and has a vital role in calcium homeostasis. These important metabolic processes are responsible for so much—including regulating metabolic pathways, such as those involved in immune response—and helping to protect the gut against toxic and carcinogen effects.

Vitamin D3 stimulates enzymes to create dopamine, and those with both VDR and COMT can have further problems tolerating methyl donors and regulating dopamine levels. Low or low normal vitamin D3 can be linked to chronic illness, neurological and immunological conditions. In addition, those carrying this gene mutation may also experience blood sugar issues and poor pancreatic activity.

Supplementing vitamin D3 may be beneficial. Some patients rotate methyl-containing supplements, some take dopamine increasing herbs like ginkgo biloba or small doses of Mucuna Pruriens (tropical legume), which naturally contains dopamine. And some, take sage and rosemary to support vitamin D receptors. It may also be necessary to support the pancreas when having a VDR mutation, using digestive/pancreatic enzymes. Nutritional support can vary, so speak to your healthcare professional.

Speak to your physician about ordering blood tests or saliva tests to detect possible genetic mutations.

CHD8 Mutations

Another mutated gene researchers have discovered is called the CHD8. According to a huge study involving thirteen institutions from around the world, it appears this gene mutation may be another link to understanding autism. All fifteen autistic children who carried this gene mutation shared the same physical characteristics (a larger head and wide-set eyes), as well as gastrointestinal problems and sleep issues. This is another clear example how people with mutations in certain genes have strong chances of developing autism. "We finally got a clear cut case of an autism specific gene," said Raphael Bernier, the lead author, an UW associate professor in the Department of Psychiatry and Behavioral Sciences and the clinical director of Seattle Children's Autism Center. "The results could lead the way to a 'genetics-first approach' that could uncover hundreds more genetic mutations and lead to genetic testing. Genetic testing could be offered to families as a way of guiding them on what to expect and how to care for their child. Currently, autism is diagnosed based on behavior," said Bernier.[8]

FOXP2 Gene Mutations

It is believed that language disorders such as speech apraxia could be due to multiple factors, including, but not limited to, medical complications during pregnancy/delivery, chronic illness, ear infections, toxicity, nutritional deficiencies and/or genetic influences. As discussed in the *Journal of Neuroscience*, scientists have discovered a speech and language gene, which, if mutated, can cause a severe speech and language disorder.[9] The FOXP2 gene located on chromosome 7 is required during early embryonic development for formation of brain regions associated with speech and language; if it goes haywire, it could begin to explain one of the causations of apraxia and other language disorders.

An article in the *PLOS Biology Journal* stated, "Genetic aberrations of FOXP2 cause developmental verbal dyspraxia (DVD), which is characterized by impaired production of sequenced mouth movements and both expressive and receptive language deficits. Brain imaging studies in adult *FOXP2* patients implicate the basal ganglia as key affected regions."[10]

Pyrrole Disorder/Pyroluria

A substantial percentage of those with ADHD and/or on the autism spectrum also suffer from pyrrole disorder, also known as pyroluria. It is genetic-based and believed to be triggered by stress or injury or by copper overload, environmental toxicity, and other environmental factors. It causes a depletion of zinc and vitamin B6, which, in turn, can lead to many neurological problems.

Symptoms of pyrrole disorder include anxiety or irritability; hypersensitivity to noise, light, smell, and touch; depression, mood swings, and/or social withdrawal; memory loss; and an explosive temper. Additional symptoms are paleness, stretch marks, white spots on the nails due to zinc deficiency, and an adverse reaction to omega-3 fish oil.

Pyrrole disorder can be diagnosed with a kryptopyrrole urine test to determine how many pyrroles the body is excreting.

Treatment typically consists of vitamin B6 and/or pyridoxal-5-phosphate (the active form of vitamin B6), plus magnesium and zinc. Treatment might also include vitamins C and E and niacinamide due to their strong antioxidant properties, and primrose oil.

This tends to be a lifelong problem. Testing eventually revealed that Evan and I both have pyrrole disorder, so we're taking the nutritional supplements on a permanent basis. To test for the disorder, contact Direct Healthcare Access II, Inc. at www.pyroluriatesting .com or a similar lab. The cost of this test is approximately $80, or you can speak with your physician or insurance company to find out if the test might be covered by your insurance policy.

Histadelia—Under Methylation Disorder

Histadelia is an inherited condition, occurring primarily in males, that is characterized by too much histamine in the blood. The elevated blood levels of histamine are caused by a metabolic imbalance known as under-methylation.

Methylation is an important biochemical process responsible for the elimination of histamine as well as the production of certain neurotransmitters. If methylation is inadequate, there is a deficiency in serotonin, dopamine, and norepinephrine. This may be why sufferers often exhibit psychological, behavioral, and cognitive symptoms such as depression, suicidal thoughts, blank mind episodes, phobias, OCD, insomnia, muscle pain, developmental delays, hyperactivity, and addictive tendencies. In fact, some people who suffer from schizophrenia are suffering from histadelia and are misdiagnosed, most likely because many doctors are unfamiliar with the condition.

Other common symptoms include rapid metabolism (hunger), asthma, excess saliva, running eyes, seasonal allergies, and frequent colds, profuse sweating, skin conditions, and headaches.

What is histamine? It's a natural chemical in the body that is involved in local immune response. It regulates physiological function in the gut and acts as a neurotransmitter.

A blood or urine test can be ordered to determine if your child has this disorder. Basophil counts greater than 50 cells/cu millimeter and histamine levels greater than 70 ng/ml (0.629umol/L) are diagnostic for histadelia.

It's also important to test for copper levels. People with this condition frequently have low copper levels since copper is part of the enzyme histaminase, which is involved in the metabolism of histamine. Copper levels can be evaluated by either 24-hour urine copper or serum ceruloplasmin tests.

The good news is that there is available treatment for this condition, which involves the amino acid methionine. This amino acid detoxifies histamine by methylating the ring structure forming N-methylhistamine. Calcium helps release the body's stores of histamine, while zinc aids the calcium-methionine program and provides sufficient relief. Typical treatment includes the following nutrients in high doses: calcium, magnesium, vitamin B6, vitamin C, zinc, and methionine. Sufferers should limit their intake of common animal proteins as well since they can spike histamine levels.

Many biomedical practitioners see progress when histadelia is treated with nutritional therapies. Improvement is usually seen within four to eight weeks, and within six months, the chemical imbalance is often corrected.

To find out more, consult a naturopath, check out the book *Mental Illness: The Nutrition Connection* by Professor Carl Pfeiffer, MD, PhD, and visit the Pfeiffer Medical Center website at www.hriptc.org/index.php

Who Is Doctor Carl Curt Pfeiffer?

Dr. Pfeiffer was a medical physician and biochemist who researched schizophrenia, allergies, and other diseases and believed that there is an undeniable connection between mental illness and nutrition, and so, created specific biomedical protocols for their treatment. He was chair of the pharmacology department at Emory University and considered himself the founder of orthomolecular psychiatry, although Linus Pauling, PhD, had first introduced the term *orthomolecular* in his 1968 article "Orthomolecular Psychiatry" in the journal *Science*. Dr. Pfeiffer has written several books on nutrition, trace metals, and biochemistry imbalances. The results of his studies have allowed some people suffering from chemical imbalances to gain stability without the use of prescription drugs.[11]

Histadelia and pyroluria are two of the more common conditions diagnosed using orthomolecular psychiatry and are not yet accepted by the mainstream medical community. Therefore, finding studies to support the validity of these conditions may be difficult. However, many integrative, biomedical physicians and physicians of naturopathy are diagnosing and treating these conditions with success.

It is understandable to question non-evidenced based medicine. However, we must consider that although a disorder or a particular treatment has not been published in PubMed, that does not make it invalid.

We must also remember that good health is not found in a pill. The scientist mentioned above, Linus Pauling, PhD, received honorable mention in the magazine *New Scientist* and has earned nearly forty honorary degrees and two Nobel Prizes. Yet, evidence based medicine still considers his work radical. Perhaps because there is no profit in good nutrition.

Type A Blood—Does Blood Type Matter?

The Link Between Type A Blood, Autism, and Low Stomach Acid

Evan and our entire family has type A+ blood. Could there be a connection? According to Donna Gates, the author of *Body Ecology Diet*,

"80% of autism spectrum persons have type A blood."[12] Peter Adamo, ND, the author of many bestselling books about eating right for your blood type,[13] believes that there is a marked prevalence of blood type A in autism. He also believes that persons with type A blood have the following characteristics.

- A more sensitive constitution. As compared to the general population, these people are more prone to take issue (mentally or physically) with stress, environmental toxins, food and other things that they are exposed to.

- A lower-than-normal level of stomach acid.

- Digestive disorders, even from birth.

- Elevated cortisol (stress hormone) because of low stomach acid.

- Mineral deficiencies due to low stomach acid.

- A body that repairs itself more slowly.

In Chapter 20, I will go into more detail about the importance of stomach acid (hypochlorhydria) as well as recommendations to enhance proper digestion of essential nutrients.

Chewing Gum Can Interfere with Digestion

Often it is suggested that chewing gun can help with focus and concentration. We must realize that when we chew gum, our brain thinks we are chewing actual food. Our stomach and pancreas work overtime getting ready to digest food by excreting the digestive enzymes and stomach acid that our brain thinks we need. Over time, the digestive organs can become overtaxed and stop producing the amount of enzymes and acid they once did.

Some harmful ingredients in gum:

Sugar, Gum Base, Dextrose, Corn Syrup, Natural and Artificial Flavors, Less than 2% of: Glycerol, Aspartame, Gum Arabic, Soy Lecithin, Acesulfame K, Color, (Titanium Dioxide, Blue 1 Lake, Beta-Carotene), BHT.

Chew all-natural gum, like Glee. Remember to use it rarely, or right before a meal, when the acid and enzyme stimulation will be beneficial.

Digestive Enzyme DPP IV Deficiency or Malfunction

Digestive enzymes in the small intestine support digestion. They are responsible for breaking down protein into smaller pieces called peptides. These smaller pieces are broken down even further into amino acids and absorbed by the bloodstream. This includes potentially allergenic proteins such as gluten and casein, as well as the morphine-related peptides that these foods produce in the gut. A lack of important digestive enzymes can inhibit the body from properly breaking down gluten and dairy products, or metabolize other proteins and fatty acids.

It is believed that individuals on the autism spectrum may not have the ability to break down proteins and morphine related peptides as well as other people, due to digestive enzyme deficiency or damage of the enzyme.

It has been reported that there is a decreased activity of digestive enzymes in children with autism. One study reported that 44 of 90 (49%) children with autism who underwent endoscopy (because they had significant gastrointestinal problems) had deficiencies in one or more digestive enzymes; all of the children with low enzyme activity had loose stools and/or gaseousness.[14]

Why does this happen? Some theories include:

- An alteration of enzyme activity due to mercury toxicity

- Altered gut flora

- Use of medication that inhibits DPP IV

- Low stomach acid. Decreased enzyme production almost always occurs together with low stomach acid. If you have low stomach acid, it's likely that you won't have adequate levels of digestive enzymes either

- Genetic deficiency

It could indicate a possible genetic deficiency of dipeptidyl peptidase IV in children with autism, according to Dr. Alan Friedman. Dipeptidyl peptidase IV is an enzyme that is also present on cells of the immune system called lymphocytes. Also, the DPP IV regulates peptides that influence many types of behavior and physiological functions including hunger, thirst, digestive function, food intake, growth, pain and touch perception, control of Candida, overall immune function, and calcium metabolism."[15]

To address digestive enzyme deficiency, it is often recommended to remove dairy and casein from the diet for a time, institute "gut healing" practices including increasing the use of probiotics, and supplement the diet with full-spectrum digestive enzymes containing DPP IV. Digestive enzymes should be taken on an empty stomach one half hour before meals. This treatment can help with the metabolism of proteins and increase one's tolerance to foods that might otherwise trigger symptoms of autism.

Some other helpful benefits of digestive enzymes:

- Stimulate the immune system
- Reduce inflammation
- Increase energy
- Reduce gut pathogens and help eliminate toxins
- Increase white blood cell size and activity
- Increase the surface area of red blood cells to help carry more oxygen to all parts of the body
- Break up cholesterol deposits
- Eliminate yeast
- Break up and dissolve uric acid crystals

A Family of Allergies and Autoimmune Disorders

According to an article titled "Your Baby's Health: All about Allergies," written by Nicholas A. Pawlowski, MD of the Mayo Clinic, either you or your spouse has allergies, your child has a fifty percent higher chance of developing them. If you and your spouse has allergies, the chances rise to seventy-five percent.[16] As written in the *Encyclopedia Britannica*, food intolerances and autoimmune disorders are seen in families throughout generations, and it appears that allergies and celiac disease are more prevalent in individuals of European descent.[17]

That was true in my European family, where many members with these sensitivities also suffered from learning disabilities, thyroid issues, asthma, skin conditions, digestive ailments, arthritic conditions, ADHD, neurological dysfunction, tic-like behaviors, and adrenal fatigue. It would be interesting to know if my extended family members who died young of cancer, multiple sclerosis, and other autoimmune disorders suffered from food sensitivities as well.

One source of this genetic predisposition is the ability to produce higher levels of IgE in response to allergens. According to the *Gale Encyclopedia of Medicine*, those who produce more of a particular immunoglobulin type E (IgE) that binds to allergens will develop a stronger allergic sensitivity.[18] It causes immediate hypersensitivity (type-1) with marked histamine release. Symptoms can include runny nose, itchiness, swelling of the intestinal lining, cramping, diarrhea, hives, anaphylaxis, asthma, or atopic dermatitis.

In an article called "Syndrome of Allergy, Apraxia, and Malabsorption," the authors stated that there are some genetic modifiers (a gene that influences the expression of another gene) that increase the likelihood of developing gluten sensitivities. For example, carrying an HLA-DQ-1, 2, or 8 allele will increase susceptibility of an individual to develop gluten sensitivity, which may contribute to inflammation in wheat-fed children.[19]

In an August 10, 2010, article in *USA Today*, Liz Szabo wrote, "Danish researchers and doctors studied children born in Denmark from 1993 to 2004, and found that many children with autism or related disorders also had a family history of autoimmune diseases. Autoimmune diseases, such as type-1 diabetes and rheumatoid arthritis, develop when antibodies that normally fight infectious organisms instead attack the body itself. In addition, children who are born prematurely have a higher risk of developing autism related disorders."

The article also noted, "Researchers found an increased risk of autism spectrum disorders in children whose parent has celiac disease, a digestive condition in which people can't tolerate gluten, a protein found in wheat, rye and barley."[20] And, on August 16, 2013, *Healthline News* published a compelling article that linked another autoimmune disorder with autism titled "Mom's Weak Thyroid Ups Baby's Risk of Autism," which highlighted a large-scale study showing that mothers with low-producing thyroid glands are four times more likely to have autistic children.[21]

It was clear, due to our family history, that Evan was predisposed to food sensitivities and autoimmune disorders, and I believe there were many other things that triggered his system to create the perfect storm.

The Expression of Our Genetic Code in a Toxic World

Studies have attempted to discover genetic etiology; however, for a genetic influence alone to create an autism epidemic would be against the basic laws of nature. A shared risk factor from the environment has tremendous biologic coherence.[22]

If we look at the unprecedented increase in the illness of our children and of autism spectrum disorders over the past twenty years, we begin to question what is different in our world. What could explain the unbelievable rise in metabolic and biological dysfunctions?

It is best expressed by Mark Sisson, an American fitness blogger and author of *The Primal Blueprint: Reprogram your genes for effortless weight loss, vibrant health, and boundless energy.*

While the DNA itself is set, the structure fixed, that's hardly the end of the story—our story. Our environment in which we live and breathe and the chemicals in the food we eat has a direct influence on the expression of our genetic code, by altering the expression of genetic information. In the study of disease, researchers in the field of epigenetics are increasingly finding, that this turning "on or off" our genes, is a key in understanding how to prevent and treat any number of conditions. It has been studied, that compounds that may not appear dramatically or immediately harmful on a cellular level nonetheless trigger significant havoc on an epigenetic level, throwing off normal methylation patterns and causing the dysregulation of microRNAs, which direct gene expression. Among the implicated substances studied, highlighted were tobacco carcinogens, asbestos, ionizing radiation, arsenic, nickel, cadmium, benzene and polycyclic aromatic hydrocarbons (PAHs—components of common air pollution). Early/in utero exposure to these chemicals appears most destructive. As one presenter noted, in utero exposure to PAHs, for example, has been identified as a significant "risk factor" for childhood asthma. Although in utero exposure has been identified as a particularly "critical period" for epigenetic impact, it doesn't mean we're out of the woods as soon as we're out of the womb. Researchers are examining the possibility of other "critical periods" and emphasize the ongoing vulnerability to epigenetic alteration throughout life. The real problem with exposure to many of these substances isn't the immediate impact on cells but the previously unseen changes to genes' subsequent activity throughout an individual's lifetime. Genes are silenced and lose their ability to manage the production of proteins for ongoing cell function and repair. Others are activated when they shouldn't be. The resulting complement of abnormal down-regulation and overexpression can set the stage for cancer, metabolic disease and neurological impairment. Researchers have already begun to identify epigenetic changes that foretell cancer development.[23]

The Inability to Detox: An Example of Faulty Gene Expression

Another issue may lie in the defective functioning of the family of proteins called metallothionein (mt), as discovered by Dr. William Walsh and Dr. Anjum Usman. This dysfunction leads to impaired brain development and extreme sensitivity to heavy metals due to the body's inability to detoxify. "This disorder is often unnoticed in infancy and early childhood until it's aggravated by a serious environmental insult such as vaccines. They believe that this malfunctioning of mt proteins may represent the underlying cause of autism."[24]

Studies show that there is nothing wrong with the genes themselves, but somehow the mt proteins have been "turned off" by other genetic or environmental factors. According to the *Pfeiffer Treatment*

Center, if we stimulate the production of mt proteins, we can restore the entire system. The body's GI track would then mature, the body would rid itself of metal, and the immune system would be repaired.[25]

Taking a Look at Possible Genetic Syndromes

Genetic testing can be extremely valuable and important in many ways. In addition to determining if your child has any genetic mutations, it appears there are a few genetic syndromes that exhibit physical, cognitive, and behavioral autistic-like symptomology. Researchers continue to identify genes that may contribute to the risk of having an autism spectrum disorder (ASD), and it appears individuals with these syndromes can be at an increased risk for ASD. In addition, there are medical issues associated with these disorders that need specific attention.

Prader-Willi syndrome is caused by a gene missing on part of chromosome 15. Patients with Prader-Willi syndrome are missing the genetic material on part of the father's chromosome. The rest of patients with this condition often have two copies of the mother's chromosome 15. It appears that genetic changes occur randomly in utero. Prader-Willi can affect both males and females. Symptoms include hypotonia (low muscle tone), lack of eye coordination, failure to thrive, undeveloped sex organs and/or undescended testicles, small stature, very small hands and feet, narrow bifrontal skull, delayed motor development, speech problems, behavioral problems, anxiety, mild to moderate impairment in intellectual functioning, such as thinking, reasoning, and problem-solving. They may also have medical complications such as constantly feeling hungry— leading to obesity, diabetes, sleep apnea, endocrine issues and hypothyroidism, osteoporosis, problems regulating body temperature, and nearsightedness. In addition, many individuals with this syndrome cannot have children (infertility).

Angelman syndrome is the sister to Prader-Willi. It is caused by deletion or inactivation of genes on the maternally inherited chromosome 15 while the paternal copy, which may be of normal sequence, is imprinted and therefore silenced. Also a neuro-genetic disorder, Angelman syndrome is characterized by a severe intellectual and developmental disability, speech apraxia, sleep disturbance, short attention span, reoccurring seizures, jerky movements (especially hand-flapping), frequent laughter or smiling, and usually a happy demeanor.

Klinefelter syndrome is a chromosomal condition related to the sex chromosomes. Klinefelter syndrome only affects males and results from the presence of one or more extra copies of the X chromosome in each cell, which interferes with male sexual development, often preventing the testes from functioning normally and reducing the levels of testosterone. It is estimated that one in every 500 males have an extra X chromosome, but do not have any symptoms. Symptoms depend on how many XXY cells a man has, how much testosterone is in his body, and his age when the condition is diagnosed.

In addition to affecting male sexual development, variants of Klinefelter syndrome are associated with intellectual disability, distinctive facial features, tall stature, small testicles, skeletal abnormalities, poor coordination, motor delays (dyspraxia), attention problems, processing issues, and severe problems with speech and language. Men with Klinefelter syndrome are also at risk for certain health issues, such as autoimmune disorders, breast cancer (abnormally large breasts), infertility (low sperm counts), vein diseases, osteoporosis, and tooth decay. Like Prader-Willi syndrome, this condition is not inherited. It appears to occur as a random event during cell division early in fetal development.

CHAPTER 9

Other Early Contributing Factors

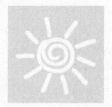

Prematurity and the NICU

Evan had a higher risk of developing sensory processing difficulties. Children born prematurely with an underdeveloped neurological system often have an inability to handle all of the stimuli presented in a busy NICU environment and are at a higher risk for sensory-based difficulties. Inevitable beeping and buzzing equipment, bright lighting, and bustling atmosphere can agitate the nervous systems of sensitive preemies.[1]

Evan fit all of the criteria explained in a 2003 study of preterm infants published in the *Journal of Developmental and Behavioral Pediatrics*.[2] He had oral defensiveness due to feeding tubes, high sensitivity to input, low muscle tone, and a preference for being alone.

We later learned that his lack of fetal movement and prematurity prevented the proper development and integration of his reflexes. The reflexes are vitally important for the proper development of the brain, nervous system, and sensory systems. Neonatal reflexes are inborn behavioral patterns that develop during uterine life. These involuntary reflexes are necessary for survival and include sucking, swallowing, and breathing. Other reflexes include the Moro reflex (or startle reflex), which should be fully present when a child is born full term.

When a child is born prematurely like Evan, pathways are sometimes underdeveloped, which can cause neurological and motor delays including apraxia/dyspraxia, poor eye-hand coordination, and an inappropriate response to stimuli. The Moro reflex has a direct link to alterations in the blood levels of adrenaline and cortisol—"the fight or flight" chemicals, as well as with blood sugar fluctuations.[3]

Patricia Lemer, cofounder and Executive Director of Developmental Delay Resources wrote an exceptional book titled, *Outsmarting Autism*. Lemer discusses how reflexes are a blueprint for motor, cognitive, and social development. "In many individuals with autism spectrum disorders, reflexes are absent, too weak, too strong, too slow to emerge, or linger past 6–24 months postnatally, and they are interfering with cortical processing and impending development. Aberrant reflexes can cause babies to become "developmentally delayed," and down the road, one or more practitioners label them as having one of the disabilities on the autism spectrum."[4] Again, Evan fit all of this criteria.

C-Section Complications—Lack of Gut Flora

When I began reading the written work of Natasha Campbell-McBride, MD, the developer of the term GAP (the gut and psychology syndrome), I learned a lot about the connection between gut dysbiosis (bacterial imbalance in the gut) and disorders such as ADHD and autism. I was convinced that I found one of the pieces of Evan's puzzle.

Who Is Doctor Natasha Campbell-McBride?

Dr. Natasha Campbell-McBride is medical doctor with two postgraduate degrees: Master of Medical Sciences in Neurology and Master of Medical Sciences in Human Nutrition.

After practicing for five years as a neurologist and three years as a neurosurgeon, she started a family and moved from Russia to the UK, where she got her second postgraduate degree in Human Nutrition. She became acutely aware of the link between nutrition and mental disorders, which spurred her to study the subject intensely.

Dr. Campbell-McBride developed the term GAP after studying and working with hundreds of adults and children with neurological and psychiatric conditions, including autism, dyspraxia, dyslexia, bipolar disorder, autoimmune conditions, ADHD, and OCD. In her book, *Gut and Psychology Syndrome: Natural Treatment for Autism, ADHD/ADD, Dyslexia, Dyspraxia, Depression and Schizophrenia*, she explains the connection in great detail. She also acknowledges that many of these childhood illnesses overlap one another. When examined in a clinical setting, it was found that psychiatric conditions in children coincide with physical ailments such as digestive disorders (abnormal stools, gas, bloating, and colic), allergies, eczema, and malnourishment. It was also found that one hundred percent of mothers had abnormal gut flora as well.

Dr. Campbell-McBride is a keynote speaker at many professional conferences and seminars around the world. She frequently gives talks to health practitioners, patient groups, and associations.

Our Gut Flora Story

Despite all of my attempts to have a healthy pregnancy, Evan was born eight weeks premature with an immature immune system and insufficient gut flora because he was delivered by C-section. In a normal delivery, I would have passed Evan my beneficial gut flora to help fight pathogens that can be responsible for gut inflammation.

A newborn infant was initially thought to be born with a sterile gut but new research suggests that the acquisition of its unique microbiota begins in the womb. It appears that colonization of the fetus's GI tract begins before delivery with ingestion of amniotic fluid containing microbes from the mother. Acccording to the *Journal of Early Human Development*, "The majority of an infant's gut flora is acquired when the baby passes through the birth canal, swallowing the mother's native bacteria."[5]

Gut flora consists of microorganisms that live in our digestive tract. Healthy microorganisms help our intestinal system to absorb and synthesize vitamin B, vitamin K, and other nutrients, including fatty acids. In fact, the metabolic function performed by these 100 trillion microorganisms act very much like an organ. Evan could survive without gut flora, but his body could not train his immune system to function properly or prevent the growth of harmful bacteria.

To add insult to injury, Evan was unable to obtain gut flora through my breast milk for more than twenty days because he was fed intravenously. Evan was never supplemented with probiotics or any "good bacteria" of any kind in the NICU. Therefore, "bad bacteria" most likely started having a party in his intestines. I believe Evan's immune system was left compromised, which contributed to him developing food intolerances.

I had the pleasure of speaking with Evan's neonatal intensive care doctor again recently, and he admitted to me that new research was helping them understand the benefits of supplementing good gut flora after a C-section birth. He confirmed that Evan wasn't given any probiotics and that the hospital is still slow to implement such practices. He also acknowledged that European obstetric care is light years ahead in some areas. "Even with the preliminary data on C-sections and gut bacteria, doctors in many other nations routinely recommend the administration of probiotic supplements to babies born via C-section."[6]

Again, I strongly believe that if Evan had been given probiotics and other remedies in the NICU to ensure better gut health, much would have been different with regard to his physical and mental health.

As stated in *Gut and Psychology Syndrome*, "The first and very important function is appropriate digestion and absorption of food. If a child does not acquire normal balanced gut flora, then the child will not digest and absorb foods properly, developing multiple nutritional deficiencies. And that is what we commonly see in children and adults with learning disabilities, psychiatric problems, and allergies. Many of these patients are malnourished. Even in the cases where the child may grow well, testing reveals some typical nutritional deficiencies in many important minerals, vitamins, essential fats, many amino-acids, and other nutrients." On top of that, people with damaged gut flora often have particular groups of pathogenic, iron-loving bacteria growing in their gut (*Actinomyces spp.*, *Mycobacterium spp.*, pathogenic strains of *E. Coli*, *Corynebacterium spp.* and many others).[7]

Why Moms Should Have a Healthy Gut During and After Pregnancy

I had always known that there were many positive aspects of breast-feeding and that Evan's immune system would benefit from it, so Evan was breastfed for approximately eighteen months. However, I didn't know about the importance of having good gut flora during pregnancy, nor did I realize that I could pass high levels of toxins and pathogens to my son through my breast milk. I wish I had been advised to complete a full detoxification regimen before conception, and I wish I had taken a heavy duty probiotic before and after conception.

I had been a low birth weight, C-sectioned baby myself. I required intestinal surgery and a feeding tube after I was born. That was 1971, and doctors didn't allow my mother to breastfeed me because I was considered too small.

I had stomach issues and constipation since birth and probably suffered with inadequate gut flora and a compromised immune system. At the advice of the doctors, I had many teaspoons of mineral oil throughout my childhood. I also struggled with anger, attention deficit disorder, dyslexia, and learning disabilities my entire life.

While I was pregnant, not one doctor ever told me about the importance of having healthy gut flora or that my son's immune system depended on it. It wasn't until I read *Gut and Psychology Syndrome* that I realized how the birth control pills I had taken for fifteen years, as well as the numerous antibiotics taken my entire life, had a devastating effect on my healthy gut bacteria and my unborn baby. It was also never explained to me that I was more predisposed to allergies, toxic buildup, mental health problems, chronic intestinal issues, and other medical problems because I had been a low-weight baby who wasn't breastfed.

A Gut Feeling

Steven Lamm, MD, from New York University School of Medicine states, "Seventy percent of the immune system is in the gut. The outer layer of the small intestine contains mucus, produced by special cells lining the digestive tract. Mucus serves as a barrier to prevent pathogens access to our blood stream. Poor food choices and improper digestion can lead to a decrease in this mucosal lining leaving us vulnerable to infection. This lining also houses antibacterial and antiviral substances that reside in your intestinal walls. When the lining of your intestines are compromised, your immunity is also compromised and there is a greater risk of becoming sick."[8] Therefore, a healthy and uncompromised gut can lead to a healthier child. A healthy gut means one free from inflammation, one with plentiful good bacteria to help the body produce immune cells to protect from toxins, bad bacteria, viruses, and fungal infections like Candida (yeast) for example. A healthy child also has a strong intestinal wall to aid in the digestion and absorption of the essential nutrients the body needs. Proper nutrients help our bodies ward off disease and illness, and they provide the brain with all of the essential vitamins needed to function properly. Essential vitamins are those that are required for normal body functioning, yet cannot be synthesized by our own bodies, thus must be obtained from dietary sources. Thirteen compounds have been classified as vitamins. Vitamins A, D, E, and K, the four fat-soluble vitamins, tend to accumulate in the body. Vitamin C and the eight B vitamins—biotin, folate, niacin, pantothenic acid, riboflavin, thiamin, vitamin B6, and vitamin B12—dissolve in water, so excess amounts are excreted.

Before conception and during the early years of a child's life, his/her gut becomes compromised by many factors besides poor gut flora, including pollutants in the air, toxic metals, chemicals the child and mom ingest, vaccinations, ultrasounds, and bacterial and viral infections. In some people the intestinal system reacts to such insults with poor immune health and malnutrition.

Are Our Hygiene Practices Making Us Sick?

We are programmed to believe that bacteria are bad and that we need antibacterial soaps and medications to fight them. We are making ourselves sicker because the body needs to be challenged to be strong. The immune system works extremely effectively "on automatic pilot" when we treat it right and feed it well. As a matter of fact, a healthy immune system is working hard all the time to prevent us from developing cancer. The name of the game is immune system strengthening!

As stated in *A Compromised Generation*, "Some doctors believe that one of the reasons for a rising epidemic of sickness in our children is due to the amount of sanitation, sterilization, chlorination, etc. and that our immune systems are no longer 'primed' to function properly."[9] We are sanitizing our water, processing our food, and using germ-killing drugs and soaps to clean our bodies. The idea is that we are killing the good bacteria along with the bad and that these are dangerous practices. We need microbes in order for our bodies to fight off illness.

I find this fascinating, as I remember scrubbing my hands for fifteen minutes with germ-killing soaps and putting on a full-length gown before I was allowed to enter the NICU to pick up my son.

Hepatitis B Vaccine

The hepatitis B vaccination has been recommended by federal health officials since 1991 for all infants and children, and there are currently mandates for children who attend daycare or school in the majority of states, including Connecticut. A pregnant mother can pass the virus on to her developing fetus. If the mother has hepatitis B, this vaccination is usually recommended within the first twelve hours of life. Otherwise, it is administered before the baby leaves the hospital. Evan received his first vaccine while still in the neonatal intensive care unit and two more before his eighteen-month birthday to complete the vaccine series. Did these vaccines contribute to Evan's autoimmune and neurological issues?

First, hepatitis B is primarily not a children's disease. It's a viral infection that attacks the liver, which is usually contracted sexually or through IV drug use or through blood products. According to the Vaccine Information Center at the Children's Hospital of Philadelphia, before the vaccine was introduced in 1984, approximately 18,000 children per year were affected with the hepatitis B virus by the time they were ten years old. Of the 18,000 children that contracted the disease, approximately half were born to drug-addicted or affected mothers through blood transfusions, while the other half caught the disease from another family member or from someone else the child came in contact with.[10] If a child contracts hepatitis B young in their lives, they are at an increased risk of more serious complications.

At first glance, this may appear to be a lot of children. However, one must consider that in 1983, there were approximately 40 million children under the age of eleven in the United States.[11] Hence, before the vaccine was introduced, only .04% of all children under eleven years old were affected by the virus.

Burton A. Waisbren, Sr., MD, a cell biologist and infectious disease specialist, enthusiastically supports vaccination where a risk/benefit ratio has been demonstrated. On the *New Yorkers Vaccination Information and Choice* website, "Dr. Waisbren hopes that federal judges will be asked for an injunction to stop universal hepatitis B vaccination, because it is an experiment that violates the civil rights of children who are put into the experiment." According to Burton A. Waisbren, "Parents of babies and adolescents who have little chance of being exposed to hepatitis B should be made aware of the potential dangers of a vaccine that can potentially damage their nervous system."[12]

A study published September 2009 in *Annals of Epidemiology* found that giving hepatitis B vaccine to infant boys more than tripled their risk for an autism spectrum disorder. This was doubly concerning because an earlier study by the same researcher group, using a different database, found the same results.

Russell L. Blaylock, MD, a board-certified neurosurgeon and vaccine expert, has written an extensive article about the dangers of excessive vaccination during brain development. In addition, a 2004 study looked at the immune reaction in newborns up to the age of one year who had received the hepatitis B vaccine to see if their immune reaction differed from adults given the same vaccine. What they found was that infants, even after one year of age, did react differently. Their antibody levels were substantially higher than adults (three-fold higher), and it remained higher throughout the study.

They found that babies reacted to the vaccine by having an intense, persistent, and completely abnormal immune response that could ultimately result in the child developing permanent brain and immune system dysfunction.

Could it be that this abnormal immune response further sets these children up for the "perfect storm" that leads to autism?

Add to this the potentially damaging effects of hepatitis B vaccine ingredients, which include aluminum adjuvant (causes inflammation in the brain), formaldehyde, and other chemicals, and you have a noxious cocktail that could have permanent negative effects on your child's health and development.[13] Adjuvants are necessary in vaccines to alert the immune response to react, but who knows what all these ingredients do to an immature brain that may not be able handle these elements.

Measles Mumps Rubella Vaccine (MMR)

The other vaccine that has become cause for concern is the combination Measles Mumps Rubella Vaccine. It is a mixture of live attenuated viruses of the three diseases, administered via injection. It was first introduced in 1988 to provide a convenient and more efficient vaccine. Yet, the safety of administering all three together was never established. Could this vaccine trigger autism? Many parents and independent researchers believe so.

There is overwhelming anecdotal evidence which suggesting that the MMR vaccine is dangerous for some children. Sensitive and gut damaged kids with compromised immune systems may be more prone to "over" reactions to vaccines. These children could be more prone to an "allergy" response to the toxic ingredients, and these kids may not respond well to live viruses being injected into their already delicate systems.

Excessive Ultrasounds

As a new parent, it was so much fun to get my first vaginal sonogram at six weeks. I received my first photo, and I was reassured that my baby was growing normally. Then, we underwent our 11–13 week ultrasound to assess risks of Down syndrome and other chromosomal abnormalities. This was estimated by taking into account numerous factors, including my age, measurements of certain hormones in my blood, the fetus's nuchal translucency, nasal bone viability, bone lengths, echogenic foci, among other markers.

At twenty weeks, I received another sonogram. I was so happy to get another picture of my baby and find out that we were having a little boy. I had an ultrasound at about thirty weeks and another the night of my emergency C-section. The doctors felt that additional ultrasounds were necessary due to the baby's breech position and the lack of fetal movement.

Women are routinely offered several sonograms during their pregnancy, and the new 3D ones are gaining even more popularity. I had always believed that just looking couldn't hurt and that this newer technology provided the doctors with a diagnostic tool to check for abnormalities and growth progress. It wasn't until I started doing the research that I discovered that these scans used to test for abnormalities aren't as accurate as we are led to believe. A study out of Brisbane, Australia, showed that the ultrasound exams used at a major woman's hospital missed about forty percent of abnormalities.[14] We must also recognize that ultrasounds are very user dependent. Factors such as a patient's body size, the equipment used, and—most importantly—the sonographer's training and experience also play a role.

In addition, current evidence suggests that routine ultrasounds during pregnancy may not be as safe as first thought, especially the vaginal ultrasound where there is little intervening tissue to shield the baby. Manuel Casanova, MD, a noted research scientist and neurologist at the University of Louisville, is sounding a warning about ultrasounds. "It's not just about taking a picture of your baby. This has physical and chemical effects, and it's poorly regulated by the government."[15] Casanova published a report in 2010 in the journal *Medical Hypotheses*, spelling out his concerns about ultrasounds. In it, he noted rising rates of autism coincident with the increased use of ultrasound in obstetrics and demanded further research.

"Even if it doesn't have anything to do with autism, it needs to be regulated."[16]

The million-dollar question is whether the ultrasonic energy used during exams is sufficient to have a possibly deleterious effect on a fetal brain? Dr. Casanova believes that this energy is known to affect cellular membranes and cell growth, as it is used as a therapy to accelerate bone growth following certain traumatic injuries. In stem cell research, ultrasound has been shown to accelerate development of cells. Could the cavalier use of ultrasounds be affecting the developing brain and contributing to the autism epidemic? One interesting Yale University study suggests that the prolonged use of ultrasounds caused brain abnormalities in mice.[17] The Center for Disease Control and Prevention is currently in the process of studying the possible effects of ultrasound on autism.

In Utero or Birth Trauma and Cranial Distortions

Another avenue to explore is the possibility of cranial distortions caused by in utero or birth trauma. It appears that some autistic children have cranial and intracranial distortions that can be treated with osteopathic manipulation (OMT), with significant positive results. In fact, Shawn K. Centers, DO, MH, FACOP, a pediatrician and internationally known expert in osteopathic pediatrics, nutrition, and natural medicines wrote an article for *Autism Science Digest* stating, "Some children make such a significant recovery that it would be difficult for anyone to ascertain that they ever had a diagnosis of autism."[18] These conditions are treated very gently with manual manipulation; surgery is not required. It has been acknowledged that the earlier the child is diagnosed and treated, the better the outcome. It is also noted that the treatment is enhanced when coupled with other therapies and modalities.

Often, traditional doctors are not trained to diagnose or treat the brainstem or cervical spine birth-related injuries, and if left untreated, these traumas can cause significant developmental and neurological problems. Robert Melillo, MD, an internationally recognized physician and expert in neurology and neurobehavioral disorders in children states, "These injuries can prevent the proper motion of cervical vertebrate and cervical muscles, which rob the brain of the necessary stimulation required to balance brain activity. This can cause learning disabilities, cognitive and behavioral problems, sensory deficits, and poor muscular abilities."[19] In addition, many experts agree that when there is a cranial strain pattern and the brain is irritable, the brain can become far more susceptible to outside adverse influences such as vaccines and other environmental toxins.

What Are the Signs of a Cranial Distortion?

- Coning of the head that doesn't resolve within one week after birth.

- Wry neck (torticollis).

- Poor latch, suck, and swallow (frequently results in biting the breast), pulls away from breast, objects to being on stomach, slow to hold head up.

- Sleep issues.

- Hypersensitive, crying that won't stop, difficult to calm, colic (check for Candida).

- Ear inflammations, temporal mandibular dysfunction (jaw issues), thrush, constipation, and tonsillitis.

- Hypoactivity (an inhibition of behavior or locomotor activity) and seizures, delayed response (no startle reflex).

- Difficulty breathing/cardiac irregularities.

- Projectile vomiting (reflux or pyloric stenosis).

- Thumb sucking, head bumping.

- Hyperactivity, developmental delays, sensory integration, poor coordination and balance, poor speech, poor listening.

- Vision problems, including clogged tear ducts.

- Excessive and constant drooling not related to teething.

What Causes Cranial Distortions?

- Prolonged push during labor.
- Interventionist obstetrics utilizing epidural anesthesia, forceps, and vacuum extractors.
- Axial pull on baby's head (connected to SIDS).
- C-section.
- Breech position.
- Fast delivery of large baby that wasn't engaged in the pelvis prior to labor.
- Severe molding that doesn't correct within three to four days (frequently caused by baby's head engaged in mother's pelvis for weeks prior to birth).
- A distortion of the maternal pelvis so that the perinatal head that comes through is basically liquid or gelatinous and takes on the form of that pelvis—much like dough coming through a cookie cutter.

These lists were created by compiling data from numerous sources.[20]

In Evan's case, the physicians who cared for him did not pick up on these issues because his birth trauma injuries were extremely subtle. Plus, most of these doctors are not trained to diagnose cranial distortions based on the symptomology noted here. It wasn't until we found a doctor of osteopathic medicine that Evan was diagnosed with cranial distortions, which the doctor believes were due to the traumatic C-section birth and breech positioning. Evan certainly had many of the symptoms, including blocked tear ducts. Unfortunately, it's well documented that these distortions are frequently not self-correcting.

Viruses and Bacterial Infections

Is there a link between infections and autism? "A population-wide study from Denmark spanning two decades of births indicates that infection during pregnancy increases the risk of autism in the child. Hospitalization for a viral infection, like the flu, during the first trimester of pregnancy triples the odds. Bacterial infection, including of the urinary tract, during the second trimester increases chances by 40 percent."[21]

The author of *An Epidemic of Absence: A New Way of Understanding Allergies and Autoimmune Diseases* writes that illness itself does not affect the fetus, but the inflammatory response does. He references a study in Denmark that discovered, "Inflaming pregnant mice artificially—without a living infective agent—prompts behavioral problems in the young. In this model, autism results from collateral damage."[22]

The measles and other infections are also believed to trigger inflammation of the walls of the GI tract, causing leaky gut. Some doctors and researchers believe that children who experience immediate deterioration after an MMR vaccination have been infected with the live measles virus.

Another contributor may be an untreated strep infection. Pediatric autoimmune neuropsychiatric disorders associated with streptococcal infections (PANDAS) wreak havoc on the immune and neurological system, causing facial tics, OCD symptoms, and other neurological problems.

PANDAS is a term used to describe children who have a rapid onset of OCD-type symptoms, and/or tic disorders that are thought to be due to an autoimmune response to a strep infection. It is believed that the body continues to produce antibodies to the strep bacteria, which mistakenly reacts in a part of the brain called the basal ganglia. The basal ganglia controls a body's movement and behavior, thus creating a host of symptoms. Most cases of PANDAS are those in which parents can clearly see a defining moment or day in which a "switch flipped" in their child, from that of a normally progressing child to that of a child who is debilitated by the symptoms below.

- Tics or abnormal movements

- Repetitive behaviors

- OCD, anxiety, irritability
- ADHD
- Sensory sensitivities
- Developmental regression
- Sleep difficulties
- Echolalia
- Dilated pupils

In the book *Healing the New Childhood Epidemics*, Kenneth Bock, MD writes, "PANDAS just cook the brains of these kids—the infection attacks the brain's basal ganglia, causing serious malfunctions of thought and behavior and the person affected could fly into uncontrollable rages and violent behavior."[23]

In addition, although controversial, there seems to be a link between late-stage Lyme disease and mental issues, including rage, psychosis, and violence. Many physicians who treat a large number of Lyme patients acknowledge that they have had patients with "Lyme rage." There are more than one hundred peer-reviewed medical journal articles linking tick-borne diseases to mental symptoms and quite a few that reference Lyme-induced rages.

CHAPTER 10

Immune System Assaults

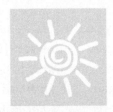

A Slew of Antibiotics

Evan was given antibiotics frequently as a small child, and so was I. In the 1970s, overuse of antibiotic treatment was common. In addition, I was put on antibiotics and treated for numerous yeast infections while carrying Evan. I used antifungal creams, including miconazole and clotrimazole, but not one doctor ever recommended more natural solutions such as acidophilus or cutting down on sugar and simple carbohydrates that feed the yeast (fungus).

I had no idea that the use of antibiotics could alter my gut flora or that the anti-yeast medications I was taking may not have been the healthiest of options. I didn't know that what my doctor prescribed could affect my baby's long-term health or that my own immune system could be compromised.

It wasn't until I recently read the article written by Claudia Morris, MD, and Marilyn Agin, MD, in *Alternative Therapies Journal* that I learned about the importance of taking a quality probiotic supplement that includes *Lactobacillus Acidophilus* during pregnancy and breastfeeding. If I had done this, Evan might have benefited more from my breast milk.[1]

Antibiotics kill pathogens, but could alter the immune system by simultaneously killing the healthy gut flora, which may also allow yeast to grow out of control. Yeast is said to be another contributor to the autism spectrum picture.

There was an interesting study in 2011 that concluded, "The common use of antibiotics must be disrupting and harming our ability to distinguish pathogens from normal cells and bacteria."[2] It isn't the immune system, as we've previously defined it, that determines what is friend and what is enemy—it's the gut bacteria that makes such decisions.

According to this study conducted by numerous researchers affiliated at various medical universities and institutions, we are seeing an enormous upswing in autoimmune diseases, and it seems to coincide with the massive misuse of antibiotics since they indiscriminately kill gut bacteria. If we wipe out the good gut bacteria that is involved with strengthening the immune system, there is nothing to stop an autoimmune response, which results in illness. So, although extremely necessary in the treatment of bacterial pneumonia and other illnesses, antibiotics are often overused today.

Taking a Deep Look at Vaccines

To vaccinate or not to vaccinate has become a much-debated discussion. I am not here to stir the debate, only to educate. I have heard from countless moms who believe that their child has had an adverse reaction to a vaccine. They have told me that their children were developing normally but developed a high fever and/or had a seizure hours after a vaccine. Within days, their children's developmental milestones started to regress, and the children slipped into behavioral patterns they had never seen before.

I have also heard from many moms that despite keeping their child away from vaccines, he/she still developed autism. So, how is this possible if we are going to blame vaccinations?

I want to go on the record as saying that I believe that vaccines are one of the triggers for autism, but certainly not the only one. I hope you recognize, after reading this chapter as well as the preceding ones, that I believe that vaccinations are only one of many immune system assaults. I believe that some children are having severe allergic reactions to the vaccines, triggering an autoimmune response. The Centers for Disease Control and Prevention (CDC) references many studies debunking the causation between ASD and vaccines; however, they do list the numerous side effects of vaccines, including severe allergic reactions, fever, seizures, permanent brain damage, and inflammation of the stomach and intestines.[3]

Some MDs do believe that vaccinations are one of the causes. According to Dr. Campbell-McBride, "Vaccines deepen the damage to these children's immune systems and provide a source of chronic persistent viral infections and autoimmune problems in these children."[4] She also makes reference to considerable research linking poor immune health in children and adults with learning disabilities and psychiatric problems.

Children can receive as many as twenty-six inoculations by age two and up to five shots at a time, and pregnant mothers are getting vaccines as well.

Interestingly, in 1999, on the recommendation of the American Academy of Pediatrics and U.S. Public Health Service, thimerosal was removed from childhood vaccines as a "precautionary" measure without admitting to any causal link between thimerosal and autism. However, despite its removal from many childhood vaccines, thimerosal is still routinely added to some formulations of influenza vaccine administered to U.S. infants, as well as to pregnant mothers.

Vaccine proponents will argue that methylmercury found in fish is different from ethylmercury used in vaccines, and that ethylmercury is harmless. Those vaccine proponents ignore, however, that studies show that ethylmercury turns into highly toxic methylmercury in the human body.[5]

Should pregnant moms be given the flu shot containing mercury? An article in the spring 2006 issue of the *Journal of American Physicians and Surgeons* reports that a study done by independent researchers point to mercury as being linked to autism, despite the government's claims to the contrary.

The consistency of the effects observed for the spectrum of NDs, including autism and speech disorders, and the agreement between the observations from two separate databases, support the conclusion that the effect is real and not a chance observation.

The magnitude of the change in the trend lines is substantial. Once mercury was removed from the childhood vaccines, the U.S. Department of Education reported a decrease of the number of new autism diagnoses recorded among children 3 to 5 years old, after years of annual increases. The biological plausibility of the present findings is further supported by recently emerging extensive toxicokinetic, molecular, and animal studies. These researchers confirmed that thimerosal crosses the blood-brain barrier and results in appreciable mercury content in urinary mercury concentration following chelation. Holmes et al. examined first baby haircuts and determined that autistics had significantly higher body burdens of mercury in comparison to non-autistic matched controls, by demonstrating that the mercury level in hair, and thus the ability to excrete mercury, was inversely proportional to the severity of autism and overall much lower in the autistic group. James, et al. have evaluated biochemical susceptibility to mercury in autistic children, in comparison of age—and gender-matched control children, by evaluating the methionine cycle and transsulfuration metabolites. They found a significant 46% decrease in the plasma concentration of glutathione, a necessary metabolite for the excretion of mercury from the body. Additionally, autistic children had significantly increased oxidative stress, as shown by a threefold decrease in the glutathione/oxidized glutathione redox ratio, in comparison to control children, which would correlate with a significant body burden of mercury.[6]

Vaccine proponents will also argue that mercury was taken out of childhood vaccines and the rate of autism has climbed, therefore, concluding that vaccines do not cause autism. However, they do not take into consideration all the other neurotoxins that immunizations contain such as monosodium glutamate (MSG), aluminum hydroxide, aluminum phosphate, and formaldehyde. Antibiotics can be added, such as neomycin and polymyxin B, to prevent the growth of germs (bacteria) during production and storage of the vaccine. These vaccines also contain many allergens such as Polysorbate 80 (an additive in food and vaccines linked to infertility, tumor growth, gastrointestinal problems, and heart conditions),[7] egg, soy, gelatin, and yeast, as well as animal byproducts such as chick embryonic fluid, guinea pig embryo cells, fetal bovine serum, and monkey kidney cells.

Could these ingredients cause unknown and unpredictable damage, elevating the risk of autoimmune disorders now and in future years? Many researchers believe that these heavy metals and preservatives do serious damage, and countless parents agree. In his book, *Cry of the Heart—Stop Hurting the Children*, Dr. Mark Sircus blames these toxins for the current epidemic of neurological disorders. He questions whether we are substituting one disease state for another. In the film *The Greater Good*, Lawrence Palevsky, MD, states, "Autism is just one piece of a bigger problem. The bigger issue today is that 1 of 6 children in America have a neuro-developmental disability."

One CDC-funded study showed a statistically significant difference in the prevalence of ADHD, autism, and tic disorders between individuals who received mercury-containing vaccines at three months and those who didn't. Analysis of data from the federal Vaccine Adverse Events Reporting System (VAERS) and the U.S. Department of Education show a linear correlation between neurodevelopmental disorders and exposure of thimerosal. Vaccine injuries continue to be reported by many parents, but it remains a very controversial subject.[8]

One case report of twins, in which one twin was subjected to the standard vaccine schedule while the other didn't receive vaccines until later, should shed strong light on this issue, since one twin is autistic and the other is not.[9]

Since 1998, Dr. Andrew Wakefield, a British former surgeon and medical researcher, discovered and reported a link between autism, digestive disorders, and the MMR vaccine. He has since been subjected to relentless personal and professional attacks in the media, and from governments, doctors, and the pharmaceutical industry. The hope is that the recent events will help to break the fifteen-year controversy and the smearing of Dr. Wakefield's reputation. In August 2014, William Thompson, a senior research scientist at the Centers for Disease Control released a formal statement that the CDC covered up data showing a vaccine-autism link. In addition, the following court rulings demonstrate the impact vaccines are having on some children.

There were two recent landmark court rulings in December 2012 that awarded money to families of children who developed "a debilitating injury to their brains, diagnosed with an autism spectrum disorder" as a result of the measles/mumps/rubella (MMR) vaccine. One family lives in Northern California and the other in Houston, Texas.[10]

The Federal Vaccine Injury Compensation Program, better known as "vaccine court," "quietly" awarded millions of dollars to the two children with autism for "pain and suffering" and lifelong care of their injuries, which together could cost tens of millions of dollars.

And on June 21, 2013, "Scientists and physicians from Wake Forest University, New York, and Venezuela reported findings that not only confirm the presence of intestinal disease in children with autism and intestinal symptoms, but also indicate that this disease may be novel. Using sophisticated laboratory methods, Dr. Steve Walker and his colleagues endorsed Wakefield's original findings by showing molecular changes in the children's intestinal tissues that were highly distinctive and clearly abnormal."[11]

Vaccinations save lives and prevent many debilitating disease states such as meningitis and polio. Therefore, flat-out refusal of vaccines may not be the answer either. We need to realize that there are safer and better ways to vaccinate. Thimerosal-free, aluminum-free, and preservative-free vaccinations are available through special order, but they require special refrigeration and care and are more expensive. Currently, many insurance companies refuse to pay for them. Therefore, clinics and doctors don't administer them unless you are willing to buy them out-of-pocket. Even then, some refuse.

It is important to make an educated decision and talk to your doctor about the benefits as well as the risks. Perhaps not all vaccines are suitable for all children.

If I had to do it all over again, I probably would have denied the hepatitis B vaccinations after learning about the risks of contracting the disease and after learning about the "benefit-to-cost ratio." Unfortunately, we do not know if a child will be sensitive to vaccinations, so perhaps we have to take greater precautions. It is my belief that giving "all" recommended vaccines may not be the answer for every child.

Can parents deny vaccines? Aren't they mandatory to enter school?

Yes, parents can deny vaccines at any time. They are medical interventions. When your child becomes part of a public setting like school, you would need to take it a step further and get a state exemption, as vaccines are mandatory to enter schools. In September 2012, *Fox News* reported, "All U.S. states allow children to be exempt from vaccination requirements for medical reasons because some children are allergic to vaccines, others have conditions that severely compromise their immune systems, and could make vaccination dangerous to a child's health. In addition, 48 states allow exemptions for nonmedical reasons (Mississippi and West Virginia do not). Nonmedical exemptions can be granted for religious reasons or philosophical reasons, though fewer states allow philosophical exemptions than religious ones."[12]

If you feel that your child was injured by a vaccine, it's important to report vaccine reactions to the Federal government through VAERS and to the NVIC Vaccine Reaction Registry by visiting the National Vaccine Information Center website at NVIC.org.

General Anesthesia

Evan had been under anesthesia many times by the time he was four years old. After learning a lot throughout this process, I believe that general anesthesia, accompanied by surgical stress, also influenced the inflammatory responses in his body and set him up for more infections. "Anesthetics have been suspected of impairing various functions of the immune system either directly, by disturbing the functions of immune-competent cells, or indirectly by modulating the stress response."[13] When the offspring of mice were tested after the mothers received a specific anesthetic gas during pregnancy they showed effects of neuroinflammation and impaired learning and memory.[14]

Research finds that exposure to anesthesia in early childhood may have long-term effects on kids' brain development. In one study involving 5,357 children born in Rochester, Minnesota, scientists found that children who had had two or more surgeries by the time they were two years old were twice as likely to be diagnosed with ADHD by the time they were nineteen years old, compared with youngsters who had had only one surgical procedure.[15]

According to author Dr. Caleb Ing, a pediatric anesthesiologist at Columbia University College of Physicians and Surgeons in New York City, a study of 2,868 Australian children revealed that children younger than age three who had gone under general anesthesia were 87% more likely to have language disabilities and abstract reasoning deficits at age ten.[16]

It certainly appears that certain young children are particularly more susceptible to the effects of anesthesia, so maybe delaying some early surgeries can possibly prevent future learning disabilities and cognitive issues in children. In an emergency, surgery may be necessary. So, make sure to talk to your doctor about your concerns so that necessary precautions can be taken. Ensuring that proper anti-inflammatories are on board may provide some relief.

In Evan's case, we later discovered through muscle testing (applied kinesiology) that Evan may have been affected by anesthesia (developed a sensitivity) that needed to be addressed through NAET (Nambudripad's Allergy Elimination Technique) for a full recovery. It was amazing; I never told the NAET practitioner that Evan had undergone anesthesia. She used applied kinesiology and then asked me if he had undergone anesthesia in his young life, because his body was telling her that he was and that affected him immensely.

What is muscle testing or applied kinesiology? The essential premise of applied kinesiology that is not shared by mainstream medical theory is that every organ dysfunction is accompanied by a weakness in a specific corresponding muscle, in what is termed the viscerosomatic relationship.[17] When this diagnostic tool was discovered by George Goodheart in 1964, it was primarily used by chiropractors. However, it has gained popularity and is now used by naturopaths, nutritionists, physical therapists, cranial sacral therapists, acupuncturists, counselors, and others to treat illness and disease.

This diagnostic tool allows the practitioner to ask the body "yes or no" questions based on a person's muscle strength or weakness. It works with the idea that a positive association or "yes" strengthens the muscles, while a negative association or "no" weakens them. Bypassing conscious thought, muscle testing accesses your intuitive and energetic systems. It is not a replacement for conventional medical diagnostics, but it can be very useful when other more conventional tests are not available. We diagnosed Evan's food intolerances using both muscle testing and conventional methods, and they both told us the exact same story.

What is NAET? It is an allergy elimination technique devised by a California-based chiropractor and acupuncturist to diagnose and treat allergies and other related disorders. It is a noninvasive procedure that uses muscle testing and acupressure to reverse the allergy or sensitivity. This technique does not require any blood draws, scratch tests, or shots. If the children are small, or if the child has a severe anaphylaxic reaction to a particular food or substance, an adult becomes the energy conduit. Autism spectrum children have been studied following aggressive allergy elimination treatment of many foods and substances including anesthesia, and the "NAET treatment is effective and well tolerated for children with allergy related autism."[18] According to Devi Nambudripad, MD, D.C. L.Ac, Ph.D. (the creator of NAET), this technique has also been used to help reverse vaccine injury with quite remarkable success.[19]

In addition to addressing inflammation, our naturopath prescribed Trehalose Complex by Genoma Nutritionals. This is one of numerous glyconutrient formulas on the market to help promote healthy brain and nerve functioning. Glyconutrients are plant carbohydrates (monosaccharides). There are over 200 carbohydrates or sugars but only eight are essential to bodily function. These are xylose, fucose, galactose, glucose, mannose, N-acetylglucosamine, N-acetylgalactosamine, and N-acetylneuraminic acid (a sialic acid).

These plant carbohydrates are believed to help prevent bacterial, viral, parasitic, and fungal infections, ease inflammation, lower blood sugar, and triglyceride levels. They can also improve brain function, inhibit tumor growth, guard against respiratory infections, inhibit allergic reactions, help wound healing, and enhance memory. It is said that glyconutrients are the key to effective cellular communication and proper cell function. This has been established by the world's leading scientists and researchers.[20]

Steroids

Evan was on many steroids to address his bronchial flare-ups, virus-induced asthma, and croup. While my little baby struggled to breathe, I knew steroids were the best course of treatment because of their quick-acting anti-inflammatory properties. However, while using a temporary fix to address his symptoms, I wish I had known that steroid use weakens the immune system. It would have been helpful to be working to strengthen Evan's immune system at the same time.

A book called *The Yeast Connection* by Dr. William Crook popularized the hypothesis that *Candida* is a major pathogen that can weaken the immune system, allowing other infections to occur. Dr. Crook also contends that toxins produced by *Candida* due to the overuse of antibiotics and steroids could contribute to the development of multiple sclerosis, rheumatoid arthritis, and other autoimmune disorders. "Steroid drugs, like Prednisolone damage gut flora. Corticosteroid therapy decreases the resistance of a host to C. albicans."[21]

Candida albicans is a common yeast; a microscopic fungal organism normally present in the mucous membranes of the mouth, intestinal tract, and in the genital area of healthy people. The *Journal of Pharmacy BioAllied Sciences* reported that under certain circumstances, it may cause superficial infections in these areas. *C. albicans* have emerged as a serious health concern for immune-compromised patients.[22] This was certainly true for Evan and explains his numerous yeast infections.

Sometimes steroids are necessary to use for the treatment of our children, they are potent anti-inflammatories, and have a place in modern medicine. We must not forget, however, that these powerful medicines also have the ability to disrupt the immune system and disrupt the normal balance of micro-gut flora in the body. So, alongside of steroidal treatments, it's important to address our immune system health simultaneously with probiotics and dietary changes.

CHAPTER 11

The Gut-Brain Connection

Many of today's conventional doctors abandon what we previously knew. The connection between the gut and the brain has been known for centuries. French psychiatrist Philippe Pinel, after working with many mentally ill patients, concluded back in the early 1800s that "The primary seat of insanity generally is in the region of the stomach and intestines." Long before him, Hippocrates (460–370 BC), the father of modern medicine, said, "All diseases begin in the gut."

As a mom, I had no idea that the state of my son's brain may be directly related to the inflamed state of his gut, nor did I realize that his symptoms of motor problems, foggy thinking, short-term memory problems, anxiety, irritability, hyperactivity, and attention problems may be potentially caused by inflammation. Apparently, the gut has its own nervous system, and that is why when we are nervous, our stomach may become upset. A wonderful resource is the book titled *The Second Brain*: *A Groundbreaking New Understanding of Nervous Disorders of the Stomach and Intestine* by Michael Gershon, MD. When the stomach is acting up and is bloated, gassy, or constipated, it may cause us to feel anxious and irritable. It's actually reacting out of the same system, and the relationship between them is intimate.[1]

If a child's inflammation in the gut is lowered, brain inflammation is automatically lowered as well. The result is a happier, calmer, and sharper thinker, without the use or need of psychotropic medications.

Naturopathic doctors and other natural health practitioners agree that ADHD and other such medical disorders arise from a combination of immunologic, allergic, and digestive dysfunction that begins with inflammation and damage to the child's immune system early in development. Some doctors agree that a few of these insults to the immune system can be transferred from the mother's toxicity, which needs to be addressed years before conception in order for the problems to be completely avoided.

The holistic belief is that every organ and every cell in the body has its own intelligence and contributes to the well-being of the entire organism. Therefore, if the intestinal tract is influenced due to stress or an environmental trigger, it needs to be restored to ensure health in the entire body.

Interesting Fact

There are actually more neurons lining the digestive tract than in either the peripheral nervous system or the spinal column. This "second brain" is known as the enteric nervous system. Dr. Michael Gershon, Chairman of the Department of Anatomy and Cell Biology at New York–Presbyterian Hospital/Columbia University Medical Center, an expert in the nascent field of neurogastroenterology, explains that ninety percent of the fibers of the vagus nerve in the neck carries information from the gut to the brain, and not the other way around. Therefore, to a large degree, our emotions are governed by the state of our intestinal system. In fact, ninety-five percent of the body's serotonin is found in the bowels.[2]

In 2013, *The New York Times* reported that one in every five school-aged boys in the U.S. have received a medical diagnosis of attention deficit hyperactivity disorder; about two-thirds of those diagnosed take a stimulant to go to school.[3] In the same year, the National Health Statistics Reports states that one in fifty have some form of autism.[4]

The American Holistic Medical Association and the American

Naturopathic Medical Association do not believe these are "psychiatric disorders" that warrant large doses of medication. They believe they are metabolic-immunologic-neurologic-digestive disorders that require a biomedical protocol.

Therefore, it's imperative that our doctors join the blossoming field of neurogastroenterology and move closer to naturopathic principles in order to treat these disorders. Our MDs need to gain some understanding of the workings of the second brain—"the gut"—and its impact on the body and mind. They need to begin to address root causes by correcting digestive problems, eliminating allergens and environmental toxins, and improving nutrition. In an emergency, we could use pharmaceuticals as a bridge to address debilitating symptoms. Ultimately, however, we need to address these underlying issues naturally.

CHAPTER 12

Malabsorption Syndrome

Food Sensitivities and Leaky Gut

Like many parents, I was concerned about food and other allergies that might be triggering Evan's asthma and chronic bronchitis. As mentioned in a previous chapter, we took Evan to an allergist. He was checked for the most common allergens by looking for histamine and leukotriene, chemical reactions on his skin. The tests didn't indicate that he had any allergies that would be contributing to his illnesses. At this time, it was the only allergy testing I believed existed.

I thought an allergy only resulted in skin flushing, itchy skin, wheezing, vomiting, throat swelling, and anaphylaxis. I had no idea my child was silently suffering from food sensitivities. His symptoms were not rashes or hives but were instead gastrointestinal, dermatological, and behavioral in nature. I had absolutely no idea at the time that food sensitivities as a result of a leaky gut and inflammation were made worse by the offending foods. It becomes another vicious cycle.

On April 11, 2012 the *Chicago Tribune* featured an article titled "Doubts Cast on Food Intolerance Testing: Allergists and Gastroenterologists Question the Use of Expensive but Sought-After Analyses." The article said, in part, "Allergists and gastroenterologists say that although food intolerance does occur—most of it involving specific food sugars like lactose or fructose—the tests being marketed to consumers don't have any scientific basis. Blood tests for food sensitivities are prone to false positives that can lead people to eliminate harmless foods from their diets, they say." It also said, "The National Institute of Allergy and Infectious Diseases does not believe that food intolerances affect or involve the immune system."[1]

According to Annette Nay, PhD, however, "More and more doctors are admitting that most, if not all; diseases are due to dietary problems and inflammation. Life-long food allergies left untreated have led to most, if not all, autoimmune diseases and a multitude of other diseases including ADHD and autism. Taking poison daily systematically destroys your body and your health."[2]

Symptoms of Food Sensitivities

In an article titled "Food Sensitivities: The Hidden Problems," by Robert J. Doman, MD,[3] and a book titled *A Compromised Generation: The Epidemic of Chronic Illness in America's Children* by Beth Lambert[4] (the founder of Epidemic Answers), both authors explain that a child exhibiting any of the following symptoms (with persistence) should look deeper into the possibility of food sensitivities. Evan had nearly all of the symptoms described:

- History of ear infections and illnesses
- Congestion; sometimes inconsistent
- Reflux or GERD
- Cradle cap
- Psoriasis and eczema
- Frequent ups and downs and/or periods of restlessness and anxiousness
- Poor attention span at times
- Night or morning coughing spells
- Dark circles under the eyes
- Variable hearing that is sometimes good, sometimes poor
- Postnasal drip
- Headaches

- Insomnia

- Frequent diaper rashes

- Red or hot ears after eating

- Vaginal or anal itching

- Colic, excessive crying, or irritability

- Distended belly

- Frequent urinary infections

- Chronic athlete's foot or thrush

Dr. Ben F. Feingold's book, *Why Your Child Is Hyperactive*,[5] includes a long list of foods and products with additives, color additives (red 40), and foods containing natural salicylates that can cause hyperactive behavior and attention deficit issues in children if they're sensitive or allergic to the substances.

It's amazing that with all that Evan suffered, not one doctor suspected gut flora issues, leaky gut, malnutrition, or food sensitivities.

Leaky Gut Syndrome

So, just what is leaky gut syndrome?

With a leaky gut, the intestinal wall breaks down due to inflammation and becomes overly permeable. Food molecules end up entering the bloodstream instead of being absorbed by the intestines. Their nutrients—including vitamins, minerals, and amino acids—should have been absorbed by the intestines, metabolized, and used in the body. Instead, they are simply lost.

This condition also alters the metabolism of proteins, carbohydrates, and lipids in the body. It can be diagnosed by the presence of lactulose in a fecal sample or by testing for food sensitivities.

The body overreacts to the food in an allergic type of way (allergies and sensitivities develop), and antibodies are created that attack the brain and the rest of the nervous system. Therefore, leaky gut can cause food allergies and sensitivities, brain damage, behavioral

LEAKY GUT SYNDROME

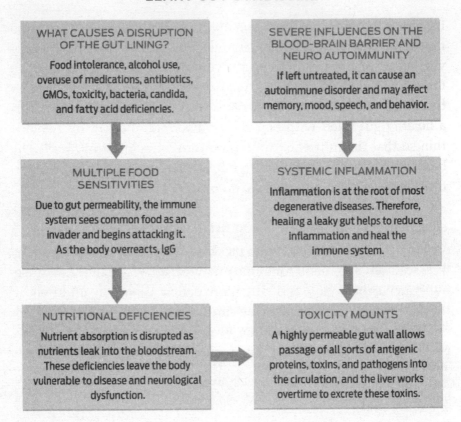

WHAT CAUSES A DISRUPTION OF THE GUT LINING? Food intolerance, alcohol use, overuse of medications, antibiotics, GMOs, toxicity, bacteria, candida, and fatty acid deficiencies.	**SEVERE INFLUENCES ON THE BLOOD-BRAIN BARRIER AND NEURO AUTOIMMUNITY** If left untreated, it can cause an autoimmune disorder and may affect memory, mood, speech, and behavior.
MULTIPLE FOOD SENSITIVITIES Due to gut permeability, the immune system sees common food as an invader and begins attacking it. As the body overreacts, IgG	**SYSTEMIC INFLAMMATION** Inflammation is at the root of most degenerative diseases. Therefore, healing a leaky gut helps to reduce inflammation and heal the immune system.
NUTRITIONAL DEFICIENCIES Nutrient absorption is disrupted as nutrients leak into the bloodstream. These deficiencies leave the body vulnerable to disease and neurological dysfunction.	**TOXICITY MOUNTS** A highly permeable gut wall allows passage of all sorts of antigenic proteins, toxins, and pathogens into the circulation, and the liver works overtime to excrete these toxins.

and mood abnormalities, and impaired speech, coordination, and memory. In addition, a highly permeable gut wall allows passage of all sorts of antigenic proteins, toxins, and pathogens into the circulation, which are driving factors in the cognitive symptoms and abnormal behaviors of ADHD and autism.

Yeast overgrowth is also a contributing cause of leaky gut because it damages the immune system, reduces the ability to produce stomach acid necessary for digestion, and damages the wall of the gastrointestinal track. In addition, gastroesophageal reflux disease (GERD) is often a result of yeast overgrowth. Jenny McCarthy states in her book *Louder Than Words: A Mother's Journey in Healing Autism* "Yeast overgrowth is a major aspect of autism—and an aspect that can be controlled."[6]

Unhealthy Biofilm

Biofilm is the slimy coating often lining the intestinal track when too much bacteria is present. This film is created by the bacteria to provide a safe and warm place to thrive. Just like the slimy coating on the teeth, if left untreated, it can prevent the good bacteria from thriving and prevent the proper absorption of essential nutrients. In a healthy gut filled with beneficial microflora, the biofilm remains thin so that the nutrients can pass through the intestinal wall. The biofilm also assists in the moistening of the intestinal tract and protects against infection, inflammation, and toxins.

If the gut is unhealthy, the film remains thick and becomes a source of inflammation. Unhealthy biofilm houses toxins like heavy metals and promotes more bacteria, parasites, and yeast overgrowth. Because nutrients cannot be properly absorbed, the thick film also causes nutritional deficiencies.

Many people who suffer from *Candida* overgrowth, gastric reflux, brain fog, attention issues, bloating, irritable bowel, Crohn's disease, ulcerative colitis, chronic illnesses, acne, arthritis, and other autoimmune problems have unhealthy biofilm that needs to be treated.

Some natural treatments that help to restore healthy biofilm include cutting out processed foods, sugars, and white flours; eating fermented foods; taking digestive enzymes; eating herbs such as cloves, black seeds, and false black pepper; drinking or making recipes that include apple cider vinegar and probiotics; and eating whole dense foods.

Malabsorption Issues Starve the Brain and Body of Essential Nutrients

Some of our kids are categorized as "failure to thrive," so malnutrition is more obvious. Evan was always categorized ninety-five percent for height and sixty-five percent for weight. I had no idea that he was so malnourished and that his brain was paying the utmost price.

"Failure to thrive" is used to describe a delay in a child's growth or development. It is usually applied to infants and children up to two years of age who do not gain or maintain weight as they should. Failure to thrive is not a specific disease, but rather a cluster of symptoms that may come from a variety of sources. Shortly after birth most infants lose some weight. After that expected loss, babies should gain weight at a steady and predictable rate. When a baby does not gain weight as expected, or continues to lose weight, he/she is considered to be "not thriving." Sometimes it implies that the baby is not receiving enough nutrients or it implies that the organs involved with digestion and absorption of food are malformed or incomplete so the baby cannot digest or metabolize the food properly.

People with ADHD/autism are usually deficient in many essential amino acids, vitamins, and minerals. Therefore, supplementation is part of an effective treatment regimen. It's imperative to keep these individuals on the prescribed supplements until all of their absorption issues clear, if they are picky eaters, or if their diets are not high in these essential nutrients.

Symptoms of a mineral deficiency may manifest as acidic blood, constipation, low blood sugar, cravings, anxiety, hyperactivity, low energy, poor digestive health, toxic buildup, low adrenal functioning (the body's chief energy producer), and depressed immunity.

Pediatrician Recommended PediaSure: Nutritious or Toxic?

Many parents struggle with feeding their children and worry about their children becoming malnourished or underweight. Some supplement their children's diet with PediaSure nutritional drinks. Should we worry about many of the ingredients used to create this product? Loaded with sugar, this product also contains **corn maltodextrin** (likely from GM corn), **milk protein concentrate** (likely from GM fed cows, antibiotics, and pesticides), **high oleic safflower oil** (highly processed), **soy oil, soy protein isolate** & **soy lecithin** (likely GM, highly processed, contaminated with **neurotoxic aluminum** and carcinogenic hexane, phytic acid, linked to malabsorbtion), **fructooligosaccharides** (a chemical sugar additive, may pose toxicological and gastrointestinal dangers), **cellulose gel** (highly processed fiber we cannot digest), **calcium phosphate, calcium** carbonate (not bioavailable), potassium phosphate (can cause allergies), potassium citrate, chromium chloride (toxic carcinogenic, has estrogenic properties, in animal studies causes issues with fertility in adulthood, aggression, sex behavior changes, inhibits liver enzymes, adverse liver changes, oxidative stress and DNA damage, genotoxicity, and adversely affects lymphocytes), monoglycerides (transfat linked to inflammation, obesity, increased LDL cholesterol), carrageenan (capable of causing inflammatory bowel disease), Sucralose (Splenda®), potassium hydroxide (toxic chemical found in drain cleaner), ferrous sulfate, artificial flavor & red#3 (linked to hyperactivity, hypersensitivity, behavioral effects), thiamine chloride hydrochloride (synthetic), pyridoxine hydrochloride (synthetic), cupric sulfate (toxic, used a used as an algicide and fungicide), sodium selenate, (synthetic selenium—not bioavailable and toxic), sodium molybdate (chemically altered sodium, linked to many ill health effects.)

Stimulant Medication Is Harmful for Malnourished Kids

Interestingly, stimulant and nonstimulant medications can cause the same side effects, such as upset stomach, decreased appetite, and weight loss. This is not exactly a good recipe for a child who is already malnourished with nutritional deficiencies.

Many stimulant and psychiatric medications deplete the body of necessary nutrients like B vitamins, magnesium, zinc, and the amino acid L-carnitine.[7]

- Certain B vitamin deficiencies are often linked to neurological dysfunction.

- Magnesium deficiency can be linked to fatigue, weakness, irritability, and sensory integration issues as well as depression, anxiety, and diabetes.

- Zinc deficiencies can be linked to sleep issues, hyperactivity, impulsivity, and emotional instability. Zinc also activates vitamin B6 to help the body produce serotonin naturally.

- L-carnitine deficiency is commonly linked to low blood sugar, anemia, muscle weakness, confusion, and decreased gastrointestinal mobility affecting proper digestion.

For more information, please refer to *Is Your Medication Robbing You of Nutrients Part 2: Getting Specific* by Hyla Cass, MD, or *Drug Muggers: Which Medications Are Robbing Your Body of Essential Nutrients—and Natural Ways to Restore Them* by Suzy Cohen, RPh.

Vitamins, Minerals and Amino Acids and the Roles They Play

Vitamins and Minerals

Vitamin A: A powerful antioxidant that boosts the immune system to combat the effects of illness and other stressors. It is the key vitamin needed for vision health and cell growth. Vitamin A deficiency is linked to night blindness, an inability to fight infections, and slow bone development. Best sources of vitamin A are sweet potatoes, green leafy vegetables, red peppers, paprika, chili powder, carrots, squash, herbs, cantaloupe, lettuce, and dried apricots. Vitamin A is fat soluble, so too much can be toxic.

Vitamin B1 (Thiamine): Helps to sharpen the mind, helps the neurological system to work properly, and metabolizes fats and proteins into energy. Symptoms of vitamin B1 deficiency include muscle weakness, nerve damage, and "pins and needles" sensations in the legs, Good sources of B1 include asparagus, crimini mushrooms, spinach, flaxseeds, tuna, green peas, and Brussels sprouts.

Vitamin B2 (Riboflavin): Helps neurotransmitters in the brain carry messages, helps balance mood, assists the adrenal gland, helps the body produce red blood cells, fights free radicals, helps with digestion of foods by converting calories from food into energy, and helps the digestive tract by aiding the absorption of iron and vitamin B6. Vitamin B2 deficiency is linked to mental confusion, slow mental processing, insomnia, dizziness, digestion issues, hair loss, and skin rashes. Foods highest in B2 are dried herbs, spices and peppers, almonds, liver, fish, sesame seeds, and sundried tomatoes.

Vitamin B3 (Niacin): Protects the nervous system, circulatory system, and the digestive system. It also helps detoxify pollutants. A deficiency of niacin can lead to irritability, poor concentration, anxiety, fatigue, restlessness, apathy, and depression. A severe deficiency can lead to a condition called pellagra, characterized by diarrhea, dermatitis, dementia, inflammation of the mouth, amnesia, delirium, and if left untreated, death. Some of the best sources of vitamin B3 are bran, fish, liver, paprika, peanuts, veal, chicken, bacon, and sundried tomatoes.

Vitamin B5 (Pantothenic Acid): A powerful antioxidant that helps fight infection and accelerates healing, B5 helps regulate the nervous system and helps treat symptoms of stress and fatigue. It helps accelerates the metabolism of nutrients into energy, maintains skin health, and helps to maintain healthy joints and ligaments. Vitamin B5 deficiency is linked to poor coordination, hypoglycemia, sleep disturbances, restlessness and irritability, numbness in hands and feet, muscle cramps and tingling sensations, fatigue, tiredness, and apathy. Deficiency can also lead to diarrhea, vomiting, and water retention. The best food sources of vitamin B5 are liver, sunflower seeds, bran, mushrooms, caviar, fish, avocados, and sundried tomatoes.

Vitamin B6 (Pyridoxine): Vital for brain health and mental clarity, vitamin B6 helps in maintaining normal nerve function. It plays a crucial role in the synthesis of neurotransmitters such as dopamine and serotonin. It also assists normal nerve cell communication, helps the immune system, helps to form red blood cells, supports sulfur and methyl metabolism for detoxification, has many anticancer properties, lowers cholesterol, and helps prevent cavities. A deficiency of vitamin B6 can lead to chronic inflammation in the body, impaired nervous system functioning, depression, irritability, confusion, cognitive problems, eczema, seborrheic dermatitis, convulsions, seizures, anemia, malaise, arthritis, anemia, fatigue, and still births. Best food sources of vitamin B6 include meat, chicken, fish, bell peppers, spinach, and potatoes with skin, yams, broccoli, asparagus, nuts, seeds, beans, and legumes. B6 absorbs better if taken with magnesium. Note: Although vitamin B6 is water-soluble, it is the one B vitamin that can accumulate and possibly lead to permanent nerve damage if taken in an excessively high dose for a long period of time. Learn more about the tolerable upper limits of vitamin B6 by visiting the Mayo Clinic's website at www.mayoclinic.com/health/vitamin-b6/NS_patient-b6/DSECTION=dosing. It's important to work with a nutritionist or naturopath when supplementing with high doses of vitamin B6. *If your child carries the pyrrole gene mutation, it may be necessary to supplement his/her diet with more vitamin B6.*

Vitamin B7 (Biotin): Plays a key role in metabolizing carbohydrates and fats properly; helps balance mood, process glucose, and protects against malnutrition. Deficiency is often linked to depression, fatigue, nausea, muscle pains, low iron levels, dermatitis, or cradle cap. Those who are constantly on antibiotics or on seizure medication need to be careful of biotin deficiency. Deficiency leads to symptoms like anxiety, depression, hair loss, anemia, and nausea. Too little vitamin B7 also reduces the ability of other vitamins in the B family to supply the nerves with the nourishment required to function normally. Eating foods such as beans, brewer's yeast, cauliflower, raw dark chocolate, avocado, egg yolks, fish, legumes, meat, molasses, nuts, bananas, oatmeal, oysters, peanuts, and poultry can boost biotin levels. Foods with higher levels of vitamin B7 include Swiss chard, nuts, chicken eggs, carrots, halibut, strawberries, raspberries, onions, cucumbers, and cauliflower.

Vitamin B9 (Folate is the natural form; folic acid is the synthetic form): Necessary for optimal brain, spine, and nerve health. It also helps produce healthy red blood cells and aids in rapid cell division and growth. Deficiency of folate can lead a host of diseases, brain defects, fatigue, headaches, diarrhea, trouble concentrating, and anemia, loss of appetite, depression, and irritability. The best sources of folate are green leafy vegetables, asparagus, broccoli, citrus fruits, strawberries, raspberries, honey, avocado, seeds, nuts, beans, peas, and lentils.

Vitamin B12 (Cobalamin): One of the most important vitamins for brain health, vitamin B12 calms the nervous system, helps the fatty acid synthesis, and helps the body produce energy to prevent fatigue. Vitamin B12 also helps regulate the nervous system and can reduce anxiety and depressive symptoms. It also plays a role in regulating our internal clock to help the brain make the transition from restful sleep to a more awake state, protects against cancer, and helps in healthy cell reproduction. Vitamin B12 is also essential for proper detoxification of toxic substances. The best food sources of vitamin B12 is dairy, fish, eggs, red meat, seafood, and liver. *If your child carries the MTHFR gene mutations, you must supplement his/her diet with more folate and the methylated form of vitamin B12.*

Vitamin C: An important antioxidant necessary for the growth and repair of tissues in the body, Vitamin C makes collagen—a protein that helps support blood vessels; supports neurological health, skin, and all of our organs; helps to strengthen our immune system to fight disease; and helps the body absorb iron. Vitamin C deficiency can lead to symptoms including fatigue, depression, rapid mood swings, irritability and a low frustration tolerance. Some early symptoms to watch for are muscle weakness, bleeding gums, gingivitis, bruising, joint pain, and anemia. Research in the *European Journal of Clinical Nutrition* suggests that some that suffer from gluten sensitivities could be deficient in vitamin C and good gut flora.[8] Some great sources of vitamin C include citrus fruits, red and hot chili peppers, red peppers, thyme, parsley, dark green leafy vegetables, strawberries, broccoli, and kiwi.

Vitamin D: An essential vitamin required by the body for the proper absorption of calcium, bone development, control of cell growth, neuromuscular functioning, proper immune functioning, and alleviation of inflammation. According to research featured in *Natural Health*, "Low vitamin D levels in the blood are directly connected to a higher incidence of cancer, osteoporosis, heart disease, depression, arthritis, and just about every other degenerative disease."[9] Lack of sunlight, gastrointestinal inflammation, darker skin, and elevated cortisol levels (cortisol is a stress hormone in the body) can cause vitamin D deficiency. Foods containing vitamin D include cod liver oil, fish, oysters, caviar, meat, eggs, and mushrooms. Also, vitamin D—especially the form D3 (the sunshine vitamin) is the only vitamin your body makes itself with the help of the sun. So be sure to get enough sun exposure to help the body make this essential nutrient.

Vitamin E: Reduces oxidative stress, boosts mental clarity and memory, reduces symptoms of mental confusion, and improves immune function. One study in the journal of *Alternative Therapies* demonstrated that "a combination of omega-3 fatty acids and vitamin E helps with speech impairments and speech apraxia. Children who were supplemented with vitamin E and omega-3 fatty acids showed improvements in speech, eye contact, behavior, and the ability to imitate others."[10] Symptoms of vitamin E deficiency are less obvious; however, some noted are muscle weakness, low iron levels, sight problems, and balance problems. Good sources of vitamin E include mustard greens, Swiss chard, spinach, kale, nuts, papaya, kiwi, red bell peppers, and olive oil.

Vitamin K: Helps blood vessels and brain cells by preventing arterial blockages and supporting brain health. It plays an important role in blood clotting and is essential for building strong bones and preventing heart disease. Deficiency of vitamin K includes bleeding within the digestive tract, easy bruising, gum bleeding, heavy menstrual bleeding, or hemorrhaging. The highest food with vitamin K include herbs, dark leafy greens, onions, Brussels sprouts, broccoli, chili pepper, curry, asparagus, cucumber, and prunes.

Choline: Enhances brain cell development and is a precursor molecule for the neurotransmitter acetylcholine, which is involved in the communication between nerves and muscles. Choline is important for reducing inflammation in the body and for metabolizing and transporting fats within the body so they don't build up in the liver. Also, the kidneys need choline to properly concentrate urine. If this does not occur properly, folate deficiency is more likely. Deficiency of this important nutrient can also cause a buildup of fat in the body and liver, insomnia, fatigue, mood instability, memory problems, and muscle and nerve problems. Foods containing higher amounts of choline are eggs, beef, pork, vegetable oil, chicken liver, fish, honey, and shiitake mushrooms.

Omega-3 Fatty Acids (EPA and DHA): These essential fatty acids play an important role in reducing inflammation in the entire body. Omega-3s boost brain function, helping to increase mental focus, reduce depression, and manic symptoms. In 2006, the journal *International Review of Psychiatry* reported, "Dietary supplementation with fish oils (providing EPA and DHA) appears to alleviate ADHD-related symptoms in at least some children, and one study of DCD children also found benefits for academic achievement."[11] Omega-3 also boosts cardiovascular health, helping to lower triglycerides and reduce blood pressure. This amazing nutrient is believed to help with numerous health conditions and is used to also treat cystic fibrosis, autism, and numerous other autoimmune disorders, including rheumatoid arthritis and lupus. Sources high in omega-3 fatty acids are salmon; sardines; eggs; pasture-raised meats; wild rice; walnuts; canola oil; hemp, chia, sunflower, flax, and other seeds; nuts; and beans.

Magnesium: Helps maintain nerve, muscle, and heart functions, and supports the immune system. According to *Autism Research Review International*, magnesium is called the antistress mineral and often helps to alleviate headaches, anxiety, and depressive symptoms, and is believed to reduce ADHD, PDD, and sensory processing issues is some children[12] by helping to send signals through the nervous system. When brain signals become disturbed and misinterpreted, sensory integration issues can arise. Magnesium also supports bowel movement regularity, healthy sleeping patterns, as well as helping the body regulate hormones. In addition, magnesium aids in digestion and acts as a natural laxative. It converts blood sugar to energy and is a natural medicine for diabetics because it helps regulate blood sugar levels. Natasha Campbell-McBride, MD, explains in her book *Put Your Heart in Your Mouth* why magnesium deficiency is such a problem today: "We have too much sugar in our diet today, and it takes 29 molecules of magnesium to digest one molecule of sugar, this sugar overload eventually leads to a magnesium deficiency." Hyla Cass, MD, explains in her book *Supplement Your Prescription: What Your Doctor Doesn't Know about Nutrition*, that many antianxiety and antidepressant medications may also deplete magnesium and calcium in the body, working against natural healing. If a supplement is required, research indicates magnesium citrate is one of the most bioavailable forms. The best dietary sources of magnesium include dark green leafy vegetables, almonds, sunflower seeds, sesame seeds, fish, beans, lentils, avocados, bananas, figs, and dark chocolate. Taking an Epsom Salt bath can help as well as the magnesium is absorbed through the skin.

Calcium: The most abundant mineral in your body, calcium is crucial for strong bones and teeth, helps promote a regular heartbeat, helps blood to clot properly, is involved in DNA synthesis, and is essential for healthy nerve and brain functioning. It plays a role in the neurotransmitter release of dopamine and carries signals in and out of the cells. Calcium deficiency leads to muscle cramping, loss of appetite, dry skin, brittle nails, bone breakage, infertility, miscarriages, headaches, common colds, allergies, heart disease, asthma, and arthritis. Those with dairy allergies/intolerances need to make sure to supplement the diet with other foods high in calcium such as dark leafy green vegetables, broccoli, sardines, fortified juices, bok choy, raw coconut, honey, tofu, and almonds.

Potassium: Maintains acid/alkaline balance in your blood and helps to build the electrical signaling panels inside the brain. Potassium deficiency is linked to confusion, fatigue, and muscle weakness, and potassium therapy has been known to prevent and treat sensory and motor dysfunction. Sources of potassium include bananas, kiwi, Brussels sprouts, almonds, avocados, apricots, tomatoes, bok choy, honey, beets, figs, Swiss chard, broccoli, and spinach.

Manganese: Assists metabolic activity in the human body and acts as a powerful antioxidant, neutralizing free radicals. Manganese is also important for bone health, the formation of connective tissue, absorption of calcium, regulating blood sugar, and ensuring proper thyroid gland and sex hormone functioning. The best sources of manganese are cloves, nuts, winter squash, dark chocolate, shellfish, pumpkin seeds, sunflower seeds, and chili peppers.

Zinc: Helps regulate blood sugar levels, boosts eye health, assists in stabilizing metabolic rate, supports immune system health, boosts digestive health, protects neurotransmitters, improves cognitive functioning, helps increase serotonin naturally, and promotes proper nerve health. According to many nutritional experts, zinc therapy has been known to reduce hyperactivity, impulsivity, and antisocial behavior, as well as help with sleep. Interestingly, stimulant medications actually deplete zinc in the body.[13] Zinc-deficient children are often suffering from frequent colds, lack of appetite, irritability, sullenness, and difficultly being sooth. ADHD/autistic individuals are often deficient in zinc, as well as magnesium, iron, and calcium. *If your child carries the pyrrole gene mutation, you may need to supplement him/her with more zinc.* The best sources of zinc include lamb, beef, scallops, sesame seeds, pumpkin seeds, nuts, oats, turkey, shrimp, and green peas.

Phosphorus: Aids in the development of bones and teeth, helps maintain heart regularity, provides energy, aids in digestion, and aids in the metabolism of fats and starches for proper nutrient absorption. Phosphorus is necessary for hormone balancing and protein formulation, as well as to properly utilize vitamin D, magnesium, and zinc. Foods rich in phosphorus include raw coconut, peanut butter, corn, broccoli, chicken, turkey, sunflower seeds, garlic, honey, legumes, and nuts.

Iodine: Iodine is a trace mineral that is crucial for the thyroid to function properly. Eating foods rich in iodine ensures the thyroid is able to manage metabolism, detoxification, growth, and development. Researchers have found that a lack of dietary iodine may lead to a weakened immune system, as well as to many health problems such as autism, neurological dysfunction, fatigue, slow metabolism, obesity, mental disabilities, infertility, non-healing wounds, infant/ child mortality, and other mental disorders such as attention issues, anxiety, and depression. Foods rich in healthy (nonsynthetic) iodine include pink Himalayan salt, sea vegetables, organic strawberries, organic navy beans, and cranberries. To learn more, read *Iodine: Why You Need It, Why You Can't Live Without It* by David Brownstein, MD.

Iron: Formation of hemoglobin to transfer oxygen to the body cells is the chief function of this important mineral. Iron is also needed to help build muscle, regulate body temperature, and aid in proper brain function. It provides energy to the body and also helps to make and transport dopamine in the brain. Iron deficiency is linked to fatigue, decreased appetite, headaches, irritability, memory problems, restless leg syndrome, and an inability to concentrate, short attention span, muscle weakness, impaired cognitive skills, and sleep problems. Anemia is also linked to many other chronic disease states of the circulatory, intestinal, and excretory system. Many doctors overlook iron deficiency until a patient hits rock bottom. Sources of iron include legumes, lentils, soy beans, dark green leafy vegetables, spinach, turnips, sprouts, and broccoli. Dried fruits also have good iron content. Eating vitamin C in conjunction with foods containing iron helps with iron absorption.

Selenium: A trace mineral found in soil, selenium is important for helping the body to make antioxidants and promote good health in smaller amounts. A deficiency of selenium is rare, but symptoms can include hypothyroidism and fatigue. Conversely, too much selenium may result in nausea and vomiting, as well as liver, kidney, and heart problems. The major benefits of selenium are that it regulates immune function, promotes a healthy heart, and assists in many metabolic processes. Most importantly, when combined with vitamin E, it fights inflammation and assists in the prevention and treatment of autoimmune disorders, including arthritis, lupus, and cancer. Selenium and iodine together help the thyroid produce hormones and function optimally and can also treat thyroid disorders. Important note: People with gluten sensitivity often have deficiencies in selenium. Some good sources of selenium include Brazil nuts, sunflower seeds, shellfish, meat, poultry, eggs, mushrooms, and onions.

Essential Amino Acids

Amino acids are organic compounds that combine together to form protein. They help to break down food, help repair body tissue, and help the body to grow. Amino acid deficiency can be another piece of the puzzle. In one study in the *Journal of Neuropsychiatric Disease and Treatment*, 85 children clinically diagnosed with ADHD were treated with amino acid supplementation; "77% achieved significant improvement and no significant safety concerns exist about their use."[14] Medication does not increase the total number of neurotransmitters in the central nervous system; it simply sets up conditions to move them around through reuptake. Meanwhile, amino acids actually help the body make more of these essential "feel good" molecules.

Amino acids cannot be made in the body, so eating a diet high enough in meat nuts, seeds, legumes, seafood, and egg protein is essential. They assist the body in making brain neurotransmitters naturally, so eating enough foods containing amino acids completes a very important biological process.

Interesting fact: Even though we are all conditioned to believe that a big turkey dinner promotes sleep because it contains the amino acid L-tryptophan, the emphasis is on the word "big," not "turkey." Although it would be nice to eat foods that contain serotonin (such as bananas) to ease depressive symptoms, the amino acids and neurotransmitters in food do not immediately cross the blood-brain barrier. Vegetarian diets often lack these essential nutrients. We need amino acids to learn, remember, and have a happy and stable mood. In addition, a deficiency of amino acids can adversely affect the lining of the gut. Are your kids eating enough protein?

If your child's body doesn't absorb these nutrients correctly, he/she can become depleted. It's essential, however, that you seek professional assistance because a delicate balance needs to be achieved. A metabolic workup would spot your child's unique imbalances, and the supplementation would be tailored specifically.

If your child is already on a selective serotonin reuptake inhibitor (SSRI) or a monoamine oxidase inhibitor (MAOI), it is important to know that amino acid supplementation could produce an adverse effect. Therefore, never experiment with amino supplementation without the help of your physician or practitioner.

L-Glutamine: The most abundant amino acid in our body. It helps to make protein our body needs for fuel. It can also be helpful for the immune system, gastrointestinal system, and for wound repair. L-glutamine was one of the remedies used to help repair Evan's permeable intestinal tract. It also provides the brain with an alternate source of fuel, helps the function of brain neurotransmitters, and improves mood, memory, and learning ability. L-glutamine is available in most meat proteins and beans.

5-HTP: A natural antidepressant. It's an amino acid produced by the body from the amino acid L-tryptophan. 5-HTP may help reduce anxiety, depression, and insomnia. Vitamin B6 converts the 5-HTP into serotonin, and magnesium prolongs its benefits. (5-HTP supplements shouldn't be taken with antidepressant medication).

GABA (Gamma-aminobutyric acid): May be a natural anti-anxiety treatment. It's a sleep-inducer and sleep-enhancer, as well as a neurotransmitter that inhibits anxiety-related messages to the central nervous system. Many children diagnosed with ADHD also suffer from anxiety and depression and often benefit from supplementation of GABA.

Glycine: When combined with GABA and glutamine, glycine can reduce anxiety, decrease cravings for sugar, help with sleep issues, improve cognitive function, and calm aggression. The body makes glycine by metabolizing many meat proteins, but a child with ADHD may greatly benefit from taking an additional supplement. Glycine has also been used to treat individuals who have had a stroke and patients with schizophrenia. It is believed that glycine may even help fight cancer.

L-tryptophan: An essential amino acid. This is one of the amino acids your body cannot produce, so you must get it through your diet. L-tryptophan is critical for the body to produce serotonin, which helps maintain a calm and relaxed mood. The body uses L-tryptophan to create 5-hydroxytryptophan (5-HTP).

Tyrosine: A nonessential amino acid the body makes from another amino acid called phenylalanine. It is a building block for several important brain chemicals called neurotransmitters, including epinephrine, norepinephrine, and dopamine. Tyrosine also helps produce melanin, the pigment responsible for hair and skin color. It helps in the function of organs responsible for making and regulating hormones, including the adrenal, thyroid, and pituitary glands. It is involved in the structure of almost every protein in the body. Some animal and human studies suggest that tyrosine supplements may help improve memory and performance under psychological stress, but more research is needed. Some practitioners use tyrosine in the treatment of attention deficit disorder to improve cognition, motivation, and mental performance.

L-Theanine: The amino acid found in green tea. It's extremely beneficial in people who experience panic attacks and "brain fog." It stimulates the production of GABA, regulating dopamine and serotonin. It produces a calming effect without sleepiness. In addition, it boosts the immune system and increases the production of alpha brain waves, which help us feel alert and calm at the same time. Some studies in *Alternative Medicine Review* have shown that supplementation can be effective in ADHD children to reduce anxiety and improve sleep patterns.[15]

L-Carnitine: A naturally occurring amino acid that plays a vital role in the metabolism of fat. It functions as a transporter of fatty acids into the mitochondria—the metabolic furnace of cells. Available through red meat, dairy, nuts, seeds, vegetables, fruits, whole grains, avocado, and tempeh, L-carnitine aids in the release of stored body fat into the bloodstream for energy. This conditional amino acid is also involved in muscle contraction and the regulation of protein balance. Research at NYU Langone Medical Center suggests that an adequate supply of L-carnitine could be instrumental in the treatment of diabetes, heart disease, infertility, chronic fatigue syndrome, and other autoimmune disorders.[16] The Department of Pediatrics at Westfriesgasthuis in Hoorn, The Netherlands, reported, "L-carnitine is being used successfully in the treatment of ADHD and is seen to decrease attention problems and aggressive behavior."[17]

Taurine: Commonly thought of as an amino acid, taurine is not a true amino acid because it has a sulfonic acid group rather than a carboxyl group, as is found in amino acids. It is often used in the natural treatment of anxiety disorders and seizures. It assists the body's neurotransmitters and has many benefits. Low taurine levels may be found in children with ADHD, anxiety, insomnia, depression, seizure disorders, hypothyroidism, digestive disorders, autism, and many other conditions. This amino acid is found in eggs, milk, meat, and seafood. To help calm ADHD symptoms, enhance brain and neurological functioning, and help eliminate toxins, children may need to be supplemented with taurine because the body cannot make it on its own. Possible reasons for deficiency include not eating meat/fish; being under high levels of physical and emotional stress; deficiency in zinc, vitamin A, B6, and other amino acids; candida or bacteria overgrowth; and eating foods that contain MSG.

Why Eating Protein Is Important

Everyone talks about how ADHD sufferers need more dopamine and serotonin, which usually translates into more meds. However, if we look at the physiology behind how neurotransmitters are made in the first place, most of them depend on an adequate intake of protein. Therefore, it's essential that we eat an adequate supply of protein daily.

Maybe you've wondered how much protein you need each day. In general, it's recommended that ten to thirty-five percent of your daily calories come from protein. Below are the Recommended Dietary Allowances (RDA) for different age groups.[18]

RECOMMENDED DIETARY ALLOWANCE FOR PROTEIN

Group	Grams of protein needed each day
Children ages 1–3	13
Children ages 4–8	19
Children ages 9–13	34
Girls ages 14–18	46
Boys ages 14–18	52
Women ages 19–70+	46
Men ages 19–70+	56

According Lauren Antonucci, MS, RD, director of Nutrition Energy in New York City, pregnant and breastfeeding woman need 20 grams more protein per day.[19]

Lots of foods contain protein; there are both vegetarian and animal sources. Some examples include meat, nuts, fish, eggs, dairy, beans, lentils, and seeds. A 3-ounce piece of meat has about 21 grams of protein. A typical 8-ounce piece of meat could have over 50 grams of protein. One cup of dry beans has about 16 grams of protein.

Why Eating Meat Is Important

Meat contains a high concentration of protein, which is essential for proper brain growth. Kid's brains need protein to function properly. A healthy diet must include quality sources of protein to allow a child's brain to grow and develop.

Proteins make up parts of brain cells and the connective tissue around them. If the brain doesn't grow, it can lead to a condition called microcephaly. Children with microcephaly can suffer from hyperactivity, dwarfism, seizures, and/or delayed motor functions or speech. Severe cases result in mental retardation.

Meat contains heme iron, which is the most absorbable form of iron. Meat is also the most concentrated form of vitamin B12 and zinc.

Grass-Fed Meat and Free-Range Eggs Are Better for Us

Eating grass-fed meats instead of their grain-fed counterparts traditionally sold in supermarkets may greatly benefit your health and the health of your child. Grass-fed animals do not need the large amounts of antibiotics that non-grass-fed animals require. The grass that is grazed by cows has higher nutritional value and is not subjected to genetically modified organisms (GMOs). Grass-fed meat contains fewer parasites and other bacteria because corn, which is fed to grain-fed animals, upsets the cow's stomach, making it unnaturally acidic. Grass-fed meat is lower in overall fat and provides more omega-3 healthy fats, beneficial linoleic acid, and vitamin E.

Free-range eggs are healthier as well. One project demonstrated that eggs sold in supermarkets are nutritionally inferior to the eggs produced by hens raised in a pasture. A 2007 *Mother Earth News* egg-testing project found that, compared to official U.S. Department of Agriculture (USDA) nutrient data for commercial eggs, eggs from hens raised on pasture contained one-third less cholesterol, one-quarter less saturated fat, two-thirds more vitamin A, two times more vitamin E, seven times more beta-carotene, and four to six times the vitamin D.[20]

CHAPTER 13

Pursuing Alternative Solutions

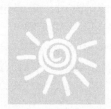

After going to the pediatric gastro doctor and getting absolutely nowhere, I was so ecstatic when my husband came home with the business card from the wife of his coworker. She is a doctor of naturopathic medicine (ND) who had just opened her practice ten miles from our home.

Doctors of naturopathic medicine attend an intensive four-year doctoral-leveled program at an accredited institution. They are trained in biomedical sciences and are considered holistic primary care physicians after passing a state board licensing exam. An ND has extensive training in areas such as clinical nutrition and nutritional science, botanical medicine, homeopathy, counseling, and laboratory and clinical diagnosis. Ultimately, they believe in the importance of supporting, enhancing, and stimulating the inherent healing power of the body.

I scheduled an appointment with Dr. Sharmilee Jayachandran the very next day because she was a naturopath who specialized in homeopathy. I then emailed her my thoughts and links to the websites I had reviewed. I wanted to know if I was possibly on the right path.

She replied almost immediately, and her uplifting email was exactly what I was hoping for. She spoke of homeopathic treatments that had proven successful with children and adults who had similar issues as Evan. She told me that I was on the right path and completely validated my ideas and concerns. She explained to me that we would do a complete metabolic workup and food sensitivity testing. She also had a test for heavy metals such as arsenic, cadmium, lead, and mercury, which could also contribute to many of Evan's symptoms. She told me it was possible that Evan had a compromised immune system and was unable to absorb nutrients because of an inflamed and permeable gut.

The initial consultation took two and one-half hours. She obtained a complete history and was more thorough than all of the other physicians we had seen combined. During the exam, the ND explained that some kids tend to have more loose stools, while others have constipation so extreme that they develop impactions. She felt Evan's abdomen, and it was so tender to the touch that he grimaced in pain. She was able to feel a huge fecal mass when she palpated his abdomen. She explained that this meant he was probably also storing large quantities of toxins. She also pointed out that Evan had tiny bumps on the back of arms—called keratosis, which may indicate a gluten sensitivity or a deficiency in fatty acids or vitamin A.

She ran lab tests on Evan that consisted of nine vials of blood and three urine tests. Lo and behold, he matched up with the issues pointed to by the Malabsorption Study of 2009.[1]

Evan had extremely low vitamin and mineral levels, including A, B-complex, D, E, zinc, and potassium, among other things. He had sensitivities to gluten, milk, mustard, eggs (severe), peanuts (mild), and almonds (mild). In addition, the tests showed that he had mercury, aluminum arsenic, and lead building up in his system.

My instincts were correct again, and the pediatric doctor at the Digestive Disease Medical Center was wrong. Even though Evan didn't test positive for celiac disease, he did have gluten and other such sensitivities.

His blood work clearly demonstrated that his intestinal tract was under attack, and the diagnosis of "leaky gut" was officially confirmed. His immune system was overreacting to certain foods that were "leaking" out of the intestines and producing antibodies to fight it. His system was completely inflamed. The body was attacking the food like it was an invader, and his intestinal walls had become weak and permeable. The nutrients (amino acids, simple sugars, vitamins, and minerals) weren't properly absorbed by his body, and his body's chemical detoxification system wasn't working properly.

The GI tract is supposed to break down and digest food into simpler parts to allow the body to absorb the nutrients, so that other organs can then convert the nutrients into proteins and energy. The vitamins and minerals are supposed to be carried across the intestinal lining into the bloodstream. In addition, the gut protects the body against infection (the immune system).

This explained Evan's vitamin deficiencies and his "bad" immune system. It finally made sense why Evan suffered from so many ear infections and sinus infections. I understood why Evan suffered from stomach issues, diarrhea, and constipation, and why he had skin inflammation like eczema/psoriasis on his arms and cradle cap.

All of the conditions I had been trying to address were part of the same "disease." Many of Evan's brain and nervous system malfunctions were a direct result of toxic insults that led to metabolic and immune system deterioration.

An Integrated Approach to Healing

In my opinion, ADD/ADHD, autistic spectrum disorders, and possibly some mental illnesses are a compilation of medical symptoms that need to be addressed. The name of the game is to identify the underlying causes, before simply placing labels. In my opinion, these are often autoimmune syndromes. The problems are biochemical and occur at the molecular level. All of these symptoms interlink with each other like Olympic rings. Getting one problem going will drive another. The important cycles that I believe to be major players include nutrition, food sensitivities, gut flora, environmental toxins, heavy metals, poor digestion, bowel toxicity, gene mutations, hypoglycemia, adrenal fatigue, and detoxification issues. Therefore, it was important for me to talk to a nutritionist, naturopath, and other such practitioners so that they could come up with a specific protocol to address and treat Evan's illness appropriately.

I want to emphasize that there was no "magic bullet," no single treatment alone that significantly reversed the effects of ADHD, apraxia, or autism. All cases are individualized, and each child needs a well-thought-out and integrated approach to move him/her along the road to improvement and recovery.

Becoming Your Child's Champion and Advocate

Helping our children becomes our mission, and it's important for us to look at their symptoms as a complicated puzzle. It's a puzzle that can be solved by putting all of the pieces together. So, take the time to uncover underlying issues and discover the many solutions that can inevitably help your child. I recommend that you find physicians and practitioners who will listen to you and address your concerns rather than dismiss them, and I encourage you to do your homework and ask your doctors a lot of questions. Most of all, I encourage you to trust your gut insticts.

During this process, I felt overwhelmed by all of the information I wanted to learn. I had to remember to take deep breaths and come to terms with the fact that it wasn't going to be an easy or fast ride. I hit many obstacles along the way, including medical professionals who wouldn't take me seriously. Never give up because there is real healing available for your child!

CHAPTER 14

Our Road to Recovery

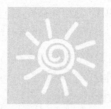

Addressing All Aggravating Factors

I've heard countless moms say, "Oh, we tried that. We eliminated dairy and gluten for six months, but there were no changes." "We took her off all processed food, gave her expensive organic foods for a year, and the only thing it did was drain my pocketbook." It's important for me to stress that in order for the entire system to recover, you must address all of the issues of malabsorption that leads to malnutrition. You must test for and address numerous food intolerances; vitamin, mineral, and amino acid imbalances; gut health; heavy metal and toxicity issues; blood sugar problems; essential fatty-acid deficiencies; pyroluria; and MTHFR and other genetic mutations. All of these things work together to heal an inflamed gut and compromised system—dietary changes are just one piece of the puzzle.

In this chapter, I will explore in more detail Evan's gut healing protocol and outline some of the available treatment options. Please note, however, that I don't endorse or promote any one modality or set of supplements for natural healing. Every child presents with his/her unique set of challenges, and it's important for each child to be tested and obtain individualized treatment.

I believed, however, that in order for Evan to heal, we needed to incorporate many Eastern medicine practices in conjunction with Western modalities to create an integrative treatment plan. We worked to address his entire system emotionally, biochemically, and physically.

Alongside the intensive speech, occupational, and other healing therapies that Evan was receiving, our naturopathic physician provided us with the framework for a proper diet. She then worked at addressing all underlying issues sequentially.

Supporting the Body to Heal Itself: Addressing Gastrointestinal Issues

Constipation issues in children like Evan often compound the problem by poisoning and inflaming the system with harmful bacteria and environmental toxins. Constipation causes food transit time to slow down and allows waste products to stay in the colon for too long. The transit time of food is the time it takes for a meal to enter the mouth and exit the rectum and should take between 18 and 50 hours and on average; children as well as adults should have at least one bowel movement per day.

Toxins enter the bloodstream through the intestinal wall and possibly settle in the tissues, leading to headaches, brain fog, fatigue, depression, obesity, indigestion, gas, bloating, and autoimmune disorders. In addition, this buildup could cause malabsorption (the lack of absorption of good nutrients into the body).

Chronic diarrhea also indicates a problem with the intestinal system and could also point to a form of bowel disease or inflammation. If a person goes two to three times a day and the stools are solid and pass easily, though, it is probably alright. However, if stools are frequent, loose, and watery, it may be a good idea to seek medical assistance. Chronic diarrhea can cause a reduced absorption of nutrients in the small intestine, which can be related to malnutrition and neurological dysfunction.

Evan's bowel movements occurred only two times a week at most. When he did go to the bathroom, he strained for forty-five minutes or more, and his stools were usually soft like diarrhea. This never made sense to me, but I started to believe that it was normal for him. After all, I had heard of many adults who complained of constipation and other ailments, so I never thought much about it.

When I brought this condition to the attention of our pediatrician, she told me to give Evan MiraLAX. For diarrhea or a stomach flu, she recommended Pedialyte.

When Evan got diarrhea, I gave him a bland diet of bananas and rice. For dehydration, I had Pedialyte ice pops in the freezer. Pedialyte is recommended by pediatricians daily, and it wasn't until recently that I discovered it's no better than Gatorade. The ingredients in Pedialyte include: sucralose (Splenda), artificial flavor, FD&C Red #40, Blue #1, dextrose (a simple sugar) made from genetically modified corn, and Acesulfame-K. Splenda is an artificial sweetener made from chlorine, a known carcinogen. Basically toxic for the brain, these ingredients can impact memory, mood, and behavior.

I knew MiraLAX was given to adults to prepare them for a colonoscopy, but I started to question the use of polyethylene glycol (PEG), an engineered chemical in MiraLAX. I looked up the ingredients and discovered that PEG is a close cousin to antifreeze. I also became aware that PEG could cause neurological and other side effects.

How many of our kids have been prescribed MiraLAX for constipation? How many of us knew it was poison or that it was never approved for use with children? According to pharmacist, medical author, lecturer, and radio talk show host, Konstantin Monastyrsky, "Technically, PEG is an osmotic laxative. Because of this property, it blocks the absorption of nutrients in the small intestine. Its extended use may result in severe malnutrition-related disorders, particularly in young children and older adults. Autism is one such disorder. It may take only two weeks of an acute iron or iodine deficiency to cause autism in a child younger than two."[1]

After talking to one mom about this, she responded by saying, "I paid good money to a pediatric gastro to give me this on long-term basis for one of my kids. It's time for big pharma to be banned from writing the textbooks for doctors!"

If you're interested in exploring the connection between autism and nutritional deficiencies related to PEG, please see the reference above. Here are two other articles of interest:

Sullivan KM. Iodine deficiency as a cause of autism. *J Neurological Science* 2009; 276 (1–2):202; author reply 203; www.ncbi.nlm.nih .gov/pubmed/18962727.

Hergüner S, Kelesoglu FM, Tanıdır C, Cöpür M. Ferritin and iron levels in children with autistic disorder. *Eur J Pediatr* 2012 Jan; 171 (1):1436; www.ncbi.nlm.nih.gov/pubmed/21643649.

Home Remedies for Treating Chronic Diarrhea and Constipation

Natural Remedies for Diarrhea

- Avoid milk or milk products, carbonated beverages, spicy foods, and wheat.
- Take probiotics such as acidophilus.
- Eat white rice (rinsed to remove arsenic) with ginger.
- Grate an apple, and eat it after it turns brown.
- Make a paste of powered ginger, cumin, cinnamon, and honey, and eat it three times daily.
- Drink pickle juice.
- Drink a glass of water with the juice of two lemons, $1/2$ teaspoon of baking powder, 1 teaspoon of sugar, and a pinch of salt.
- Mix 1 teaspoon of cinnamon in a cup of warm water and add a little bit of organic sugar.
- Eat crushed chia seeds because they absorb water in the colon. Be careful because a little goes a long way, and too much can cause colon upset.
- Eat shelled hemp seeds.
- Drink blackberry leaf iced tea.
- Make a pineapple and blueberry smoothie.

Replenish Electrolytes

Drink Coconut Water

Coconut water is all natural, and children love it! Try naturally flavored varieties. It is a well-balanced fluid loaded with minerals such as iron, calcium, potassium, and manganese; amino acids; B vitamins; vitamin C; and cytokinins, which have an anticarcinogenic (anticancer) effect.

Make Your Own Pedialyte-type Drink

Lemon-Watermelon drink is rich in potassium, phosphorus, magnesium, calcium, and more. It is healthier than store-bought varieties and can be made with this simple recipe:

- 3 cups natural spring water
- $1/3$ cup freshly squeezed lemon juice
- 1 cup fresh watermelon juice
- $1/3$ cup raw honey* or molasses
- Pinch of natural sea salt
- $1/2$ to 1 teaspoon aluminum-free baking soda (sodium bicarbonate)

*WARNING: Honey is not safe for children under one year of age.

Natural Remedies for Constipation

- Avoid milk and milk products.

- Take probiotics such as acidophilus.

- Eat foods high in magnesium such as flax seeds, kidney beans, black beans, lentils, quinoa, millet, spinach, and oatmeal (if not sensitive). A magnesium supplement is often helpful in chronic situations. Taking vitamin B6 in conjunction with magnesium can help the body absorb it better.

- Talk to a naturopath about the homeopathic remedies, Calcarea Carbonica 30c and Nux Vomica.

- Eat high-fiber foods such as fruits and vegetables, apricots, prunes, organic (non-GMO) corn, quinoa, and rhubarb sweetened with honey.

- Eat hemp seeds.

- Eat an apple or raisins one hour after a meal.

- Cut back on processed and refined foods.

- Eat blackstrap molasses and honey.

- Snack on flaxseeds, pumpkin seeds, and sesame seeds.

- Cook with olive oil and coconut oil.

- Massage organic/pure essential oils on the abdomen or take a drop orally. The best oils for constipation are peppermint, ginger, lemon, fennel, and lemongrass.

- Exercise.

- Become aware of medications and over-the-counter remedies that can cause constipation. Many prescribed medications warn about constipation, especially those containing calcium or aluminum, which are binding.

    Warning: Honey is not safe for young children under one year of age.

There are also many herbal and homeopathic remedies for diarrhea and constipation, so please check with your naturopath.

The Body on the Mend with Homeopathy and Natural Treatments

Gut rehabilitation can be a slow process, and I remember feeling impatient some days. This is certainly not the quick fix that the current pharmaceutical companies promise, but there's real healing taking place. We addressed not only Evan's symptoms, but began digging deeper to address the causes.

Evan's Treatment Plan

Our naturopath recommended digestive enzymes with DPP IV (Dipeptidyl peptidase IV) to help Evan break down his food so that absorption would be easier on his digestive tract, and she gave us a pediatric encapsulation product called G.I. Fortify and colostrum powder to help restore Evan's gut. This particular product contains licorice extract, marshmallow root, lemon balm, L-glutamine, and chamomile extract. She also started him on his first round of homeopathic treatments for constipation, cradle cap, and eczema, which included Calcarea Carbonica 30c (calcium carbonate from an oyster shell) and a magnesium/B6 supplement (IN-GEAR) by Metabolic Maintenance. Both treatments proved successful. Calcarea Carbonica 30c has also been used to treat speech disorders, and we certainly saw a difference almost immediately.

Once Evan's gut was on the mend, the naturopath started detoxifying his liver and kidneys. She used constitutional remedies to reverse the vaccine side effects and the many other insults to his immune system.

After that, she continued him on many other homeopathic remedies for a specified period of time. She gave him Nux Vomica to treat irritability, impatience, digestive ailments including constipation, insomnia, and sensory integration issues. She gave him cell salts such as Kali Phos 6x (potassium phosphate) to provide his brain with the nourishment it needed to relax, recover, and strengthen. She also provided him with Ferrum Phos 6x (iron phosphate) to strengthen his blood cells, which had been stressed due to systemic inflammation.

Here are some other homeopathic remedies used in the treatment of ADHD and related disorders:

- Stramonium: Used for the treatment of posttraumatic stress disorder (PTSD), and for individuals who experience night-terrors, extreme anxiety, rage, and/or aggression.

- Tarentula Hispanica: Used for the treatment of individuals with a noise sensitivity, and who are hyper and hurried. Some individuals who experience the feeling of powerlessness and a low self-esteem are also treated with this remedy.

- Cina: Used to calm excessively irritated individuals who may have an aversion or to being looked at or touched, cradled, and loved. The individual treated with this remedy is often feeling agitated or aggressive.

- Hyoscyamus Niger: Used for the treatment of poor impulse control, as well as clowning around and acting and/or laughing inappropriately. This remedy also relieves many of the symptoms relating to persons who are considered oversexual in thought or action.

- *Withania somnifera* (Ashwagandha): Used for the treatment of inflammation, immune system strengthening, stress reduction, improving mental concentration, and providing nourishment to the brain.

  Do not self-treat. Be sure to find a practitioner who specializes in homeopathy. Homeopathic remedies are quite affordable, however, it is important to find the correct remedy and to ensure that the correct doses are given and at the correct times.

For more information about homeopathy in the treatment of ADHD please refer to: http://nationalcenterforhomeopathy.org/; http://adhdhomeopath.com/what-to-expect-from-a-homeopathic-consultation.

For more information about homeopathy in the treatment of autism and to review case studies please refer to: http://homeopathyplus.com.au/reversing-autism-part-1/ and the *Internet Journal of Alternative Medicine,* http://ispub.com/IJAM/7/2/8801 to read "New Dimensions in the Treatment of Autism with Homeopathy."

Treating Parasites

Many of us carry intestinal parasites that are virtually harmless, but some parasites can cause gastrointestinal problems, malnutrition, acute diarrhea, and constipation. Our little ones can pick up these parasites anywhere, including salad bars, buffets, cafeterias, daycare centers, school, grocery stores, and on vacation in exotic locations.

These little critters are quite common and are an unsuspected cause of many illnesses.

You should have your child tested for two types of parasites. The first consists of tapeworms and roundworms that attach themselves to the lining of the small intestine, causing internal bleeding and the loss of essential nutrients. The symptoms of these parasites may not be obvious, such as slowly losing iron.

The second type are protozoa, tiny one-cell organisms that can cause acute or chronic diarrhea, constipation, fatigue, joint pain, dizziness, and/or hives.

There are numerous medications that can remove these parasites from the intestines, and naturopathic doctors have a toolbox of natural remedies. Evan was treated for parasites with grapefruit seed extract and pumpkin seeds. Please speak with your healthcare professional before starting any regimen, however.

Adding Friendly Bugs

We then needed to address Evan's gut bacteria. In a healthy body, yeast cohabitates in a friendly balance with probiotic bacteria (the "good" bugs such as *Lactobacillus acidophilus*, *Bifidobacterium bifidum*, and *Lactobacillus rhamnosus*). Adequate probiotic populations promote good digestion and immune function, and they improve resistance to infections, allergies, and eczema.

Evan was given a quality probiotic supplement that didn't contain any dairy products to provide his gut with good bacteria. Our naturopath explained that some physicians overprescribe medications to treat yeast infections without addressing the root cause of the infections. That was certainly true in our case. Medication was used numerous times to treat Evan for excessive yeast. Never once was the idea of naturally healing his gut introduced. Even when I asked if I should give him probiotics to combat an antibiotic, I was merely told, "Yeah, I guess, that's probably a good idea—it couldn't hurt."

Evan was tested for candida about six months after he had been on probiotics, a revised diet, and homeopathic remedies. His tests came back negative, and he no longer suffered from chronic thrush, athlete's foot, or other fungal infections. Teachers, therapists, and family members saw drastic improvements in his cognitive functioning, mood, speech, and motor coordination, too.

My mother-in-law, Carol, is a huge fan of yogurt and raw milk kefir and had insisted that it would help Evan's gut. Kefir is a cultured dairy product produced by fermenting milk with kefir grains. A cousin to yogurt, it is believed to have many health benefits including immune system enhancement and the ability to stabilize gut flora and rid the body of any bad bacteria in the gut. I learned from the naturopath and the books I was reading, however, that many children on the autism spectrum are sensitive to milk protein (casein). Evan was no exception.

So, before supplementing your child's diet with yogurt or kefir, have your child's blood tested for possible milk protein antibodies. You can make kefir with water or coconut milk or simply use a quality nondairy probiotic powder. We tried making coconut kefir, but Evan didn't like the taste. So, we put him on a quality probiotic to assist in the rebuilding of his intestinal tract and help him achieve a healthier gut balance.

Probiotics & Prebiotics 101

Probiotics are defined as "live microorganisms, which, when administered in the adequate amounts, support gut health." The microorganisms found in probiotics are known as "friendly bacteria" or "good bacteria" and are, for the most part, microorganisms naturally found in the human body. The most commonly used probiotics come from two groups known as *Lactobacillus* and *Bifidobacterium*.

Buy a high-quality, extra-strength probiotic supplement that needs to be refrigerated and is free of gluten, dairy, and other allergens. Also, get one that provides a high amount of live units per capsule. Do not take with warm liquids, give it to your child daily for best results, and store it in the freezer for extended life.

Feed probiotics with prebiotics. Prebiotics are defined as non-digestible dietary fiber that triggers the growth of healthy gut bacteria. The most common type of prebiotic is the soluble fiber inulin. It is important to get plenty of inulin from plants containing fructan. Some of these sources include asparagus, chicory, garlic, leek, onion, and artichoke.

"Adequate intake of dietary fiber is increasingly being recommended by governmental public health agencies as a means to maintain and increase health and well-being. Some epidemiological studies have shown support for an inverse relationship between dietary fiber consumption and risk of some chronic diseases. Developing evidence suggests that dietary fiber protects against cardiovascular disease, obesity, type 2 diabetes and many digestive disorders; inflammatory bowel disease and colon cancer."[2]

That said, there are concerns by some health experts that prebiotics may also feed the bad bacteria in our gut. So, with individuals with an unbalanced digestive tract, such with those with chronic digestive symptoms like diarrhea, flatulence, stomach pains, reflux, and leaky gut syndrome, food allergies, or food intolerance, doctors may suggest "starving out" good and bad bacteria initially by removing certain fiber from the diet. Although this sounds like a contradiction, if fiber is not limited symptoms may become worse.

If there is an overgrowth of pathogenic bacteria, yeast, and/or fungi, the good microbes cannot do their job of properly digesting fiber, which causes the very symptoms we are trying to eradicate. Natasha Campbell-McBride, MD, provides all the necessary details for the GAPS protocol in her book *Gut and Psychology Syndrome*.

Nurture a Happy Gut

Here are some tips for creating a healthier, happier gut:

1. **Cook with flavor-enhancing herbs and spices** such as turmeric, rosemary, ginger, basil, bay leaves, cumin, dill, cilantro/coriander, garlic, oregano, pepper, chili peppers, black seeds, and sage. These are natural digestive aids that reduce inflammation, prevent gas and bloating, improve asthma, purify the blood, and assist with the management of many autoimmune disorders.

2. **Serve plenty of colorful fruits and vegetables** such as grapes, blueberries, strawberries, and leafy greens. This allows your family to get essential anti-inflammatory antioxidants with every meal in order to reduce gut inflammation. Be careful about eggplant, potatoes, and tomatoes, however. They contain chemical compounds called alkaloids, which can actually trigger inflammation.

3. **Provide your child with enough healthy fatty acids** from foods such as cold-water oily fish like salmon, walnuts, pumpkin seeds, sesame seeds, ground flaxseed, ground chia seeds, grape seeds, and coconut oil. Ensure that omega-3 supplements are distilled, filtered, and free of mercury, pesticides, PCBs, and other contaminants. Getting enough fatty acids helps with digestion and absorption of nutrients and is even thought to possibly reduce the severity of allergies. Taking evening primrose oil is also recommended because it is high in the essential fatty acid gamma-linolenic acid (GLA), omega-6. It is recommended to take fatty acid supplements in the morning because it of its brain-sharpening and mood-enhancing effect that could disrupt sleep if given to late in the day.

4. **Use honey as a natural sweetener in lieu of refined sugar (but only if your child is older than one year).** Honey is an amazing food that helps heal the gut and provides good gut bacteria, helps the colon, boosts the immune system, stabilizes blood sugar, and helps fight off bad viruses, bacteria, and yeast. Buy honey from a local farm stand or local store you trust to ensure that it is pure and contains a plentiful supply of pollen. Many store brands of honey are simply imposters for the real thing, and some companies feed sugar water and high fructose corn syrup to their bees instead of allowing them to graze in pastures. In other cases, the honey is ultra-filtered, highly processed, and watered down so that it contains little to no pollen.

5. **Drink organic aloe vera juice.** High-quality, raw organic aloe vera can be a phenomenal digestive aid. It seals the gut wall, aids in digestion, has anti-inflammatory properties, helps the immune system, and detoxifies the liver, skin, and colon. Too much aloe can cause the kidneys to work too hard, so proceed cautiously.

6. **Cook with more black pepper** to help the body absorb nutrients better. Black pepper contains a compound called piperine, which increases the bioavailability of food by decreasing activity in the intestinal tract and inhibiting the metabolism of certain enzymes. Better still, cook with lots of turmeric and black pepper together. The combination helps the body absorb more curcumin, the active ingredient in turmeric. This ingredient can heal gut wall permeability due to its amazing anti-inflammatory properties. An article on CNN iReport.com discussed how turmeric also aids in digestion, strengthens the immune system, improves asthma, heals wounds, prevents the progression of memory loss, controls diabetes, improves liver function, lowers cholesterol, and fights cancer.[3]

7. **If you or your child gets a stomachache, avoid an over-the-counter antacid** laced with aluminum and artificial ingredients. Instead, try drinking two ounces of raw organic aloe vera juice with the juice of half a lemon mixed in water.

8. **Don't throw away the core of the pineapple; eat it.** Bromelain is powerful enzyme that is used as a medicine that heals the gut wall, aids in digestion so that nutrients absorb better, helps with constipation naturally, treats irritable bowel syndrome, and reduces inflammation. It also helps to thin the blood naturally, so use caution with anyone who is taking blood-thinning medications. Cooking the pineapple core can reduce the bromelain content, so use it to make a delicious smoothie instead.

Yummy Pineapple Smoothie

$1/2$ cup fresh pineapple juice   6 ice cubes

1 cup coconut milk   1 cup crushed pineapple core

3 teaspoons honey* $1/2$ teaspoon vanilla extract

Blend the ingredients together, and enjoy.

*WARNING: Honey is not safe for children under one year of age.

CHAPTER 15

Addressing Food Sensitivities and Diet Modifications

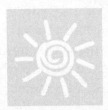

Evan had many of the symptoms of a child who suffered from dietary triggers, including congestion, history of ear infections, reflux, poor attention span, coughing spells, dark under eye circles, insomnia, and sinus issues. Evan also suffered from psoriasis (an autoimmune disease that causes new skin cells that grow deep in your skin to rise too fast and pile up on the skin surface). Psoriasis is often related to arthritis (an autoimmune disease in which the immune system attacks the lining of the joints throughout the body). It just so happens that arthritis is very prevalent in my family. Evan had a form of eczema and cradle cap on his arms, which I found out later were related to the psoriasis (another autoimmune disorder).

I asked one of Evan's conventional doctors why Evan had such skin issues, and he said, "No worries; he's of Italian decent and has an overexcretion of oil. He will probably develop acne as a teenager." Was he kidding me?

After getting back the results of our IgE and IgG food allergy and food sensitivity tests, our first line of defense was to immediately eliminate the worst food offenders from Evan's diet. His list included all dairy products, wheat, eggs, and mustard, and we needed to be very careful with peanuts and almonds. The naturopath reminded me that even though Evan tested negative for celiac disease, it didn't mean that he didn't suffer from a gluten sensitivity. I was happy that she went further in her testing. She also explained that we needed to restore his gut to its normal healthy state before reintroducing the foods to his system. There was a possibility that Evan could eat some of the foods again after his gut made a full recovery in a few years. It would depend on whether or not the food sensitivity was genetic.

The Most Common Food Sensitivities

While we can be allergic to most anything, the most common foods that aggravate the delicate balance of our kids' systems are:

- Wheat
- Dairy products, including cheese and yogurt
- Eggs
- Yeast
- Shellfish
- Tree nuts
- Peanuts
- Garlic
- Soy
- Preservatives
- Artificial color and flavoring
- Phenols/Salicylates

What Is a Phenol/Salicylate Intolerance?

Managing food sensitivities can be a challenge, especially since some of them fail to show up on blood tests. One such sensitivity is salicylates, a subgroup of phenols. These are naturally occurring chemicals in many plants, acting as natural pesticides, protecting them against diseases, fungi, and bacterial infections. There are also synthetic chemicals that mimic natural salicylates in food dyes, preservatives, and medications like aspirin, acne products, detergent, lotion, skin cleansers, hair products, shampoo, mint-flavored toothpaste, gum, makeup, sunscreen, and foods containing artificial color/flavoring.

Toxic to everyone in large doses, salicylates cause sensitive people to experience toxic symptoms when they eat even a small amount. Some symptoms include gastrointestinal distress, asthma, fatigue, nasal congestion, memory loss, inattention, ADHD, depression, anxiety, inappropriate laughter, extra self-stimulatory behaviors, waking up during the night, and dark circles under the eyes.

Almost all foods have phenols, but in varying amounts. Foods high in natural salicylates are tomatoes, apples, peanuts, oranges, chocolate, red grapes, coffee, berries, and peppers.

One way to test for an intolerance is to dramatically reduce the exposure of the substance from diet and the environment to see if symptoms improve. Muscle testing through applied kinesiology is another method that can work.

Food sensitivities are especially important to address in order to repair the intestinal lining and improve immune function. Each time a person eats a food they are sensitive to, the body's immune system reacts. This overreaction to the food particles breaks down the intestinal lining and taxes the immune system even further, potentially setting the body to react to more and more foods, as well as other seemingly benign substances.

Our naturopath also explained that food sensitivities alone can disrupt healthy blood sugar levels, cause brain fog, and cause many psychiatric symptoms, including some that mimic ADHD. Doctors and psychiatrists often jump to prescribe stimulants instead of addressing the real issues, and as I noted before, these drugs are only designed to improve symptoms.

The puzzle pieces began to fit. Evan hated macaroni and cheese, and now I knew why. My "picky eater" may have been trying to tell me something.

Author Kelly Dorfman, MS, LND, confirmed what I was thinking. In her book, *Cure Your Child with Food*,[1] she explained that picky eating can be a sign that certain foods may be irritating to your child's body. Also, constipation and mucus caused by this irritation can lead to a dampened appetite.

It was recommended that Evan eat cooked, as opposed to raw, vegetables, and high-quality (grass-fed) protein containing cysteine (an essential amino acid often deficient in children with ADHD and other disorders). We also learned that ground meat is easier to digest.

It was important to limit seafood consumption to anchovies, krill, and sardines because of the high mercury levels in larger fish, and it was better for him to eat rinsed white rice instead of brown because it's easier to digest and contains less arsenic than brown.

We limited foods with unfermented soy because soy is considered a hormone disruptor. We were careful with foods high in sugar and tried to stay away from as many processed foods as possible. Many of these foods contain high fructose corn syrup, dyes, artificial flavors, pesticides, fungicides, and preservatives such as BHT, BHA, and TBHQ. These preservatives are, simply put, poison. They may make our kids hyperactive, aggravate allergies and asthma, and cause dermatitis/rashes. They affect hormone balance and can even cause cancer. These preservatives are often found in non-organic cereals, butter, low-quality meats, chewing gum, snack foods, pre-packaged meals, and boxed processed foods.

Acrylamide is also a dangerous substance that is linked to neurological disorders and cancer. It occurs naturally when we brown starchy food because the sugars in the food react with the protein and create a chemical reaction, says Joseph Mercola, MD.[2] Therefore, it's recommended to only lightly brown our food, take crusts off breads, and bake instead of fry.

The Dietary Changes: A Challenge and a Test to My Own Resolve

When I was first introduced to the idea of changing Evan's diet, I was overwhelmed to such a degree that I sat down and cried. How were we going to do this? No wheat, no dairy, no eggs? Is that possible? Doesn't everything contain those ingredients? And—oh no!—peanuts, too? Peanut butter and jelly on wheat bread was Evan's staple!

Our food companies today certainly do not make it easy for us to eat healthy. What we call organic now was just what my grandparents called "food." But to my surprise, although a huge inconvenience at times, it wasn't as difficult as I originally imagined. Supermarkets and restaurants are becoming more and more accommodating. I actually started to look at the offending foods as though I was poisoning my son, and that helped me to forge ahead.

Buying allergy-free cookbooks helped me to recognize this didn't have to be as difficult as initially imagined. A great place to start is a book written by nutrition blogger Tracy Bush of Nutrimom.

The Stepping Stones to Food Allergies is a step-by-step resource guide with a complete list of allergy-friendly companies, taste-tested allergy-friendly products, kitchen must-have's, substitution lists, and recipes. A couple other great books that helped me tremendously were *Special Diets for Special Kids* by Lisa Lewis, PhD, and *Healing Autism in the Kitchen* by board-certified pediatrician Dr. Annette Cartaxo and Dr. Garima Jain, ND. These books provided me with explanations and recipes that helped me implement a dairy-free, egg-free and gluten free lifestyle.

One of the most frustrating parts of this new diet for us, however, was the need to continuously plan Evan's meals. We no longer had the luxury of stopping by the local fast food restaurant on a long car ride, on our way to T-ball practice, or on the way home from a swim lesson.

Over time, we adjusted, and it became easier. There was also some relief in the knowledge that this change in diet might not necessarily be a "forever thing," but only for a while as we restored his gut and repaired his immune functioning.

I learned quite fast how to substitute flaxseed meal for eggs in baked goods. I felt happy when Evan welcomed millet bread, flax milk, and coconut ice cream. Quinoa pasta and buckwheat pancakes just became our new normal. The entire family started to eat healthier, and a lot of the foods were quite tasty.

I started reading all labels and noshing naturally. We tried to avoid all foods and consumer products that contain Blue 1, Blue 2, Citrus Red, Green 3, Red 3, Red 40, Yellow 5, and Yellow 6. We switched to organic foods colored and flavored with natural ingredients such as beet juice and turmeric spice.

It was fascinating. My "sometimes" picky eater started to welcome the new foods almost immediately. My sweet and grateful little boy thanked me when I fed him gluten-free, egg-free, and dairy-free food. I was honest with him about what was happening to his body and why we needed to change what he ate. I reminded him on many occasions how much we loved him and how we wanted his body to heal. I would tell him that I understood how hard it was for him to watch other kids enjoying McDonald's French fries. He'd frown for a moment and say, "Mommy, I know you love me, and my tummy is happier. Thank you."

One night when we sat down to eat together as a family, Evan very nonchalantly said, "I don't really want to eat this tonight. I think I want to eat 'crap.'" We all chuckled; I guess he listens to us when we talk.

Kids watch our reactions. If we get excited about something, they will often have the same reaction. When we go to the dentist, I say, "Guess what? It's a great day because the dentist is going to shine your teeth all up and give you the brightest smile and a brand-new toothbrush." My children say, "Yay, and we get to play games there and win prizes."

When Will You See Real Changes in Your Child's Health?

Of course every child is different. We started to see improvements within a few months after beginning the gut-healing treatments and after starting the dietary changes. Evan was on the way to recovery from his autism and related conditions. His constipation issues began to improve. We had noticed in the past that when he was constipated, his anxiety worsened. Without constipation, he was calmer.

His immune system began to improve as well. He no longer suffered from colds, flu, or asthma. His body was able to utilize the nutrients, and it was becoming obvious that his brain was also appreciating the changes.

Evan appeared more present. He was no longer in a "brain fog." His "staring off into space" episodes decreased, and his anxiety eased. He was able to pay attention for slightly longer periods. He was looking healthier, and the dark circles under his eyes began to disappear. His motor planning was also a bit better. His speech improved, and his cradle cap and psoriasis lessened.

What About Dairy/Casein and Gluten?

As we conducted research about the benefits of a dairy-free and gluten-free diet, we recognized that this lifestyle just might benefit everyone's health. Processed milk has been robbed of its goodness.

Some enzymes and probiotic properties have been stripped. Raw cow's milk from a reputable farm or goat's milk or non-homogenized milk are better choices if you do not have a cow's milk protein allergy or intolerance.

Gluten is found in wheat, barley, rye, and oat. Some individuals can eat oat without an issue, because it contains a different type of gluten. Wheat seems to be the worst offender because it contains a particular gluten—the gliadin type, which can irritate the gut wall.

Gluten sensitivities have skyrocketed throughout the world. Gluten is a complex of proteins that often inflames the intestinal track in at least thirty percent of the population. This inflammation makes the intestinal tract more permeable, allowing gut bacteria and toxins to enter the body, which triggers antibodies.

According to one website created in collaboration with the American Celiac Disease Alliance, "Three million Americans suffer from celiac disease, and another 18 million from non-celiac gluten sensitivity."[3] Notably, autism rates have skyrocketed as well during this same time period. Some speculate that the reason for the jump in allergies is that the wheat we are eating today is a genetically modified creation of the 1960s and 1970s. Neurologist David Perlmutter, MD, concludes in his book *Grain Brain: The Surprising Truth about Wheat, Carbs, and Sugar—Your Brain's Silent Killers* that our ancestors ate gluten for many millennia, but that recent changes to crops have transformed a once-safe food into a something that causes great suffering.[4] This "new" wheat contains gliadin, which binds to the brain's opiate receptors and stimulates our appetites to want to eat more. Also, we as a culture are eating more of it than ever before. It is found in many processed foods in alarming amounts. To learn more, please refer to the book by William Davis, MD, *Wheat Belly: Lose the Wheat, Lose the Weight and Find Yourself Back to Health* or the article, "Why Are So Many Allergic to Wheat Now?"[5]

Why Our Kids Do Better Without Dairy

Dairy is very offensive to many children and causes allergic symptoms such as chronic ear infections, constipation or diarrhea, colic, astmma, frequent illnesses, and headaches.

Dairy inflames the gut lining and contributes to leaky gut and food intolerances. In addition, casein (a milk protein present in cow, goat, sheep, and human milk) has a direct effect on the brain because when digested, it releases a chemical that mimics morphine. In the book *Breaking the Food Seduction* by Neal D. Barnard, he explains how these opiates called casomorphins are histamine releasers that can cause allergies and intolerances. High levels of opiates are often found in the bloodstreams of children with autism. In 1991, Dr. Kalle Reichelt observed that autistic children had elevated levels of peptides (protein breakdown products) in their urine not found in the urine of non-autistic children.[6] These opiates act much like heroin, slowing the bowels and causing constipation. In addition, it can also increase autistic symptoms like mental confusion, irritability, and less desire to communicate socially.

Important note: Human milk does contain casein, so if you are breast-feeding a baby with a milk allergy or sensitivity you should avoid milk products in your diet. Talk with your healthcare provider and make sure to eat a healthy diet. In addition, continuing to take prenatal vitamins and extra vitamin D and calcium may be necessary.

Important anecdote: we have recently tested our six-year-old daughter, Elaina, for food sensitivities due to increasing anxiety and fits of rage. Looking back, I remember how she cried excessively due to colic and acid reflux, and how many trips we took to the pediatrician for chronic ear infections. Lo and behold, testing revealed she too was sensitive to gluten, dairy, and egg. We immediately eliminated these foods from her diet and began a gut-healing protocol. It was certainly difficult for her at first to remove her favorites, like cheese, yogurt, and bread, until she started to feel better. Within a few weeks, we saw a dramatic difference in her mood. She said, "Mom, I feel happier, and I am talking more with friends because I am not afraid." She also said, "Mom, I didn't know my tummy wasn't supposed to hurt."

My dad has a similar story. At age 71, he writes, "I have been Dr. Jekyll & Mr. Hyde all of my life. My moods could turn on a dime. I appeared depressive or manic at times during Jennifer's entire childhood. I also suffered from a slight case of paranoia. I had so much anger inside of me and a very low frustration tolerance. I suffered with learning issues, dyslexia, and although I had a high IQ, I suffered with attention issues my entire life.

"There were many times I appeared normal, and I always had a great sense of humor so my family was perplexed. After Jenn began her healing journey and was having so much success in treating Evan, and after I was diagnosed with thyroid cancer, I got tested. I have discovered I'm intolerant to eggs, gluten, dairy, and mustard. Since staying away from these foods and healing my gut, I am much more stable. I can't help but wonder how many of the kids out there who are angry and even murderous can be helped by learning what our family has learned—it's worth investigating!"

10 SIGNS OF POSSIBLE GLUTEN SENSITIVITY

1. You have been diagnosed with an autoimmune disorder. There are over 80 identified, including multiple sclerosis, rheumatoid arthritis, lupus, celiac disease, Crohn's disease, and cancer.

2. Mood swings, anxiety, ADHD

3. Digestive issues such as constipation or diarrhea, bloating, and gas

4. Always tired, memory issues

5. Joint and/or knee inflammation

6. Migraine headaches

7. Keratosis (tiny bumps on the back of arms)

8. Fibromyalgia/chronic fatigue

9. Hormone imbalances

10. Unexplained infertility

10 POSSIBLE SIGNS OF DAIRY SENSITIVITY

1. You have been diagnosed with an autoimmune disorder. There are over 80 identified, including multiple sclerosis, rheumatoid arthritis, lupus, celiac disease, Crohn's disease, and cancer.

2. Mood swings and behavioral changes

3. Digestive issues such as constipation and diarrhea, smelly stools, bloating, and gas

4. Always tired, moody, memory issue

5. Asthma or other breathing problems

6. Nausea or vomiting

7. Skin rash and/or acne or hives

8. Bad breath

9. Hormone imbalances

10. Runny nose that won't quit, chronic cold, flu, and sinus/ear infections

Are GF/DF Diets Really Effective in the Treatment of These Disorders?

More research is needed, but scientific studies have shown that many autistic patients have significantly lower intestinal permeability and improve dramatically when put on a diet free of gluten and dairy foods.[7]

One particular study of twenty autistic children reported a reduction of autistic behavior and an increase of social and communicative skills after casein and dairy were removed from the diet. It was also noted that with a reduction of autistic behavior and increase of communicative abilities, the children were able to learn in a more effective way.[8]

The Department of Physical Medicine and Rehabilitation at Chang Gung Memorial Hospital, Taiwan, released a case study report in 2007 after studying the effects of a gluten/casein free diet in the treatment of a 42-month-old autistic boy. The case study reflected that the autistic child exhibited improvements in his daily behavior. Although he still had autism, he showed improved emotional reactivity, social communication, and fewer gastrointestinal–associated symptoms such as postprandial vomiting and constipation. After two and one-half months, interpersonal relations including eye-to-eye contact and verbal communication improved. At five and one-half months, the boy was capable of playing and sharing toys with his sibling and other children, behavior noted to be closer to that of an unaffected child. In addition, the decreased frequency of postprandial vomiting led to a significant increment in body weight, body height (from below the third percentile to the tenth percentile), and vitality after eleven months on the diet.[9]

Another study was done by researchers at the University of Rome. Their results lead them to hypothesize a relationship between a milk/casein sensitivity or allergy and the disturbance of the central nervous system.[10] There was a "marked improvement (after an eight week period on an elimination diet) in the behavior of autistic children who were taken off dairy products." And this was certainly true for Evan.

Yummy and Healthy Alternatives to Cow's Milk

Drink almond milk for brain, body, and digestive health. If your child is not sensitive or allergic to tree nuts, this "super food" contains vitamin E, folate, riboflavin, and L-carnitine. These nutrients boost brain activity, nourish the nervous system, and reduce the risk of neurological impairment. Almond milk also regulates blood sugar levels, alkalizes the blood, reduces heart attack risk, lowers bad cholesterol, and contains phosphorus for strong bones and teeth.

You can make your own almond milk that is free of refined sugars, preservatives, and food additives like carrageenan (a sneaky, dangerous and common "natural" food additive made from processed red seaweed). It is believed to be linked to chronic inflammation of the intestinal system, i.e., irritable bowel syndrome (IBS). Making your own is also cheaper than buying it off the shelf.

Make homemade almond milk: Start with 1 cup of raw almonds. Soak them overnight in water (5–8 hours). Drain the water, and give it to your house plants for nourishment. Blend the almonds and 4 cups of water in a blender for 2 minutes. Add pure vanilla extract, dates, and honey to sweeten. Pour the milk through cheesecloth or a nut milk bag. Refrigerate and enjoy. This milk will last about 3–4 days in your refrigerator, or you can freeze it.

Drink flax milk as a heart-healthy no-nut alternative. If someone in your family has a nut allergy, try flax milk. This dairy-free milk is made from cold-pressed flax oil. Loaded with many healthy nutrients such as omega-3 essential fatty acids, vitamin E, zinc, iron, beta-carotene, and phosphorus, and vitamins A, D, and B12, it has a smooth texture and is easily used as a milk substitute in smoothies, desserts, puddings, and ice cream. If you don't want to make your own, you can find organic flax milk that is certified GMO-free in original, vanilla, and non-sweetened varieties.

Make homemade flax milk: Start with ¼ cup of raw whole flaxseeds, 6 cups of water, 5 pitted dates, and 2 teaspoons of pure vanilla extract. Place the flax seeds in your blender, and add the water. Blend for one minute until all of the seeds have been broken down but are still visible. Place cheesecloth or a nut milk bag over the blender jug, and slowly pour the mixture into a large bowl. Strain the mixture again, and pour it back into the blender. Add dates, vanilla extract, and any other spices you would like for flavor, including cinnamon, cloves, nutmeg, or ginger. Add any fine protein powder or probiotic powder you would like as well. Blend together for about 2 minutes. Gently remove any froth from the top with a spoon or sieve. Pour the milk into an airtight container. It will keep in the refrigerator for 3–5 days. Natural separation will occur, so just shake it before serving.

Drink coconut milk for all of its amazing health benefits. Many of us are going dairy-free these days because it can contribute to mucus, allergies, asthma, and digestive issues. Coconut milk is another nut-free solution. Most people with nut allergies can consume coconut, coconut water, and coconut milk. Coconut is related to the palm family, which is not related to nuts or peanuts.

Like other alternative milks (almond, hemp, oat, and flax), coconut milk is vegan, easy to digest, and easily absorbed thanks to its balanced macronutrient and micronutrient ratios. Coconut milk is the least allergenic of all of the milks and full of delicious nutrition. Coconut is an amazing food used in many cultures as a natural cure for gastritis, Crohn's disease, irritable bowel syndrome, gut permeability, yeast and bacteria overgrowth, inflammation, eczema, psoriasis, dermatitis, glucose imbalances, and constipation. In addition, coconut contains healthy fatty acids to support mood and mental health, and it contains antioxidants and lauric acid for brain and immune health. If that isn't enough, it also gives you magnesium (a natural healthy laxative), iron, phosphorus, and potassium.

Make homemade coconut milk: Start with 2 cups of organic, unsweetened dried coconut or the meat of one fresh young coconut, $3^1/_2$ cups of filtered water, and a pinch of sea salt. In a high-speed blender, mix the ingredients together. Let the mixture soak for 30 minutes if using dried coconut. Pour the milk through a nut milk bag or cheesecloth, and pour it into a glass jar. It keeps well for about a week, or you can freeze it for a longer life. The extra pulp can be used to make smoothies or added to oatmeal or quinoa. You can also add pure maple syrup, vanilla, cinnamon, dates, or honey to sweeten and flavor it a bit.

Homemade (Non-Dairy) Chocolate Brownies

$2^1/_4$ cups coconut cream, coconut butter, manna, or coconut oil

$3/_4$ cup raw cacao powder

$1^1/_2$ tablespoons vanilla extract

$1/_3$ cup raw honey* or molasses

Pinch Celtic sea salt

3 tablespoons shredded coconut

Nuts (if not allergic)

Use organic ingredients if at all possible

*WARNING: Honey is not safe for children under one year of age.

1. Grease a small glass or stainless steel pan (about 8-inch square) with virgin coconut oil. Set aside.

2. Heat a medium-sized saucepan over low heat. Add 1 cup of the coconut cream, coconut butter, or manna, and allow it to melt.

3. Add the cacao powder, 2 tablespoons of the shredded coconut, the vanilla extract, and the salt. Slowly add the honey until combined, and add chopped nuts, if desired.

4. Pour the mixture into the greased pan, and sprinkle the batter with shredded coconut.

5. Place the pan in the freezer for about 1 hour to cool and set.

6. Cut into squares, and store the brownies covered in the refrigerator for up to 2 weeks (if they last that long) or in the freezer for up to 6 months.

What About Raw Goat Milk?

The use of goat milk as a hypoallergenic food or as a milk substitute in children allergic or intolerant to cow milk has often been debated over the past decades. Goat milk has been used in many cultures and is believed to be easier to digest and have a different protein composition than cow's milk. However, a study confirmed what my naturopath had told me. Both cow milk and goat milk contain casein (phosphoprotein) and lactalbumin protein. A very interesting article titled, "Goat Milk and Its Use as a Hypo-Allergenic Infant Food," in the *Goat's Milk Journal* stated, "The distribution of the different components of goat milk protein are similar to that of cow milk and that the casein fraction is nearly the same elementary composition as bovine casein."[11] I needed to keep Evan away from both to avoid an allergic immunological response.

What About Soy Milk?

Although soy milk was first thought to be a healthy alternative to cow's milk, its benefits may be outweighed by its risks. As stated in *A Compromised Generation—The Epidemic of Illness in America's Children*, processed soy consumption has been associated with impaired iodine absorption (an essential mineral to prevent hypothyroidism and developmental delays).[12] Soy is also known to be a hormone disruptor. In addition, it is estimated that approximately ninety percent of soybeans grown in the United States are genetically modified (GMO).

Raw, non-GMO soybeans, including edamame, are high in isoflavones and provide us with high amounts of protein, help prevent certain cancers, and may be especially helpful for menopausal women. But it is clear that more studies are needed to determine the impact of raw soy on people in different age groups, how soy affects different disease states, and how the health benefits of soy foods differ from supplements.

The issue of whether or not soy is a poor or good choice is debated quite heavily. Many Asian cultures have been using soy as a staple for thousands of years of healthy living. However, we need to realize that they only eat fermented soy products such as miso, tofu, and natto, and the fermenting process reduces the high level of phytates (and phytic acid) found in raw soybeans. Phytates are also found in many other whole-grain foods such as bran, rice, beans, nuts, and sprouted beans. Soaking these foods in water for 24 hours significantly reduces the phytic acid content.

Phytates and phytic acid are considered to be potent anti-nutrients because they bind to certain dietary minerals such as calcium, magnesium, copper, iron, and zinc. This is a significant problem because these nutrients are necessary for the proper functioning of the central nervous system and immune system.

In an article written for NaturalNews.com, the author Barbara Minton said, "Writings about the soybean dates back to 3000 B.C., when the Emperor of China suggested that Chinese recognized that soybeans in their natural state were not fit for human consumption."[13]

Don't We Need Dairy Products to Get Enough Calcium?

Again, calcium is crucial for strong bones and teeth, helps promote a regular heartbeat, helps our blood to clot properly, is involved in

DNA synthesis, and is essential for healthy nerve and brain functioning. It also plays a role in the neurotransmitter release of dopamine and carries signals in and out of the cells. Supplementation of calcium citrate may be necessary for non-dairy kids.

There are also many non-dairy foods with high amounts of calcium. Some options are broccoli, bok choy, pumpkin seeds, sesame seeds, kale, collards, turnip greens, onions, leeks, Brazil nuts, artichokes, celery, green beans, avocado, coconut meat, butternut squash, Brussels sprouts, and Swiss chard.

Why Our Kids Do Better Without Gluten

Gluten is the protein found in wheat, rye, spelt, barley, and sometimes oats. It is present in cereal grains, pastas, and breads and is the substance that gives elasticity to the dough. Gluten is also sometimes found in cosmetics, including hair and skin products.

As described by the Autism Spectrum Disorders Health Center, in the bodies of children and adults whose guts are compromised, gluten proteins are not digested properly, causing an allergy or sensitivity. Just like casein, gluten may produce and exacerbate autistic symptoms.[14] When the offending food is eaten, the immune system sends out an alarm, triggering a response that can damage the intestines and prevent them from absorbing much-needed nutrients. Food intolerances can lead to inadequate hydrochloric acid production in the stomach, inadequate pancreatic enzyme release, and an unhealthy small intestine lining.

In addition, the brain reacts to these proteins like false opiate-like chemicals because gluten turns into substances with similar chemical structure to opiates like morphine and heroin. There has been quite a substantial amount of research done in this area showing that, "gluten and casein peptides (incompletely broken down pieces of protein) called gluteomorphins and casomorphins were detected in the urine of schizophrenic patients and autistic children who exhibited speech apraxia, as well as cognitive, social, and behavioral issues."[15]

Incidentally, these substances were also found in patients with depression and rheumatoid arthritis. These substances derived from wheat and dairy products can penetrate the blood-brain barrier and bind with opiate receptors in the brain, just like morphine or heroin. As a result, they may cause various neurological and psychiatric symptoms.

As a psychotherapist for drug abusers, I can attest that my son had similar symptoms to a person on opiates. He was frequently spacey, irritable, lethargic, and severely constipated. The opiate-like effect is known to slow down the entire body, including the bowels.

The effectiveness of a gluten and casein-free diet in the treatment of autism spectrum disorders has not been one-hundred percent supported by medical research. However, there are thousands of moms, naturopathic doctors, and even some MDs who back this theory because it has indeed helped certain children when followed.

Yummy and Healthy Alternatives to Wheat/Rye/Barley

Eat quinoa, the "brain grain." Quinoa, which originated in the Andes of South America, is a grain-like crop grown primarily for its seeds. It is a complete protein containing all nine essential amino acids, and is also high in fiber. It's our natural anti-anxiety/anti-depressant remedy. It's loaded with iron, which assists in the production of neurotransmitters such as dopamine, serotonin, and norepinephrine. It is high in B vitamins to keep the mind sharp, and it stabilizes mood. It contains lots of minerals, including magnesium, which helps with the transmission of nerve impulses, energy production, and detoxification. It also improves colon health and is a natural laxative. Quinoa can be made as a side dish and can be used to make gluten-free pasta or as a substitute for wheat flour.

Eat buckwheat, the "healthy seed." Despite its name, buckwheat is not related to wheat and can be eaten instead of rice or the usual breakfast cereal or wheat pancake. It contains a rich supply of flavonoids, which are the phytonutrients that help prevent against disease. Buckwheat is also a highly digestible protein that reduces cholesterol, helps regulate blood sugar, cleans and strengthens the intestines, improves chronic diarrhea, and improves appetite. It is also nonallergenic and is grown quickly, which means it doesn't require a lot of pesticides. Be careful when buying buckwheat pancake mix, as many brands also add wheat to their product.

Eat shelled hemp seeds, the "smart seed." Hemp seeds have a light, nutty flavor and can be added to anything, including gluten-free/dairy-free pancakes, to give a carbohydrate breakfast a zap of protein. These seeds are great for the body and the brain, as they are high in protein and contain all nine essential fatty-acids. They reduce inflammation, boost the immune system, relieve constipation, and promote learning and memory. Hemp seeds come from a plant similar to marijuana with lower levels of cannabinoid compounds, and they are also rich in vitamin E, zinc, phosphorus, magnesium, and iron.

Evan & Elaina's Gluten-Free/Dairy-Free/Egg-Free Chocolate-Chip Walnut Pancakes

1 cup gluten-free pancake mix (buckwheat or other; we love Bob's Red Mill brand)

$1/2$ cup coconut, hemp, or almond milk

1 teaspoon pure vanilla extract

$1/8$ cup dairy-free chocolate chips

$1/8$ cup walnuts

1 tablespoon organic coconut oil

1–2 tablespoons shelled hemp seeds

1. In a large bowl, mix all ingredients until you reach the desired pancake batter consistency, adding a little water, if necessary.

2. Place a few drops of coconut oil on a hot griddle. Pour the batter onto the griddle to make the size of pancakes you prefer.

3. Cook until golden brown on both sides.

We make extras of these on the weekend and throw some in the freezer for school days.

Substitutions: blueberries and/or other fruit for chocolate chips and walnuts

Other Gluten-Free Options:

- Amaranth grain has anti-inflammatory properties, lowers triglycerides, and lowers bad cholesterol. It has been shown to help prevent cancer, heart disease, and hypertension.

- Millet is more than just bird seed or an interesting alternative to more common grains. It is an excellent source of some very important nutrients, including manganese, phosphorus, fiber, vitamin E, and magnesium. Millet promotes heart health and is also used to prevent certain cancers, type 2 diabetes, and childhood asthma. I have found millet bread to taste delicious and have a similar texture to its whole-wheat bread counterpart, making it great for sandwiches.

- Sorghum, a cereal grain originated in Africa over 5,000 years ago, can be eaten as porridge or turned into flour and baked into breads and cakes. Sorghum is more nutritionally dense than ordinary white flour. It contains a lot of dietary fiber, protein, phosphorus, potassium, calcium, and iron.

- Corn, rice, and potatoes are also acceptable for those needing a gluten-free lifestyle, as long as there are no sensitivities to these foods.

Quick tips:

1. As I mentioned earlier, gut-compromised individuals tend to do better with white rice than brown rice because it is easier to digest. Brown rice is also known to contain more arsenic.

2. Buying your rice from American companies may be better for you. It was found that many rice and rice protein products sourced from other countries contain harmful metals. A California rice company, Lundberg Family Farms, was put to the test and came out clean for mercury, cadmium and lead.[16]

3. Corn that is not certified organic or not locally grown could be genetically modified (GMO). Nice to know: blue corn/corn chips are not GMO.

Sources of Gluten and Casein

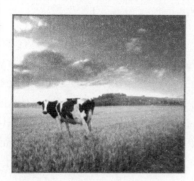

GLUTEN	DAIRY / CASEIN
Wheat	All milk products (cow, goat, sheep)
Rye	Yogurt
Barley/Malt	Kefir
Spelt	Butter/buttermilk
Wheat Flour (flour)	Casein/caseinate
Kamut	Sour cream
MSG	Cheese, ice cream and other dairy products
Dextrin	Sherbet (sorbets are ok)
Artificial flavoring	Cool whip
Oats (commercial)	Artificial butter
Citric Acid	Seasoned potato chips & other snacks
Soy sauce (unless specified GF)	Whey/whey protein
Sauces/gravies/broth/soup	Galactose
Beer (unless GF)	Lactose/Lactulose
Hotdogs / lunch meat	Curds
French fries (may contain a flour coating)	Probiotics (unless specified DF)
Wheat Pasta Orzo / Couscous	Mineral supplements such as magnesium and calcium (unless specified DF)

Any non-whole food item (processed food) could conceivably contain gluten and dairy, so always double-check the ingredients.

When dining out, be careful! Many restaurants and fast-food chains add gluten and dairy to many of their dishes. Make sure to ask a lot of questions.

Source: www.healingwithouthurting.com

CHAPTER 16

Say *No* to Processed Foods

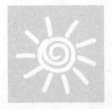

"Toxic load consists of past and present physical, chemical, biological contaminants in food, air and water, as well as the emotional state of the individual. You can compare total body burden to a container—you can only fill it to capacity. Anything above capacity causes spillover or, in other words, allergic symptoms and ultimately sickness."

—JOZEF J. KROP
HEALING THE PLANET: ONE PATIENT AT A TIME (2002)

I'm sometimes asked if there is a link between processed foods and ADHD. From my personal experience, the answer is yes, and there is research to back up this view.

In a 1997 study, for example, 486 parents of hyperactive children were surveyed along with 172 parents of normally active kids. Sixty percent of the parents of the hyper group reported that their children's behavior grew worse after consuming artificial colors and flavors, preservatives, select other chemicals, and/or cow's milk. In contrast, only twelve percent of the parents of the normally active kids reported a connection between food chemicals and bad behavior.[1]

In the same study was a subgroup of hyperactive children with known sensitivities to synthetic colors found in everyday foods. After the researchers gave twenty-three of these children a beverage containing the coloring called tartrazine, eighteen responded by becoming overactive, sixteen became aggressive, four became violent, and several developed eczema, asthma, poor speech, or poor coordination. Two other food colorings—sunset yellow and amaranth dye—also led to significant negative behavior. In contrast, only one child from the normally active group showed even minor behavioral changes after drinking the beverage with tartrazine.

One explanation for these results may be that the hyperactive children started out with lower zinc and iron levels than the normally active kids, and after the hyperactive children consumed the food colorings, their zinc levels plummeted. Other earlier studies show zinc deficiency leads to greater stress and aggressive behavior.

The bottom line is that if your child already has behavioral issues, processed foods laced with chemical additives and pesticides could make those issues significantly worse. This is a great reason to buy organic and natural foods instead of mainstream products.

In my home, we've eliminated processed foods as much as possible. We've replaced cookies, crackers, and chips with whole-food snacks such as fresh fruit and vegetables. I have also tried to return to my grandmother's generation, making more homemade meals. I took what I call "the Grandma pledge," which states, "I promise to buy whole foods and cook meals for my family as much as possible."

Due to the price of healthy food and our hectic modern lifestyles, homemade meals have too often been replaced with boxed, frozen, and canned foods. This needs to end. The processed foods often worsen our children's symptoms because they typically contain high levels of refined sugar, artificial colors and flavors, chemical preservatives, and genetically modified ingredients. Buying whole food and organic ingredients for preparing your own meals can help protect your child's health and the health of everyone else in your family.

Healthy food does not have to cost a fortune, however. Going back to basics is essential. Preparing meals with a meat and/or other protein, a starch and a vegetable is all it takes. Nutritionist Kelly Dorfman wrote a wonderful article in the *Huffington Post* called, "Eating at Whole Foods for Less Than $11 a Day."[2] In the article, she demonstrates that if meals are planned and budgeted for, it is relatively easy to eat healthy on a strict budget and without adopting an unusual diet.

The Dangers of Refined Salt

A scientific study conducted by scientists from Yale University in the U.S. and the University of Erlangen-Nuremberg in Germany indicated that "excess refined salt used in fast food restaurants and the over-consumption of sodium from other processed foods may be one of the environmental factors driving the increased incidence of autoimmune diseases."[3]

Health experts recommend that adults consume no more than 2,300 mg of sodium (i.e., salt) per day. During the study, they discovered that United States fast food chains often use more than twice as much salt as chains in other countries. While there have been campaigns against such usage, the U.S. government has been reluctant to press the issue. The highest "hidden salt" was found in the bread. For example, a six-inch roasted garlic loaf from Subway—just the bread without the meat, cheese, and other ingredients—contains 1,260 mg of sodium, which is about as much as fourteen strips of bacon.

It is believed that refined table salt encourages Th17 cells in the body to multiply, and it has been found that an increase in Th17 cells leads to increased inflammation and autoimmune responses. At Yale University, a study of rats found that too much salt in their bodies led to diseases like multiple sclerosis (MS).

In 2012, *Nature International Weekly Journal of Science* published an article revealing that refined salt exposure increases the levels of cytokines released by Th17 cells to ten times more than usual. Cytokines are proteins used to pass messages between cells. When there are too many, the immune system may overreact and mistake the nerve fibers in the brain and spinal cord for invaders. The immune system then begins to strip myelin from the nerves fibers, which disrupts the messages passed between the brain and the body, causing problems with speech, vision, and balance.[4]

Again, these are not diseases of bad genes alone or diseases caused solely by the environment. They are diseases created as a result of a bad interaction between genes and the environment.

In moderation, salt is critical for our health, but many researchers believe that the quality of the salt is what matters. Unlike refined table salt, Himalayan rock salt, Celtic salt, and sea salt are loaded with trace minerals that our body craves, and they also contain the natural iodine that is necessary for immune health and thyroid functioning.

Mineral salts help the body heal itself and help to balance all of the body's functions, including pH levels. Although Speleo/Halotherapy is not widely practiced in the U.S., it has been thoroughly researched and used as a popular alternative respiratory therapy in some regions of Central Europe, Russia, the Balkans, and in Turkey. These are drug-free treatment in underground salt mines and caves. The patient is exposed to microclimate dry saline aerosol inhalation to provide systemic relief of respiratory diseases. The dry saline aerosol is believed to go deep within the respiratory system and have amazing health benefits: mucolytic, antibacterial, anti-inflammatory, and immunomodulating.[5]

Haloaerosol therapy was studied in Russia for its effectiveness in the treatment of asthma. The results were assessed by physicians on the basis of clinical symptoms, functional parameters, and medication dosages with the use of standard questionnaires. Haloaerosol therapy resulted in improvement of clinical state in eighty-five percent of mild and moderate asthma cases, seventy-five percent of severe asthma cases, and ninety-seven percent of chronic bronchitis and bronchiectasis cases. Long-term examination of patients (for one or more years) demonstrated the effect of HT on reduction in the frequency of exacerbations and reduction in chronic symptoms.[6]

In addition, mineral ions conduct electrical nerve impulses that drive muscle movement and thought processes. Many scholars and scientists believe that it is not only our salt intake, but also our low mineral consumption that causes problems. We need to consume foods with adequate minerals, such as organic vegetables, nuts, and fruits rather than convenient processed foods and carbonated beverages.

Of course, too much salt, regardless of its source, is harmful, as the content of sea salt is still mainly sodium chloride.

To read more, see the "Autoimmune Disease Fact Sheet" on the website of the American Autoimmune Related Disease Association. www.aarda.org/autoimmune-information/autoimmune-statistics/

Instant Ills from Instant Foods

Instant foods have been found to cause and aggravate ADD/ADHD symptoms. The ingredients in foods like instant potatoes and instant stuffing mixes affect the nervous system and often make brain fog and hyperactivity worse. They tend to be loaded with preservatives such as sodium bisulfate, BHA/BHT, MSG, hydrogenated "GMO" soybean oil and corn syrup, maltodextrin (sometimes wheat-derived, causing concern for people with gluten intolerance), dairy products, and sometimes sodium acid pyrophosphate and dipotassium phosphate.

Silicon dioxide is sand you find at the beach, but it's also added to some instant foods to prevent them from forming clumps during storage. Instant mashed potatoes include high sodium content and artificial flavors. Instant noodles contain MSG and preservatives. Check the packaging of instant rice products as well. Some varieties pretend to be healthy when they are actually packed with sodium and chemical additives. Some researchers believe consumption of these foods is linked to cancer, diabetes, and heart disease.

Artificial Food Dyes and Flavoring

> *"The pigments that make grapes purple and pumpkin orange protect brain cells, while the artificial ingredients that mimic these colors in processed foods can impair brain function."*
>
> —TYLER GRAHAM AND DREW RAMSEY, MD,
> *THE HAPPINESS DIET* (2011)

Artificial dyes and flavoring are made from everything, including bugs, to chemicals derived from petroleum. These are typically produced by chemically manipulating naturally sourced chemicals, crude oil, or coal tar. The FDA allows "permissible" amounts of contaminants like mercury, lead, arsenic, and certain carcinogens such as benzidine in the foods we eat and the products we use regularly.

In the United States, there are products on the market that contain large amounts of artificial dyes and flavors. It is vital to read labels every time you buy a product, even if it's a product you have used for years, because you don't know when they will sneak a new ingredient into your favorite food, cosmetic, or medication.

Homemade Strawberry Roll-ups

Did you know that the ingredient list for commercially produced strawberry fruit roll-ups doesn't even include strawberries? What's more, you can avoid corn syrup, refined sugar, food dyes, and the chemicals in commercially produced fruit roll-ups by making your own. Here's an easy recipe:

1. Purée organic strawberries in a food processor.
2. Add some honey* and lemon juice to taste.
3. Heat the mixture for 10 minutes in a saucepan until it thickens.
4. Spread the mixture on a cookie sheet lined with parchment paper.
5. Bake for 3 hours in a 170-degree oven until dehydrated.

When done, cut it into strips.

*WARNING: Honey is not safe for children under one year of age.

Concerns in Europe about the negative behavioral and health effects of dyes and artificial flavors led many European manufacturers to stop using them. Many of these ingredients have been banned in Norway, Finland, Austria, France, and the U.K. Yet, in the U.S., companies are still using these dyes and flavors because they make the food look and taste more appealing. These substances are actually low-cost substitutes for real food extracts.

Many parents report that removing food dyes from their children's diets alone dramatically reduces impulsivity, hyperactivity, and angry or violent outbursts. Both of our kids are sensitive to food dyes. I know almost immediately if they eat a red ice pop. They begin bouncing off the walls. Evan gets "brain fog," and our daughter, Elaina, starts to act aggressively.

A statement from the FDA says that it does not believe that artificial food dyes cause hyperactivity in children in the general population. However, the FDA does admit that food dyes may exacerbate problems in susceptible children diagnosed with ADHD because they may have a unique intolerance to them.

Sports Drinks Are Poison: Dyes and Brominated Vegetable Oil

Bromine is a naturally occurring element found as a salt in nature, especially in oceans. At high temperatures organobromine converts to free-bromine, which was originally created to be used on children's clothing as a fire retardant.

Elements of free-bromine have been bonded to vegetable oil to create something called brominated vegetable oil (BVO), which is used in many sports drinks and soda manufacturers in the U.S., to prevent the color from separating in their products.

More than a hundred countries have banned this very dangerous chemical that has been known to cause many health and behavioral problems. There are safer alternatives to this practice, and we need to put more pressure on the companies and change the laws at a Federal level. Some companies are feeling the pressure from consumers and are finding alternative methods, but many continue using the oil.

So, what does BVO do to us? It is believed that drinking too many servings of soft drinks that contain BVO can cause abdominal cramps, anxiety, blurred vision, diarrhea, dizziness, headaches, weakness, nausea, memory loss, and fatigue. In addition, BVO is believed to contribute to reproductive, learning, and behavioral problems.[7] Jorge Flechas, MD, speaks internationally to medical doctors on the topic of thyroid and iodine. "Bromine actually replaces iodine in the body and depletes the stores of iodine which creates issues in the brain. When a person is treated with iodine and stops using BVO-containing soft drinks, many behavioral and learning symptoms resolve within a few weeks."[8]

Instead of consuming these soft drinks, hydrate naturally; drink coconut water. Coconut water strengthens thyroid activity instead of weakening it and contains vitamins, minerals, electrolytes, enzymes, amino acids, cytokine, and phytohormones.

Potassium Bromate (Bromated Flour) and Azodicarbonamide

Potassium bromate is a food additive that is often used as a low-cost and fast-rising baking flour. The breads and bakery goods you find in local supermarkets typically contain it. It is believed to be safe because the potassium bromate turns into potassium bromide, a harmless byproduct, after the bread has been baked. In 1982, however, Japanese researchers published studies that linked this chemical to cancer, kidney damage, and nervous system damage.[9] The FDA has acknowledged that it is a potentially dangerous additive, but it has still not yet been banned in the U.S., even though it has been banned in Australia, Canada, China, England, and most European countries.

Azodicarbonamide is a food additive made of carbon monoxide, carbon dioxide, and ammonia gases. It can be found in the breads of many fast-food chains and in the bread and baked goods at local supermarkets. It is also found in foamed plastic-like exercise mats and the soles of our sneakers. This chemical has been banned in other countries because it is believed to be linked to cancer, allergies, and asthma. Yet, in the United States, azodicarbonamide has been recognized as safe because it decomposes upon baking. One step in the right direction was that Subway recently removed azodicarbonamide from their bread because of social pressure from the petition created by Vani Hari of FoodBabe.com.

Sodium Nitrates/Nitrites

Sodium nitrates and nitrites are preservatives that are found in some processed meats. They are considered to be harmful carcinogens that wreak havoc on the liver, pancreas, and the lining of the stomach. They also promote the growth of cancer cells. They are found in bacon, ham, hot dogs, luncheon meats, corned beef, smoked fish, and other processed meats.

In a 1998 article, "How Additives Turn Your Little Angel into the Devil" published in the *Daily Record* of Glasgow, Scotland, the author lists sodium nitrates as among the foods that can provoke hyperactive behavior (ADHD) in children.[10]

The USDA tried to ban nitrates and nitrites in the 1970s but was vetoed by food manufacturers who needed a chemical to turn meats bright red so that old meat could appear fresh and vibrant.

My family buys nitrate-free products and brands, and we ask a lot of questions at food establishments and restaurants before we place our orders.

Monosodium Glutamate (MSG): Is It Harmful?

MSG, a sodium salt used to enhance food flavor, is made from a naturally abundant amino acid (L-glutamic acid). Glutamate can be found in literally any natural food. In fact, the digestive system breaks down the natural glutamic acid, which is then delivered to the glutamate receptors in the body and brain. These are neurotransmitters in the brain that play a key element in learning and memory. So, why should MSG pose any real danger?

The glutamic acid broken down the natural way is harmless. In a factory, however, the bound glutamic acid is refined/broken down or made "free" by various chemicals and other processes, making it more dangerous. In addition, we are consuming more and more MSG than ever before. Eating too much processed food with MSG added can be problematic.

On the Center for Science in the Public Interest website, MSG is on the list of foods to avoid. "MSG has been shown to overstimulate and damage neurons (nerve cells) in the hypothalamic region of the brain."[11] There is research that points specifically to high levels of MSG in the brain as a contributing factor in ADHD, autism, anxiety disorders, and others, because it throws off the natural balance of GABA and glutamate and causes the dopamine levels to drop.

In December 2003, the American Medical Association summarized research from the *Journal of Neuropsychiatry and Clinical Neurosciences* in a press release. It was reported that researchers found increased levels of glutamate in the brains of children who suffered from ADHD. In those same children, levels of the essential amino acid gamma amino butyric acid (GABA) were decreased.[12]

Here are some types of foods that often contain MSG, so read labels carefully: snack foods, prepackaged and boxed foods, frozen meals, canned soups, dry soup mixes, frozen pizza, soy sauce, jarred gravies and dipping sauces, seasonings, artificial sweeteners, processed cheese, and everyday condiments like mayonnaise and ketchup. Unfortunately, the labels will not always list it as MSG. Watch for these unassuming names: whey protein concentrate, soy protein concentrate, hydrolyzed vegetable protein, plant protein extract, potassium glutamate, and calcium caseinate, to name a few.

It is also important to be careful at fast-food chains and Asian-style restaurants. Evan and I, like many of you, are very sensitive to MSG. We experience numerous side effects after eating it, such as headaches and nausea, as well as other allergic reactions.

Microwave Popcorn:
One of the Unhealthiest Snacks!

If you want to eat popcorn, stick to kernels that you can prepare on your own stove using healthy ingredients such as coconut oil or Earth Balance organic dairy-free/soy-free butter.

Microwave popcorn is unhealthy because of the preservative chemicals and refined salt it contains. Many popcorn varieties contain diacetyl, a chemical used to create the buttery taste and smell. This chemical is also used in margarine, snack foods, candy, baked goods, pet foods, beer, and chardonnay, and it is known to cause lung damage and neurological problems.

Recent research as found in the *Chemical Research in Toxicology* journal has linked this common food ingredient with Alzheimer's disease. These findings were submitted by the Center for Drug Design at the University of Minnesota.

Also, perfluorooctanoic acid (PFOA) lines microwave popcorn bags. When heated, the compound leaches into the food. PFOA has been linked to infertility, increased cholesterol, and elevated uric acid levels. Recently, higher serum levels of PFOA were also found to be associated with an increased risk for chronic kidney disease.

Air-popped corn and popcorn made the old fashion way (on the stove) is best. If you decide to make popcorn in brown paper bags, it is best to purchase eco-friendly bags free of chemicals. White paper bags and paper products are bleached with chorine.[13]

The Dangers of "Fat-Free" Olestra/Olean

Olestra is a chemical substitute for fat. It was created by the food industry as a low-fat substitute for cooking oil. This food additive can be found in processed foods such as potato chips, corn chips, and French fries and can be found under the brand name Olean. Critics call such a chemical concoction "risky." It is believed that foods containing this additive prevent the absorption of particular vitamins, such as vitamins D, E, A and K. Also, Olestra has the ability to prevent the absorption of important antioxidants called carotenoids, from fresh fruits and vegetables. Diarrhea, cramps in the abdomen and loose stools are only some of the most common side effects. Some experts believe it can also create leaky bowel syndrome. Countries such as the U.K and Canada have already banned this additive due to its negative health effects.

Stay Away from TBQH—Tertiary Butylhydroquinone

TBHQ is a byproduct of petroleum, basically butane lighter fluid, and is used as a cheap food preservative. It is found in many cosmetics and processed foods, including McDonald's chicken nuggets in the United States, as well as the "cheap" value foods that Walmart carries. It is also sprayed on many fast food cartons. The Food and Drug Administration says that small amounts are allowed in our food supply despite many toxic effects of this preservative. It is believed TBHQ contributes to the symptoms of attention deficit disorder. It can also cause hyperactivity, asthma, extreme anxiety, night terrors, and rage in some individuals. Other symptoms of TBHQ toxicity include liver damage, DNA damage, biochemical changes in the body, tumor growth, reproductive effects, diarrhea, and irritable bowel syndrome. This ingredient is banned in Japan, Canada, and in many products in Europe.

BHA and BHT

BHA and BHT are preservatives to prevent food from spoiling or becoming rancid. They can be found in cereals (including gluten-free Chex cereal), gum, butter, dehydrated potatoes, and non-organic meats. Known to cause cancer in rats, they are banned in the U.K., Japan, and many European countries.

Side Effects of Sulfur Preservatives

Sodium sulfate and sulfur dioxide are preservatives that extend the shelf life of fruit juices, dried fruits, vinegar, and wine. These sulfates inhibit the growth of microorganisms and prevent discoloration. Many people are extremely sensitive to them. Some common effects are migraine headaches, asthma, wheezing, and life-threatening respiratory conditions. The U.S. government requires that foods containing sulfur preservatives are labeled as such, but it has made no attempt to ban these chemicals.

Be a Careful Vitamin Shopper!

Before having Evan, I never paid attention to the ingredients in children's vitamins, assuming they were all pretty much the same. The truth is they are not. It's vital to read labels carefully, buying only vitamins that test for purity and don't include aluminum, heavy metals, dyes, or chemicals. When purchasing quality supplements it is always a good idea to find ones that are sourced from natural "whole food" concentrates. Synthetic ingredients do little to help and can sometimes be harmful.

Here are some of the ingredients commonly found in mainstream children's vitamins that you may want to avoid:

- **Stearic acid:** Saturated fatty acid linked to cancer, as well as brain and nervous system disorders.

- **Magnesium stearate:** The FDA considers the additive as generally safe. However, some experts agree it can weaken the immune system and harm the intestinal wall, which prevents the proper absorption of nutrients.

- **Magnesium orotate or magnesium malate:** Minerals derived from rocks with iron fillings.

- **Magnesium oxide:** A substance that is useless to the body's cells.

- **Microcrystalline cellulose:** Provides texture but adds nothing nutritionally and may have undesirable effects.

- **Artificial flavors:** They may make vitamins more interesting to swallow but add nothing nutritionally. Plus, they may have undesirable effects.

- **Artificial food dyes:** Blue 1, Blue 2, Citrus Red, Green 3, Red 3, Red 40, Yellow 5, and Yellow 6: these can inhibit cell respiration and have been linked to ADHD, allergies, and asthma.

- **Maltodextrin:** A candy additive produced from starch that may have undesirable effects.

- **Aspartame, carbonate, corn starch, and/or dextrose monohydrate:** Sugars and sugar substitutes that are added in excess to vitamins and are often harmful.

- **Sodium ascorbate:** Salt for flavor, which isn't appropriate for vitamins and potentially harmful.

- **Hydrogenated soybean oil:** May have undesirable effects.

- **Pregelatinized starch:** Hidden gluten.

- **Aluminum Lake:** Chemical concoction derived from aluminum and coal tar. Used in the industrial production of colorants, the term "lake" is applied to pigments or dyes that are precipitated with metal salts such as aluminum, calcium, barium, or others. Aluminum Lake is linked to sensory processing and speech disorders, folic acid uptake disruption, depression, fatigue, gastrointestinal issues, confusion, Alzheimer's disease, dementia, neuromuscular disorders, and hypoglycemia.

If this list makes it seem as if no vitamin is safe, don't despair. There are actually a number of companies that make excellent children's vitamins, including Source Naturals, Jarrow, Metabolic Maintenance, and Kirkman.

What About Aspartame?

Aspartame is an excitotoxin. During digestion it breaks down to phenylalanine and aspartate methanol, then breaks down further into formic acid and formaldehyde. It is believed to cause inflammation to the nerves. Children's brains are much more susceptible to damage from excitotoxins like aspartame than adults. It is believed by many that too much aspartame/phenylalanine in the daily diet can trigger ADD/ADHD-type symptoms. Such symptoms include seizures, impaired learning, depression, fatigue, headaches, memory loss, diarrhea, stomach pains, and marked behavioral and/or personality changes.

What About Sucralose (Splenda)?

Many food companies have replaced aspartame with sucralose, another artificial sweetener that is the primary ingredient in Splenda. Is it any better? It's made by adding chlorine molecules to sugar, rendering the sugar indigestible while still maintaining a sweet taste.

Unfortunately, "indigestible" doesn't actually mean indigestible. "Numerous studies have shown that we digest an average of fifteen percent of the sucralose we consume."[14] When metabolized in the body, sucralose has been shown to form chlorocarbons because of the presence of chlorine. Some research, as described in the *Journal of Toxicology and Environmental Health*, shows chlorocarbons can cause gastrointestinal problems, allergy reactions, seizures, headaches, depression, and genetic and reproductive problems. In addition, it is believed to be linked to metabolic syndrome. These are a cluster of risk factors such as weight gain, high cholesterol, high blood sugar, and high blood pressure, all of which can raise your risk of heart disease and diabetes.[15]

Many deceiving marketing campaigns are claiming that their product is "all natural," even though sucralose is on the ingredients label. Take Del Monte peaches and V8 Strawberry Kiwi Splash, for example. Many products on the supermarket shelves contain it, so read labels carefully. Sucralose can be found in baked goods, salad dressings, fruit waters, jams and jellies, fruit juices, frozen desserts, milk products, and others.

What About Sugar?

Although sugar is believed to be better than many of its artificial counterparts like aspartame, Splenda, and saccharine, we all need to consume it in moderation. Refined sugar overload can make us angry and depressed and is addictive.

When Evan ate foods with too much sugar, he would get a quick boost of energy and become hyper. Then, within a short while, his sugar levels would plummet, and he'd become irritable and easily frustrated.

Sugar of all kinds affects our health in many, many ways. Sugar inflames the body, which suppresses the immune system, causes chromium deficiency (which leads to hypoglycemia), causes hormone imbalances, and interferes with the absorption of vital vitamins and minerals. Sugar contributes to dysfunctional bowel movements, feeds yeast in the gut, and is a contributing cause of inflammation

and autoimmune diseases. Sugar can also cause a spike in triglycerides, which can cause cravings for more food. It can also affect
insulin production, affect mood, cause hyperactivity, increase brain
fog, and increase fatigue, among many other things.[16]

Is High Fructose Corn Syrup Dangerous?

High fructose corn syrup (HFCS) is a man-made sweetener. Derived
from corn stalks, the sugars are extracted through a chemical enzymatic process. It is used in almost all processed foods—and in every
school cafeteria across America. Soup, ketchup, yogurt, salad dressings, BBQ sauce, soda, and much more are sweetened with it.

Chemically, HFCS is "virtually" identical to table sugar (sucrose),
which is fifty percent fructose. Some believe that our bodies break
down HFCS and sugar the exact same way, so blame the abundance
of sugar in our food and beverages for playing a major role in our
national health and obesity epidemic, not HFCS.

They believe, from a biochemical standpoint, that drinking soda
with HFCS is no worse than too much fruit juice or home-brewed
iced tea with nine teaspoons of table sugar or an equivalent amount
of honey.

However, we cannot ignore what other researchers, professors,
and medical leaders from Harvard and other such institutions are
saying about HFCS.[17] Websites such as www.cornsugar.com and
www .sweetsurprise.com contain numerous quotes from esteemed
people about the dangers of this syrup. They agree that sugar is
sugar and that quantity certainly matters, and they also agree that
HFCS is "virtually" the same as cane sugar. However, they argue
that there are distinct and important differences between them:

- Regular cane sugar (sucrose) is made of two sugar molecules
  bound tightly together—glucose and fructose—in equal amounts
  (50/50 ratio). The enzymes in the digestive tract must break down
  the sucrose into glucose and fructose, which are then absorbed
  into the body.

- HFCS also consists of glucose and fructose, but in a 55/45 ratio of fructose to glucose in an *unbound* form. There is no chemical bond between them and no digestion required. This fructose is referred to as "free fructose."

High Doses of Free Fructose Cause Damage in the Body

Free fructose:

1. Is quickly absorbed in the bloodstream, goes straight to the liver, and triggers triglycerides and spikes cholesterol, which damages the liver.

2. Depletes the energy fuel source in the gut that is required to maintain the strength of the intestinal lining. It contributes to gut permeability and the triggering of immune system reactions and inflammation. "Since HFCS was introduced there has been an explosion of leaky gut syndrome."[18]

3. Research done by a group at the Children's Hospital Oakland Research Institute found that free fructose "literally punches holes in the intestinal lining allowing nasty byproducts of toxic gut bacteria and partially digested food proteins to enter your blood stream and trigger the inflammation."[19]

4. In a 2012 UCLA study published in the *Journal of Physiology*, researchers found that a diet high in fructose over time can damage your memory and learning ability. The study also suggests that omega-3 supplementation can offset damage.[20]

   As Mark Hyman, MD a family physician and internationally recognized leader in the field of Functional Medicine points out, "Naturally occurring fructose in fruit is part of a complex of nutrients and fiber that doesn't exhibit the same biological effects as the free high fructose doses found in corn sugar."[21]

I have learned that too much sugar of any kind is not the healthiest choice, but I have discovered that some alternatives to white sugar or HFCS are healthier because they have a lower glycemic index, which means that they break down more slowly and release glucose more gradually into the bloodstream. There is substantial scientific evidence to support that low GI foods may be beneficial for the prevention and treatment of a number of chronic diseases and conditions, including diabetes, autoimmune disorders, heart disease, and obesity. In addition these alternatives are known for their gut-healing properties and nutrient value.

These include:

1. **Raw honey.** After your child's first birthday, raw honey is the sweetener nature intended. Honey heals the gut wall, provides good bacteria, builds resistance to certain allergies, boosts energy, helps the body rid itself of toxins, boosts the immune system, contains antioxidant properties, helps the colon, stabilizes blood sugar, and fights off viruses, bad bacteria, and yeast. Raw honey contains eighteen vitamins, including B, C, D, and E. It also contains twenty-five minerals, including iron, iodine, phosphorus, calcium, manganese, magnesium, zinc, selenium, and potassium. Bee pollen has twenty-two amino acids and fifty-nine trace elements, as well as folic acid, choline, and inositol.

2. **Real maple syrup.** We should get in the habit of cooking and baking with real maple syrup. It's an antioxidant powerhouse that reduces inflammation and helps keep blood sugar levels in check. It settles digestion issues and is an excellent source of manganese, which helps repair muscle and cell damage. It is filled with other important nutrients like zinc, iron, calcium, and potassium. To begin to cut white sugar out of your child's diet, try real maple syrup in baked good recipes. Just be sure to reduce the amount of liquid the recipe calls for by about a half-cup.

3. **Sorghum blackstrap molasses.** Did you know one tablespoon of blackstrap molasses has as much iron as one chicken breast? Molasses is the leftover liquid "goodness" after the raw dark sugar is extracted from real sugar cane. Swap molasses for sugar, and reap the benefits. It provides us with vitamin B6, magnesium, iron, calcium, copper, and selenium.

CHAPTER 17

I'm Saying *No* to GMO

So, what does GMO mean, and why should we care? A genetically modified organism (GMO) is an organism with genetic material that has been altered using genetic engineering techniques. These are foods produced in the laboratory like we might see in any science fiction movie. In 1994, genetically modified tomatoes (to delay ripening) hit the market in the U.S. as the first commercially available genetically modified crop. Genetically modified tomatoes have since disappeared, because they did not meet expectations. Yet, this relatively newer technology continues to spread like wildfire with little research to determine its long-term effects.

Due to current climate changes on this planet, many argue that we need to grow GMO plants to survive. Crops today are struggling to flourish. Perhaps a better solution would be to use hydroponic technology to create indoor habitats with controlled climates and organic fertilizers and plant nutrients, rather than using genetically engineered technology to create plants, animals, and bacteria with biological characteristics that would never occur in the natural world. Scientists insert genes into or delete genes out of the DNA of plants and animals. They are inserting certain genes into vegetables so that they can resist cold temperatures. They are injecting corn plants with a bacterial gene that tolerates increased herbicide use.

The Alliance for Natural Health, which is a group of well-respected natural health practitioners, and many watchdog groups believe that GMOs are dangerous and extremely harmful to our bodies. Many long-term risks are still unknown, but GMOs are believed to adversely affect brain health and alter the digestive system, leading to leaky gut, increased allergies, and adverse immune system responses. Sadly, it is estimated that about eighty-five percent of the foods sold in the grocery stores contain these GMOs. We are messing with "mother nature," creating mutant foods, and we're likely to suffer the consequences.

At a Glance: Processed Food Ingredients to Avoid

- Food Dyes: Blue 1, Blue 2, Citrus Red, Green 3, Red 3, Red 40, Yellow 5, and Yellow 6
- Artificial flavoring
- Sugar & high-fructose corn syrup
- Aspartame and other artificial sweeteners
- Azodicarbonamide
- Brominated vegetable oil
- Potassium bromate
- TBHQ
- BHA & BHT
- MSG: hydrolyzed vegetable protein, plant protein extract, potassium glutamate, calcium caseinate
- Refined salt
- Artificial sweeteners
- Diacetyl (found in artificial butter)
- Nitrates/Nitrites
- Olestra/Olean
- Sodium sulfate
- Sulfur dioxide

Don't Be Fooled by Tricky Food-Marketing Gimmicks!

1. **Low Fat:** Instead of fat they add a chemical cocktail that is more harmful than fat ever would be.

2. **Natural Flavoring:** A tiny drop of something healthy has been mixed with a list of chemicals.

3. **No Sugar Added:** Instead they have included sweet-tasting carcinogens linked to brain damage, seizures, depression, memory loss, and insomnia.

4. **An Essential Source of Vitamins and Minerals:** They add a few non-absorbable vitamins and minerals to hide the chemicals and trick us into thinking we are eating healthy.

Become Informed:

- Check out this wonderful website, www.labelwatch.com, to compare food additives, ingredients, and nutritional facts about more than 25,000 brand name foods.

- Look into Fooducate and Buycott. These are a couple of the available healthy food smartphone apps that will allow you to scan your food to check for GMOs, processed ingredients, sugar, and dangerous chemicals while grocery shopping. They even recommend healthier alternatives.

- Eat Out/Eat Smart: Find Me Gluten Free is a free smartphone app that helps you find gluten-free restaurants. It allows you to view local business ratings and reviews, browse gluten-free menus, get directions, and call a restaurant right from the app. Also, you can easily view gluten-free menus and allergen lists from restaurant chains and fast food restaurants.

- Check out the wonderful smartphone apps, including Food Additives Checker and E Food Additives, to help you identify over 500 food additives (E numbers).

In addition, most GMOs require massive amounts of pesticides, herbicides, and fungicides. If we are eating GMO foods made with Roundup (trade name for glyphosate), we are also ingesting a broad spectrum herbicide used to kill weeds. Glyphosate is scientifically shown to wreak havoc with the immune system, and it is sprayed on our commercially grown food. "Two recent studies published reveal a disturbing finding: glyphosate-based herbicides such as Roundup® appear to suppress the growth of beneficial gut bacteria, leading to the overgrowth of extremely pathogenic bacteria."[1]

Toxicity problems are only the start. A newer study reveals how glyphosate in Monsanto's Roundup inhibits natural detoxification in human cells.[2] So, not only are we poisoning ourselves, but we are inhibiting the enzymes in the body that assist in the detoxification of those very poisons.

Alfalfa, canola, corn (cornmeal, corn syrup, corn flour and grits), cottonseed, rice, peas, papaya, soy, sugar beets, rapeseed (canola), and summer squash are the eleven crops that are currently genetically engineered. This list does not include the animal protein products we eat that have been feeding on these crops. If a product contains these ingredients and it isn't labeled as non-GMO Verified or Certified Organic, there is a good chance it is genetically modified.

In our home, we avoid foods containing genetically modified organisms (GMOs) and try to only purchase food with fewer than five ingredients. We learned that the many neurotoxins in foods were potentially contributing to Evan's poor health by impairing his gut and neurotransmitters, increasing ADHD symptoms, and aggravating allergies. Since there are currently no labeling laws requiring a manufacturer to inform us if their produce is GMO or produced using GMO ingredients, the only way to avoid them is by purchasing certified organic foods or foods that are specifically labeled "GMO-Free" or "Non-GMO." If a product is not labeled certified organic or GMO-Free, we can assume it most likely contains GMO ingredients.

Help raise GMO and related pesticide awareness. Join the coalition of unstoppable moms at MomsAcrossAmerica.com for health, freedom, and the future of America! MomsAcrossAmerica's mission is to empower millions and improve the health of our children by insisting on GMO labeling, and offering GMO-free and organic food solutions.

CHAPTER 18

How Food Sensitivities & Nutritional Deficiencies Can Lead to Rage and Violence

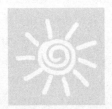

There was a very interesting article published on December 15, 2012, right after the Sandy Hook, Connecticut massacre in which twenty children and six adults were killed with a semi-automatic rifle by a young man with Asperger's, PDD, OCD, and sensory issues. The article, "School Shootings: How Can American Food Lead to American Blood," by DyeDiet draws our attention to the possible link between the American diet and food dyes and the dramatic increase of violent crime by intelligent young people who appear emotionally unattached, socially awkward, and without empathy.[1]

Could all the chemicals we are eating be contributing to the autism epidemic, increased OCD, and violent behavior? Is there more we can do to help prevent such senseless tragedy? I believe so. The above article mentions, "There are more than three thousand chemicals allowed in the American food and drink supply. Many of them are harmless, but others such as artificial colors, flavors, preservatives, emulsifiers, hydrogenated vegetable oil, etc. are not compatible with human bio-chemistry, to say the least."

Thanks to several national campaigns, school food programs are under pressure to expand their healthy options for kids, but more needs to happen.

Evan can't have ice cream during recess, for example, so the school offered him the only popsicles they had available. When I found out what they were serving him, I was appalled. The popsicles were made of high fructose corn syrup, corn syrup, sugar, yellow 5, blue 1, and red 40. The large amounts of sugar and chemicals are blamed for contributing to cancer, allergies, autoimmune disorders autism, ADHD, and other mental illnesses. Needless to say, I started bringing in homemade meals and one hundred percent fruit bars for his school to store in the lunchroom freezer.

Before schools suggest medication for their kids who are acting out or having attention issues, they might want to look at the food served in their lunchrooms. They are often serving processed foods full of preservatives and other harmful ingredients.

School Children vs. State Prisoners

Whose lunch is more nutritious?

Hard to say! These highly processed lunch options are loaded with chemicals, preservatives, excess salt, and artificial color & flavor.

Inmates may actually fare a bit better with more whole food and more vegetable options.

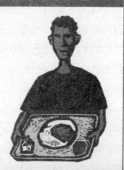

	Monday	Tuesday	Wednesday	Thursday	Friday
Connecticut School	Chicken tenders, brown rice, gravy, carrots and pears, milk or juice	Hamburger, lettuce, tomato, corn, French fries, fruit or juice	Sloppy Joe on a bun, potato puffs, baby carrots, apple, milk or juice	Mozzarella sticks, three bean salad, or bagel lunch, fruit or juice	Nachos, cheese, black beans, salsa, sour cream, fruit, milk or juice
Connecticut Prison	8 oz. Chicken & gravy, mashed potatoes, peas, carrots, bread, milk	8 oz. Roast beef, mashed potatoes, green beans, bread, milk	3 Hot dogs, grilled cheese, broccoli, sauerkraut, bread & milk	Soup de jour, chicken bologna, cheese, coleslaw, egg salad, pasta salad, milk	Chicken patty, fish patty, baked potato, zucchini, tomatoes, bread milk

Some improvements have been noted since the Hunger-Free Kids Act of 2010.

Is the average prison meal more nutritious than the average school lunch?
Christopher Reinhart, Chief Attorney, "Food Service in Prisons," OLR Research Report. Connecticut, Dec. 3, 2010. www.cga.ct.gov/2010/rpt/2010-R-0502.htm
School lunch menu data has been cross-referenced between several Connecticut public school systems.

According to the DyeDiet article: "These chemicals are not going to kill your child right away, but in the long run, the health effects of junk food can be quite devastating. The U.S. Food and Drug Administration (FDA) has done nothing to protect children from food additives that affect children's behavior."[2]

New studies published in the journal *Food and Chemical Toxicity* warn us that blue dyes (FD&C Blue No. 1) in foods such as kids' blue popsicles, sports drinks, and lollipops, as well as on our clothing, in our cosmetics, and on our textile leathers, could be entering the bloodstream. Even through our clothing, these dyes inhibit cell respiration and have been linked to ADHD, allergies, and asthma.[3] The studies recommend that these dyes be banned to reduce consumer risk.

We can learn something from certain European countries such as Italy and France. They are committed to avoid childhood epidemics and U.S.-style obesity. In addition, they recognize that well-balanced and healthier school meals help improve a child's concentration in class, increase educational performance, and reduce absenteeism.[4,5] In fact, Italy started serving their children only fresh, organic, and locally grown lunches in 2010. A typical lunch in France or Italy consists of fresh organic fruit, grilled chicken with a beet compote, sautéed vegetables, a baguette, and a glass of water. Also important to note: Most European countries, including France and Italy, understand the importance of banning artificial color, pesticides, growth hormones, chlorinated chicken, food containers containing neurotoxic chemicals, and Monsanto's GMO seed.

Poor health and nutritional deficiencies are common among young criminals, and research indicates that treating food intolerances and changing the diet might be one key to preventing behavioral problems, antisocial behavior, and even criminality. In a study published in 1997 in the *Journal of Nutritional and Environmental Medicine*, the study inferred that "many symptoms exhibited by the offenders are linked to food allergies or food intolerance."[6]

In a study published in 1998 in the same journal, physicians tested the effects of nutritional interventions on young criminals. The research involved nine children between the ages of seven and sixteen with histories of "persistent anti-social, disruptive and/or criminal behaviors." The nine subjects were found to have collectively committed sixty-seven crimes, and "all of the subjects regularly displayed irrational aggression and violence."[7]

Physicians identified nutrient deficiencies and food allergies in all nine of the subjects and elevated levels of cadmium, a neurotoxic heavy metal, in four of the subjects. The researchers provided treatment for all subjects, including dietary restrictions and allergy desensitization therapy.

The health and behavior of all of the subjects improved during treatment. Three children later discontinued the dietary intervention, and two of those reoffended. Of the six other subjects, two reoffended, "but with much reduced frequency and violence than before the project." In all, of the nine subjects, five did not reoffend during the two years following the intervention.[8]

In the *British Journal of Psychiatry*, results from an experimental, double-blind, placebo-controlled, randomized trial of dietary supplements on 231 young adult prisoners concluded, "Antisocial behavior in prisons, including violence, were much reduced after vitamins, minerals and essential fatty acids were administered."[9]

According to a University of Southern California study, researchers followed the nutritional, behavioral, and cognitive development of more than 1,000 children and discovered that malnutrition in the first few years of life leads to antisocial and aggressive behavior throughout childhood and late adolescence. Compared to those in the control group, malnourished children showed a 41 percent increase in aggression at age eight, a ten percent increase in aggression and delinquency at age eleven, and a 51 percent increase in violent and antisocial behavior at age seventeen. The study concluded that poor nutrition and deficiencies in key brain nutrients such as zinc, iron, vitamin B, and protein can lead to a lower IQ and antisocial behavior.[10]

Research in the *Journal of Nutritional and Environmental Medicine* also demonstrates that nutritional deficiencies and sensitivities to certain foods and additives can cause hyperactivity—a strong risk factor for criminality.[11] In one particular study, hyperactive children were exposed to synthetic colorings and flavorings, preservatives, cow's milk, and certain chemicals. When 486 parents of these children were surveyed with 172 non-hyperactive controls, the parents of the hyperactive children reported that more than sixty percent of the children exhibited increased behavioral problems. In contrast, only twelve percent of the parents of the controls reported a connection between food additives or colorings and worsened behavior.[12]

Although a highly controversial topic, I know food and other sensitivities had a huge impact on Evan's entire system. When he ate certain foods or was exposed to food dyes, he became a child we did not recognize.

CHAPTER 19

Neurotoxins
and Heavy Metals

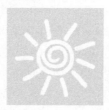

How can such small children accumulate heavy metals in their bodies? I certainly wondered. As revealed by the Environmental Working Group (EWG) cord blood testing has revealed that toxic metals and other environmental toxins are often passed through the placenta from mother to child. "It is truly amazing how many chemicals and toxic metals can pass from the mother into the developing fetus—it really does explain how the prevalence of chronic disease in younger people is escalating quickly as these toxins are capable of damaging many tissues and organs of the body."[1]

In addition, these children are exposed from a very young age to vaccinations and other environmental toxins and chemicals. When tested, many of these kids have high levels of metals and other toxins in their bodies.

When we tested Evan at age five and one-half, levels of lead and other metals were found. When I was tested, I also had lead and other metals in my system. I may have passed it to him in utero.

One source of lead is gasoline fumes. I have always loved the smell of gasoline. When I was a kid, I purposely got out of the car to inhale the fumes every time my mom filled up. My mother was also a heavy smoker with the car windows always rolled up. That could have contributed to the lead cadmium poisoning in my body. Who knew it would contribute to my own ADD symptoms or that

I would pass the poison on to my unborn child twenty-five years later?

Environmental toxins can trigger an autoimmune disease. Toxins disrupt normal immune function and can alter tissue proteins, making them look foreign to the immune system cells. In a 2001, Dr. William Walsh and Dr. Anjum Usman discovered that defective functioning of metallothionein protein (MT) is a distinctive feature of autism. "99% of the autistic children studied had (mt) protein deficiencies which were caused by environmental triggers." As explained by Amy S. Holmes, MD, this abnormality results in impaired brain development and extreme sensitivity to toxic metals and other environmental substances. This disorder is often unnoticed in infancy and early childhood until aggravated by a serious environmental insult.[2]

To add insult to injury, our kids do not have the ability to bind and remove heavy metals in the same way that other children do. They appear to be deficient in minerals, may have difficulty transporting minerals in and out of cells, and may have problems with binding and removing the heavy metals due to malfunctioning methallothionein (mt) proteins, as mentioned in Chapter 8. In a 2001 study, the researchers found that "99% of the autistic children studied had (mt) protein deficiencies which were caused by environmental triggers."[3]

Neurotoxins Crossing the Blood-Brain Barrier

Not only is it important to recognize the many environmental toxins in the air, water, and food, but we need to take a look at the different neurotoxins in the gut that are passing through the damaged gut lining and then crossing the blood-brain barrier.

Normally these nasty bugs that produce damaging neurotoxins do no harm, because they can't get through the healthy gut wall and are controlled by the beneficial bacteria. Unfortunately, many patients, whom we are talking about, don't have a healthy gut wall or enough healthy gut flora, due to the overuse of many broad-spectrum antibiotics and for other reasons mentioned earlier.

Clostridia

"Clostridia may be involved in a wide variety of human infections or illnesses."[4] Some include digestive disorders, tetanus, lock jaw, seizures (due to buildup of ammonia), and blood pressure problems. According to Dr. Campbell-McBride, in gut dysbiosis this powerful neurotoxin can pass through the damaged gut lining and then cross the blood-brain barrier, also affecting the person's mental development and well-being.

Although *Clostridia* can be present in neurologically typical people, it appears that the dangerous neurotoxins produced can cause neurological symptoms in some people. Dr. Campbell-McBride states, "There are many different *Clostridia* species known so far. They are present in the stools of people with autism, schizophrenia, psychosis, severe depression, muscle paralysis and muscle tonus abnormalities and some other neurological and psychiatric conditions."[5]

Research by Dr. Sidney Finegold compared the gut flora of children with regressive ASD to neurotypical children. The results show that clostridial counts were higher in the children with autism. The number of clostridial species found in the stools of children with ASD was greater than in the stools of neurotypical children. Children with ASD had nine species of *Clostridium* not found in the neurotypical group. The neurotypical group showed only three species not found in children with autism. In all, there were twenty-five different clostridial species found. In stomach and small intestine specimens, the most striking finding was total absence of *Clostridia* from neurotypical children and significant numbers of such bacteria from children with autism.[6]

Hydrogen Sulphide

Low levels of hydrogen sulfide occur naturally in the body, the environment, and the gut. It is often tolerated, because it is detoxified by enzymes into harmless sulfate.

The methylation cycle and glutathione are both parts of the overall sulfur metabolism in the body. When functioning normally, the sulphates (sulfur) we consume through our diets help us detoxify and assist in normal metabolism and brain functioning.

If the sulphates are consumed by an influx of toxins and bacteria in the gut, the sulfur is unavailable for use. The body then turns the sulphates into substances like hydrogen sulphide. This "toxic" gas often smells like "rotten eggs" and can be present in the stool of autistic and hyperactive children. Higher levels of hydrogen sulphide in the body is believed to poison several systems, especially the nervous system.

When hydrogen sulphide builds in the body due to the overgrowth of harmful, pathogenic bacteria as occurs during inflammation, the intestinal barrier breaks down further. "In addition, it stimulates the production of destructive compounds called ROS, which inhibits mitochondrial function. As stated in a research article titled "Gut Inflammation in Chronic Fatigue Syndrome," an increase in ROS caused by an imbalance between antioxidant defenses and ROS results in tissue damage and, eventually, cell death. Thus, there is evidence that hydrogen sulphide is involved in chronic (long-term) inflammation of the gut."[7]

Living in a Toxic World

Robert Melillo, MD, states in his book *Disconnected Kids* that "four out of five children diagnosed with autism and ADHD are boys. For one, boys are more susceptible to environmental toxins during prenatal development and during the first two years of life."[8]

There are thousands of toxins in our environment and among the most prevalent are:

Polychlorinated Biphenyls (PCBs). Widely used in coolant fluids, these toxins were banned by Congress in 1979. However, they are persistent pollutants in our environment and found in lakes and in our drinking water in small amounts. Farm-raised salmon and tilapia have absorbed PCBs, so it's best to avoid them. Buying smaller, wild-caught deep sea fish are best to avoid PCBs and mercury toxicity. Risks: impaired fetal brain development and cancer.

Perfluorinated compounds (PFCs). A family of manufactured fluorine-containing chemicals. They have unique properties to repel oil and water from clothing, carpeting, furniture, cookware, and food packaging to make these materials stain and stick resistant. People are most likely exposed to these compounds by consuming PFC-contaminated water or food, or by using products that contain PFCs. A research study in the *Environmental Health Perspectives* journal outlines the harmful effects of PFCs. "PFCs are extremely resistant to environmental and metabolic degradation and have been detected globally in the environment and wildlife."[9] The National Institute of Environmental Health Sciences reports, "In animal studies, some PFCs disrupt normal endocrine activity; reduce immune function; cause adverse effects on multiple organs, including the liver and pancreas; and cause developmental problems in rodent offspring exposed in the womb."[10] Studies have also explored the relationship between PFC compounds and behavior problems, specifically attention-deficit/hyperactivity disorder (ADHD), memory problems, and impulsive behavior; the researchers found "increased odds of ADHD in children with higher serum PFC levels."[11] There are many forms of PFCs, but the two most commonly found contaminants are PFOA, or perfluorooctanoic acid, used to make Teflon products, and PFOS, or perfluorooctane sulfonate, a breakdown product of chemicals formerly used to make Scotchgard products.

Pesticides. Herbicides, fungicides, and insecticides are often detected in foods in the U.S. "Within the past three decades, pesticide use in agriculture and for home and industrial purposes has increased by 50 percent and according to monitoring by the FDA, pesticide residues were detected in 50 percent of our foods."[12] The major sources are in commercially sold fruits, vegetables, and meats. This is why it's best to buy organic food or to buy from local farms that only use naturally sourced/biological pesticides. Risks: cancer, Parkinson's disease, ADHD, nerve damage (neurotoxicity), neurological dysfunction, birth defects, and the blocking of absorption of nutrients.

Chlorine. This highly toxic gas/chemical is widely used in household cleaners, drinking water, in the air in industrial areas, and in swimming pools. Risks: asthma; eye and skin irritations.

Chloroform. A colorless man-made toxic liquid made from chlorine and methane. Until the mid-1900s, chloroform was used as an anesthetic to reduce pain during medical procedures and was used in many consumer products. Due to its harmful effects it has been banned for these purposes. Yet, it is still used as a solvent for lacquers, floor polish, and adhesives, and is used in the production of paper, pesticides and other chemicals. This toxin is found in the air, drinking water, and food. Risks: cancer, dizziness, birth defects, fatigue, headaches, and liver and kidney disease. Chloroform also is toxic to the central nervous system.

Phthalates. A family of man-made chemical compounds developed in the last century to soften plastic and lengthen the life of fragrances. According to the United States Consumer Product Safety Commission, six types of these harmful chemicals have been banned for use in children's toys and certain child-care articles. Yet, phthalates are still used in the manufacture of many other plastic products such as solvents, household products, and personal-care products. They are colorless, odorless, oily liquids. They can be found in air fresheners, plastic wrap, plastic medical tubing, plastic shower curtains, plastic bottles, plates, and food storage containers. In addition, they are also found in nutritional supplements, enteric-coated pharmaceutical tablets, and many other products. Sadly, our diet is a main source of phthalate exposure. They leach from food storage containers and food wrap into foods (particularly those foods that are oily or that have a high fat content) such as milk, butter, and meat. Phthalates are especially dangerous, because they are linked to asthma and allergies, and also mimic hormones and damage the endocrine system. A 2009 study in Korea also showed a strong positive association between phthalates metabolites in urine and symptoms of ADHD and other neurological dysfunction.[13]

Bisphenol A (BPA). An industrial chemical used primarily to make plastic and resins. It is widely used in the production of plastic linings for metal cans and for the storage of beverages (soda cans) and plastic water bottles. BPA can leach xenoestrogens (hormone disruptors) into the water. The FDA has banned the use of BPA in baby bottles and toddler cups (as of July 2012), so the discussion has started. However, we need it taken out of all food packaging. We are exposed to this chemical daily, especially when we consume canned foods. Risks: causes adverse effects of the endocrine system and damages brain synapses, resulting in an increased risk of depression, memory problems, ADHD and other neurological disorders, asthma, aggression, thyroid dysfunction, and cancer. A 2013 study of school-aged children, aged eight to eleven years, was conducted to investigate the relationship between environmental exposure to BPA and childhood neurobehavior. The results demonstrated that urinary levels of BPA were positively associated with an increase of learning problems, anxiety/depression, and attentional issues.[14]

To prevent the leaching of this harmful chemical into your food, it is very important to avoid microwaving food in plastic. In addition, buying canned foods without BPA and purchasing stainless steel, glass, and non-BPA plastic containers are good ideas. Companies that use BPA-free cans are Eden Organics, Wild Planet, Trader Joe's, Native Forest, Native Factor, Oregon's Choice, and Eco Fish. Drinking from plastic water bottles, promotional water bottles, and baby bottles that are not BPA-free can be harmful, especially when they are left in a hot car or used over and over again. You can usually identify a plastic bottle containing BPA by the recycling codes "3" and "7" on the bottle.

Polyvinyl Chloride (PVC) and Polystyrene (PS) are harmful chemicals found in styrofoam and plastics. They release carcinogens when heated in the microwave and in the dishwasher and are found in bottles and packaged foods, as well as party plates, cups, and utensils. The PVC recycle code is "3," and the PS recycle code is "6." PVC is a harmful carcinogen and is the third most widely used chemical in the production of plastic. It is used in clothing, upholstery, vinyl flooring, and shower curtains. The production of PVC releases harmful chemicals into the air, endangering people who work and live near PVC-manufacturing plants. PVC produces dioxin and causes many ill effects, including cancer, immune disorders, and reproductive problems, to name a few. Polystyrene, which is used to produce Styrofoam cups, packing material, and the like, can also cause health problems such as respiratory issues, GI problems, depression, fatigue, muscle weakness, and possibly cancer.

Dioxins. Formed as a result of the combustion process, such as commercial waste incineration and from burning fuels like wood, coal, and oil, dioxins are chemical compounds found in commercial animal fats. Risks: cancer, developmental disorders, ADHD, learning problems, acne, skin rashes, excessive body hair, and mild liver damage. A 2007 Korean study demonstrated a correlation between dioxin exposure and learning disorders and attention deficit disorders.[15]

Mold and Fungus. Many people have allergic reactions to these mycotoxins. Sources include contaminated buildings, peanuts, wheat, corn, and alcohol. Risk: respiratory illnesses, cancer, heart disease, asthma, multiple sclerosis, diabetes, and nervous system disorders. A study out of Brown University showed a link between airborne mold spores and depression.[16]

Volatile Organic Compounds (VOCs). Organic chemicals that include both human-made and naturally occurring compounds. They are a major contributor to ozone air pollution. Levels are often higher inside than outside because it is present in so many household products like carpets, paints, dry-cleaned clothes, air fresheners, and drinking water. VOCs can cause eye and respiratory irritation, dizziness, and memory issues. In a study of the effects of indoor residential chemicals, it concluded that VOCs can cause respiratory distress and allergy symptoms in children.[17] Buying organic, non-chemical household cleaning supplies and air fresheners is best. A house full of plants such as spider plants, Boston ferns, English ivy, areca palm, aloe vera, Chinese evergreen, snake plants, and the peach lily act as living air purifiers.

Toxic Heavy Metals. These include mercury, lead, cadmium, aluminum, and others. They have no known function in the body and are harmful in large quantities. Today, humankind is exposed to the highest levels of these metals in recorded history. They affect everyone and are a major cause of illness, aging, and even genetic defects. The problems with toxic metals are rarely emphasized in medical schools, and for that reason, they are often not treated by mainstream doctors.

TOXIC HEAVY METALS

Heavy Metal	Where It Is Found	Linked to:
Aluminum	Cookware, glazes on plates, foil, cans, over-the-counter medicines such as antacids, vaccines, baking powder, refined foods, processed cheese, table salt, soy-based infant formula, antiperspirants	Alzheimer's disease, dementia, neuromuscular disorders, hyper-sensitivity, diarrhea, interference with the uptake of folic acid, depression, fatigue, gastro-intestinal issues, confusion, speech problems, hypoglycemia
Arsenic	Pesticides, chicken feed to make meat look fresher and pinker, apple juice, rice, cleaning supplies, pesticides, well water	Confusion, digestive disorders, drowsiness, seizure disorders
Cadmium	Potatoes, grains, sunflower seeds, contaminated water, cigarette smoke, hydrogenated oils found in commercial peanut butter, margarine, soy margarine, vegetable shortening, shellfish and bottom feeders, mining industry and environmental pollution	Learning disabilities, ADHD, and other neurologic dysfunctions
Copper*	Avocados, seeds, nuts, copper cooking pots, oysters, cocoa powder, dried herbs, copper pipes, water	Birth defects, miscarriages, acne, adrenal fatigue, hyperactivity, allergies, anxiety and nervous-ness, panic attacks, arthritis, autism, candida, depression, dyslexia, inflammation, insomnia, schizophrenia, thyroid dysfunction, vitamin deficiencies

*Some copper is essential for good health, but too much is toxic.

Heavy Metal	Where It Is Found	Linked to:
Fluoride	Water and, thus, into the food chain; baby foods; reconstituted fruit juices; fluoridated toothpaste	Alzheimer's disease, brain abnormalities, and functional changes to the neurological system that can affect the brain tissue of babies in utero
Lead	Lead-based paint, leaded gasoline, some hair dye, cleaning supplies, contaminated water from lead pipes, rubber products, kids' toys from foreign countries, pesticides	Abdominal pain, adrenal insufficiency, ADD, constipation, depression, dyslexia, epilepsy, fatigue, inflammation, learning disabilities, violent behavior
Mercury	Fish, flu shots, dental amalgams, health and beauty products such as cosmetics, pesticides	Adrenal gland dysfunction, bipolar disorder, birth defects, depression, dermatitis, hyperactivity, immune system dysfunction, insomnia, kidney damage, loss of self-control, memory loss, mood swings, nervousness, thyroid dysfunction, muscle weakness

This chart was adapted from the work of Lawrence Wilson, MD, a specialist in nutritional balancing science.

Evan exhibited many of the symptoms of mercury poisoning. He was frequently clumsy, easily distracted, slow in his physical development, sensitive to light, displayed an abnormal gait, had delayed speech, was verbally inarticulate, had poor cognitive processing, suffered from bowel disorders, and had many allergies.

In the *International Journal of Risk and Safety of Medicine*, "Animal studies show mercury poisoning can cause autistic-like behavior and existing scientific literature provides grounds for strong suspicion that mercury plays a causal role in the development of autism."[18] The article "How autism is linked to mercury toxicity—and what to do about it" spoke volumes to me. I learned that mercury poisoning can lead to social withdrawal, fear, anxiety, OCD, anger, brain fog, sound sensitivity, repetitive movements like flapping or spinning, gut problems, decreased serotonin levels, low sulfate levels, and low glutathione levels. Plus, it is believed to be a major cause of thyroid disease.[19]

Testing for Toxic Metals and Other Minerals

Evan was tested for heavy metals through a blood test and was treated by the naturopath. However, I have since learned that some naturopaths and physicians prefer hair testing or baby teeth analysis over blood tests because they believe blood tests only show the last thirty days of heavy metal exposure. Teeth and hair are supposedly closer to tissue sampling. Blood tests and hair sampling testing can be ordered by your physician, or you can order one online from the Great Plains Laboratory, Analytical Research Labs, Inc., or the Canadian-based company, CanAlt Health Laboratories. Check with your insurance provider about possible coverage.

How Can You Avoid Toxic Metals and Chemicals?

Here are some tips:

- Buy organic foods as much as possible to avoid pesticides.

- Have your tap water tested. If toxic elements are identified, consider a reverse osmosis water-filtration system.

- Avoid cooking in aluminum foil or using aluminum cookware.

- Avoid hydrogenated oils, as they contain cadmium.

- Stay away from chemical sources such as fresh paint, food additives, and food dyes.

- Avoid Bisphenol A (BPA) by drinking and eating from glass containers or BPA-free plastic, reduce your use of canned goods, and never microwave in plastic wrap or in plastic containers.

- Limit "big fish" consumption such as tuna and swordfish. Only buy quality omega-3 supplements that are made from smaller fish like sardines and krill.

- Avoid fire-retardant clothing, and wash all new clothes before wearing.

- Use only fluoride-free toothpaste.

- Purchase nontoxic cleaning supplies and air fresheners, and get rid of all toxic chemicals previously used for cleaning the house.

- Ditch dryer sheets and chemically laced clothing detergents.

- Avoid antiperspirants, and use only organic and natural hair products, skin products, and cosmetics.

- Please check out the Environmental Working Group at www.ewg .org to learn more about the toxic ingredients in bug sprays, beauty supplies, and hair products. Another great resource is *The Green Beauty Guide: Your Essential Resource to Organic and Natural Skin Care, Makeup, and Fragrances* by Julie Gabriel.[20]

Also, check out Katiebugproducts.com. Katiebug's handmade body products were created by Danielle, a mom on a mission, who was determined to create natural bath products to help her daughter Katie and the rest of her family heal from many health ailments, including asthma, eczema, ADHD, and ASD. Danielle began creating bath soap, lotion, skincare products, diaper rash cream, sunscreen, and shampoo without chemicals, dyes, and other harmful ingredients. She uses healing herbs, essential oils, and oxide minerals for color to create her amazing products. Her products have become extremely popular in numerous locations across the world and are even distributed at Akron, Ohio's Children's Asthma and Allergy Center.

Detoxification and Our Sensitive Kids

As I've discussed earlier, our sensitive kids have more difficulty detoxifying toxic substances than their neurologically typical peers. This may be due to inadequate gut flora and other biological causes. It can become a vicious circle.

Microflora play a role in sulfation. When sulphates and intestinal defenses are low in these children, it can lead to yeast overgrowth, which, in turn, can lead to sulfur-reducing bacteria and even lower sulphate levels. If sulfur is unavailable for appropriate use, the process by which the body eliminates toxins fails. Toxins then get absorbed into the bloodstream and can be carried across the blood-brain barrier, causing different neurological and psychiatric symptoms.

Yeast overgrowth in the gut can cause fermentation of food in place of digestion and cause bloating and gas. Candida can contribute to leaky gut syndrome—thus, in turn, can lead to the production of toxins that may affect the brain and nervous system. Yeast overgrowth can produce alcohol as its byproduct, acetaldehyde, giving these kids a "hangover" feeling. It can also lead to liver damage, and it prevents the proper detoxification of other pollutants, increasing the toxicity of other toxins.

One study in the *Journal of Biological Psychiatry* suggests that one component of autism could be expressed as a chronic metabolic imbalance that impairs normal neurodevelopment and immunologic function and that the inability to effectively metabolize certain compounds, particularly phenolic amines, toxic for the central nervous system, could exacerbate the wide spectrum of autistic behavior.[21]

It is so essential to add detoxification regimens into your daily practices. Here is a simple, yet effective recipe for Detox Water:

Lemon/Cucumber Detox Water

2 liters water in a glass container

1 medium cucumber, sliced

1 lemon, sliced

10–12 mint leaves

Combine all ingredients in a glass container, and steep overnight in the refrigerator. Drink daily.

Sulfur-Based Homeopathic Remedies

Once Evan's gut was on the mend, our naturopath began to detoxify him with sulfur and other homeopathic remedies. She introduced mineral supplementation and detoxifying foods that would assist in the process. She stressed that it was essential to restore the gut before starting an aggressive detox regimen. If we released the toxins from his tissues into his body without the ability to eliminate them effectively, it could wreak havoc with his entire system.

The road to recovery was very much like a roller-coaster ride. While on certain homeopathic treatments and detoxification regimens, Evan's symptoms often got much worse before they got better. I know this seems backward, but it's just part of the detoxification process. Our naturopath reassured us that once Evan's body was detoxed, we would see a noticeable jump in his cognition and social functioning. She was right; we definitely did!

Glutathione Fights Free Radicals and Toxins

Glutathione is the body's main antioxidant that combats free radicals (atoms with an odd number of electrons that cause damage in the body). It is synthesized from the amino acids L-cysteine, L-glutamic acid, and glycine. However, if the body is not digesting properly or if there is an overload of toxins, the body may not metabolize glutathione correctly.

Low glutathione levels reduce the body's natural ability to detoxify itself of environmental toxins and heavy metals through the process of methylation. Deficiency also increases allergic responses, causes autoimmune attacks on the body, and prevents brain cells from communicating appropriately.

If the toxins coming into the body are more than the body can eliminate through detoxification, this leads to a buildup of the toxins. As a result, the toxins create more free radicals, which, in turn, deplete glutathione stores.

Researches also believe that taking acetaminophen such as Tylenol during pregnancy and beyond lowers glutathione levels, which could also be contributing to the rise in ADHD and other neurodevelopmental disorders in children. One study in *JAMA Pediatrics* analyzed over sixty-four thousand children and their mothers, following them from pregnancy till the children were adolescents. More than half of the women took acetaminophen at some point while pregnant. By the time the children were, on average, eleven years old, those whose mothers had taken acetaminophen were nearly thirty percent more likely to exhibit ADHD behaviors and be taking medications for the disorder than were children whose mothers had not taken the painkiller.[22]

Sulfur-rich foods such as garlic, onions, and cruciferous vegetables like broccoli, spinach, parsley, kale, collards, cabbage, cauliflower, and watercress are required for the synthesis of glutathione. So, eating more of these can be extremely helpful.

Other effective ways to raise and maintain glutathione levels are to exercise regularly and provide the body with the raw materials and cofactors to make it.

When autistic children are biomedically treated, they are often supplemented with an antioxidant called N-acetylcysteine (N-AC) to support the immune system—in the form of a liposome capsule or an effervescent tablet for better absorption. They may be given vitamin B12, folinic acid, alpha-lipoic acid, trimethylglycine (TMG), and vitamin C in tandem, to help raise glutathione levels and combat toxic free radicals. TMG supplementation is believed to be especially beneficial for those who carry a MTHFR genetic mutation.

In 2012, the effectiveness of oral N-acetylcysteine in children with autism was studied in a twelve-week randomized pilot trial of oral N-AC in children with autism. "When examining all participants, oral N-AC treatment significantly improved irritability in children with autism spectrum disorders (ASD). Additionally, oral N-AC treatment resulted in a significant improvements in social cognition and a trend toward significance in improvement of stereotypic/repetitive behavior."[23] More and more parents agree, reporting a decrease in many symptoms including stimming and self-injurious behavior when their child took N-AC, such as high-quality PharmaNAC.

Dr. Jon Grant, MD, of the Department of Psychiatry at the University of Minnesota also believes that N-acetylcysteine significantly helps those suffering from addictions, nail biting, skin picking, hair pulling, and other compulsive behaviors.[24]

Taurine

Taurine is also an important sulfonic amino acid that helps detoxify the liver and body by playing a vital role of enhancing cellular anti-oxidizing activity. Taurine is also involved in processes involving metabolism, nervous system, brain, and visual pathways. Supplementing with taurine may be important in cases where an individual is deficient in this important nutrient.

Drink Enough Water

Drinking adequate amounts of water daily aids in the detoxification process. In a world of sugary soft drinks, sports drinks, and coffee, we often forget to drink enough water.

To deeply cleanse the body of free radicals, drink lukewarm purified water with the juice of $1/2$ organic lemon squeezed into it. Lemons contain more than twenty anticancer compounds and help cleanse your liver, kidneys, and colon. Lemon also boosts the immune system and aids in digestion. For the best results: drink lukewarm lemon water on an empty stomach and wait about 20 minutes before drinking or eating anything else.

Washing Away Toxins

Natural is always better. Be careful of commercial detoxification remedies. They can be ineffective or, in some cases, even dangerous, as some brands contain harmful ingredients such as aluminum. In addition, a detox program should always be under advisement of a clinician or physician. They will often test your liver and kidneys to determine if they are efficient enough to handle a detox.

One natural detox remedy, which is an excellent way to rid the body of heavy metals, is as follows: Toss a bunch of organic cilantro, ice, and pineapple in a blender. Or try cilantro, pears, banana, ice, and a few dates. It's delicious, and the kids love it.

Here are additional tips for getting rid of toxins:

1. *Eat organic green foods containing lots of minerals* such as chlorella (algae), kelp and other sea minerals, aloe, kale, spinach, Swiss chard, arugula, parsley, and cilantro. All of these contain high levels of chlorophyll, which boosts the digestive tract to rid itself of harmful environmental toxins from toxic metals, herbicides, cleaning products, and pesticides. They assist the liver in detoxification, alkalize the body (restore pH balance), reduce inflammation, fight infections, and promote healthy intestinal flora. According to Dr. Weston Price, author of *Nutrition and Physical Degeneration*, primitive man ate five to eleven times the amount of essential minerals as we eat in today's diet.[25] When food is low in essential minerals, the body absorbs and makes use of more toxic metals.

   Here's one mom's story: "My thirteen-month-old son went silent after five months of simple noises and a tiny vocabulary. Then I started him on chlorella tablets by Source Naturals. My veggie and fruit–hating son just chewed the tablets with minimal prompting (I was shocked) and within two weeks, he was speaking in full sentences." (Sirah Morgan)

   Warning: Some people are sensitive to chlorella and/or oral cilantro, so discontinue use if any nausea or discomfort develops after eating it.

2. *Make a lot of fruit salads with citrus fruits like lemons, grapefruit, oranges, and limes.* They assist the body by flushing out toxins and jump-starting the digestive tract with enzymatic processes. They support the detoxification of the liver, alkalinize the body, and help rid the intestinal tract of viruses, bacteria, and parasites. Lemon juice and warm water is a great remedy. The vitamin C in these fruits also transforms toxins into digestible material for quicker elimination.

3. *Cook with garlic.* It is one of the best detoxifying foods known to man. It stimulates the liver into producing detoxification enzymes that filter toxic residues from the digestive system.

4. *Familiarize yourself with mung beans.* Native to China, mung beans have been used by Ayurvedic doctors in Asian and Indian cultures

for thousands of years. They are incredibly healthy and an easily digestible bean. They're delicious in soups, help with natural weight loss, and absorb toxic residue from the intestinal walls.

5. *Juice and eat certain vegetables containing high levels of sulfur.* These include carrots, spinach, onions, broccoli, asparagus, kale, beets, cauliflower, parsley, radishes, tomatoes, grapes, and cabbage. The combination of these foods can help your liver purge toxins during the cleansing process because they are high in naturally occurring sulfur, which is essential for the synthesis of glutathione. Additionally, sulfur-rich foods like garlic, egg yolks, and onions are rich in beneficial minerals such as calcium, iron, zinc, iodine, chromium, and selenium.

6. *Add more of the easily digestible seeds and nuts into your diet* such as flaxseeds, pumpkin seeds, sunflower seeds, walnuts, almonds, hemp seeds, sesame seeds, and chia seeds. *Salvia hispanica*/chia seed is in the mint family, and it binds with toxins in the digestive system to help eliminate waste. It's also the richest and only unprocessed, whole food source of pure omega-3 fatty acid, is high in fiber, and slows the absorption of sugar. It is important that chia seeds are crushed, however, in order to prevent colon distress, and bear in mind that consuming too many can cause constipation. Add to smoothies, salads, or to your next meatloaf. Also, great when used as an egg replacer in baked recipes. Simply mix one tablespoon of chia seeds to three tablespoons of water mix and let gel; ground flaxseeds also work well.

7. *Lubricate the intestinal walls with omega-3 oils* such as avocado, coconut, olive, and flaxseed oils. The toxins can be absorbed by the oil and more readily eliminated from the body.

8. *Drink plenty of water, preferably filtered water with minerals.*

9. *Eat adequate amounts of organic animal protein* for sulfur-containing amino acids that help eliminate toxic metals and support liver detoxification pathways.

10. *Eat plenty of fiber-rich foods* to reduce toxic metals by speeding bowel transit time. Certain fibers such as modified citrus pectin

also bind with some toxic metals and reduce their absorption.

11. *Eat sea kelp*, a great source of minerals that our diet frequently lacks. It removes heavy metals, aids in digestion, helps metabolize amino acids, improves immunity, and reduces yeast.

The Power of Taking a Bath

Take a quality Epsom salt bath for a minimum of twenty minutes a few days a week. Soaking in water that contains a half cup of Epsom salt is important for detoxification pathways. Epsom salt (magnesium sulfate) is easily absorbed into the skin. It allows the body to cleanse of heavy metals and other pollutants, relieves constipation, and relaxes the body, which can help you sleep better.

Additionally, take a calcium bentonite clay bath every five to seven days. This powerful clay is composed of aged volcanic ash. This clay is believed to hold a negative charge, which bonds to the positive charge of many toxins.

This successful treatment regimen is being used as a natural and safe way to eliminate heavy metals and environmental toxins from the body through the pores of your skin. It's being used in many autism treatment centers to rid the body of mercury, cadmium, and lead, and it can also be used to detoxify yeast, parasites, chemicals, and pesticides. To have a strong drawing effect, it's important to use high-quality clay without impurities.

It is also essential to consume an electrolyte drink such as Emergen-C or coconut water to help replace any lost vitamins, minerals, and electrolytes after the bath. To purchase bentonite clay baths, please visit www.evenbetternow.com, and search for their "Kids Clear" product.

Calcium bentonite clay can also be ingested. It has been used in many cultures for thousands of years as a detox regimen. It is believed to be a magnet for parasites, yeast, and environmental toxins because it has a negative ion charge and attaches itself to positively charged pathogens. Please speak to your naturopath or alternative healthcare provider about the benefits of bentonite clay as part of your child's (or your own) detoxification protocol.

CHAPTER 20

A Deeper Look at Other Issues Plaguing Our Kids

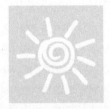

Liver Stress and Pancreatic Dysfunction

Leaky gut syndrome can also cause liver and pancreas problems. The liver of leaky gut patients works overtime to excrete toxins. When the body does not detoxify adequately, it synthesizes free radicals, which wind up in the bile. It then becomes more toxic and can damage bile ducts in the liver and reflux back into the pancreas, causing damage there also. The toxic bile, rich in free radicals, further damages the small bowel mucosa and exacerbates hyperpermeability in the intestines. In an effort to eliminate toxic oxidation products, the liver depletes its reserves of sulfur-containing amino acids, which would aid in the detoxification process. It is yet another vicious cycle.

Adrenal Fatigue

After a great deal of reading, I became convinced that Evan was also suffering from adrenal fatigue. It is a term coined in 1998 by Dr. James Wilson, the author of *Adrenal Fatigue: The 21st Century Stress Syndrome*. Evan was chronically tired and lacked the appropriate energy of a small child. He also suffered from sleep disturbances and many of the overlooked symptoms of adrenal fatigue such as morning tiredness, behavioral problems, memory problems, anxiety, OCD, occasional hyperactivity, asthma, allergies, food sensitivities, recurrent illnesses, excessive thirst, sleep issues, sensory issues, hypoglycemia, sweet cravings, and salt cravings.

The writing of Georgia Davis, MD, who specializes in the diagnosis and treatment of complex neuropsychiatric conditions and holds board certifications in psychiatry, neurology, and forensics, tied it all together for me. "Adrenal dysfunction coexists with imbalances of the hormonal and immune system; and hypersensitivities and toxicities are the underlying causes of chronic illnesses and autism spectrum disorders."[1] Although not always recognized by physicians, many autism spectrum children have problems with their adrenal glands. Stressors are cumulative, and if they persist over time, adrenal insufficiency or even an adrenal crisis may result.

Evan's food sensitivities were clearly a profound stress on his adrenals. The adrenal fatigue made it more difficult for him to produce the additional amounts of the anti-inflammatory hormone cortisol to adequately counteract his inflammatory allergic reactions. Dr. Wilson puts it this way: "When the adrenals are fatigued, it is more difficult to produce the additional amounts of cortisol necessary to adequately counteract the inflammatory allergic reactions. People going through times of adrenal fatigue may notice that they seem to have more allergies or their allergies seem to get worse."[2] Conversely, the more histamine released, the harder the adrenals have to work to produce enough cortisol, the more fatigued they may become. It is therefore not surprising that people with food and environmental allergies commonly tend to experience adrenal fatigue as well. This can set up a vicious cycle of reduced cortisol, allowing histamine to inflame the tissues more, leading to deepening adrenal fatigue as well as to bigger allergic reactions."[3]

Evan's cortisol tests revealed that his levels were extremely low indicating that he was indeed suffering from adrenal fatigue. It explained many of his symptoms. Cortisol is supposed to peak when a person wakes up to give them "get up and go" and then gradually decline as the day wears on. This important hormone makes the brain more alert and better able to cope with a changeable environment. It may have explained why Evan needed routine and had an aversion to change. When we treated Evan's low cortisol with herbs, he started to sleep better and appeared less anxious. Also, he stopped asking about the plan for the day as much, which had been a repetitive behavior.

Hormone and Neurotransmitter Imbalances

While blaming hormones for all of life's problems has become a habit for most of us, it's important to recognize that hormones really do play a very important role in regulating many functions within the body. The hormone levels of kids on the autism spectrum are often out of balance, and there are many dietary recommendations, supplements, and herbal and homeopathic remedies that can treat the imbalance without the use of potentially harmful medications.

A blood test to determine possible COMT and MAO-A genetic mutations, along with simple urine tests will determine hormonal imbalances, amino acid deficiencies, and much more. One leader in nutritional testing is Great Plains Laboratory. Their menu of tests include an Amino Acid Urine Test and an Organic Acids Test (OAT). Testing reveals a person's essential and non-essential amino acid levels and provides information about hormone/neurotransmitter imbalances. The OAT test also checks for other nutritional markers, glutathione status, oxalate metabolism, and provides an accurate evaluation of intestinal yeast and bacteria. Another option is to get a blood test to check the levels of different hormones and amino acids (which help make up these neurotransmitters) before coming up with a treatment plan.

It's controversial, as much of the medical community does not think that neurotransmitter testing is reliable. However, many people, including my father, believe that these tests are indeed credible. For my dad, his test results matched his symptoms, and the natural treatment plan to address his imbalances proved to be successful. My dad has always been an anxious person with a bad temper. Once he was treated with the help of his integrative physician, he couldn't believe how much better he felt. He was sleeping soundly for the first time in years, he had more energy, and his mood improved immensely. I needed to see this for myself.

After approximately one year of gut rehabilitation and doing continued research, I consulted another naturopath, Jared Skowron of Harvest Park Naturopathic Medicine. Dr. Skowron is a DAN (Defeat Autism Now) practitioner and author who specializes in the biomedical treatment of children with ADHD and autism.

He ordered a random urine test for Evan to determine all of his amino acid and neurotransmitter levels. Even though he was improving drastically, he still was having trouble sleeping soundly and was still very anxious. He would ruminate about many things and he would ask the same questions repeatedly. He would still get upset if his plan was disrupted and was often frustrated. He also had difficultly staying on task and staying in the moment. He was driving us crazy, and I believe Evan was driving himself crazy too. When I asked him why he needed to ask me the same question one-hundred times, he said, "Mom, there is something wrong with my head." My heart sank. I reassured him with a huge hug that he was okay, and told him that we were going to get to the bottom of this.

The testing revealed what I had suspected: Evan carried the COMT gene mutation. His GABA (amino acid) levels were very low and his neurotransmitters were not in normal range either. Our naturopath started Evan on GABA supplementation, NA-C, and B-complex spray in the morning, added 5-HTP, and increased his magnesium dose at bedtime. Within hours of giving him GABA, he presented much calmer. Within days, he was a bit more focused. He was no longer repeating himself, and his sleep patterns improved, as well.

The second urine test (six months later) revealed that many of the levels were starting to correct. However, his epinephrine (adrenaline) level was still at zero, possibly due to his being a fast metabolizer, or because of his suffering from some adrenal fatigue. Low epinephrine very possibly explains Evan's low stamina, hypoglycemia, and poor concentration at times. The naturopath suggested continuing with the GABA and starting taurine, L-theanine, and Myo-Inositol (a carbohydrate found in higher plants and animals) to raise epinephrine levels. Again, within days we saw amazing improvements. When I asked him if he was feeling better, with a big infectious smile he said, "Mom, my head stopped making noise. I feel so much better, thank you." My heart sang.

The following table shows a list of some of the most important hormones/neurotransmitters that should be tested and the roles they play in the body:

IMPORTANT HORMONES AND NEUROTRANSMITTERS

Hormone/ Neurotransmitter	Role in the Body
Melatonin	This hormone is made "naturally" in the brain by converting tryptophan, vitamin B3, B6, and B9 into serotonin. The serotonin then triggers the production of melatonin. Vitamin B12 helps regulate our alertness and turn off melatonin, signaling the transition from sleep to a more active awake state.
Serotonin	Serotonin controls mood, appetite, and sleep cycles. Too little serotonin can make us feel depressed, sad, and socially withdrawn, and can affect attention span.
Epinephrine	Our "fight or flight" response. Also called adrenaline. Too much can create severe anxiety, sleep difficulties, attention issues, and heart palpitations. It regulates attentiveness and mental focus; so too little can create low stamina, fatigue, low mood, lack of motivation, weight gain, and poor concentration.
Norepinephrine	Controls heart rate and blood pressure and contributes to sleep, arousal, and emotions. Too much can make you feel anxious and hyper and increase blood pressure, while too little can affect focus, leave you feeling depressed or numb. It can also induce hot flashes and headaches.
Dopamine	Dopamine is a pleasure-producing neurotransmitter in the brain and is also responsible for muscle control and GI issues. At correct levels, it helps a person feel happy and is important for cognition, motor movement, and cognitive stability. Elevated dopamine can cause poor intestinal function, developmental delays, attention issues, OCD, impulsivity, and pleasure-seeking and repetitive behaviors such as the compulsion to play video games or an obsession with violence. Reduced levels can contribute to fatigue, irritability, and the inability to carry out simple tasks.

Hormone/ Neurotransmitter	Role in the Body
Cortisol	Produced by the adrenal gland, cortisol regulates the body's stress response. High levels of cortisol can make you feel anxious and often causes sleep issues and low immune activity. Low levels of cortisol can cause you to feel anxious or fatigued.
Corticotrophin-Releasing	Releases cortisol in response to stress.

Our bodies function like a well-oiled machine when working properly. If these important hormones are out of balance, there can be physical, emotional, and behavioral consequences. Speak to your naturopath about testing and about all of the possible natural treatment options because there are plenty. Also, remember that protein is the body's building blocks of neurotransmitters and that amino acid levels can play a role.

Many foods and herbs that naturally raise serotonin levels and lower dopamine levels can be found in organic health food stores. You can buy them in supplement form or grow them in your own garden. They include oat straw, dandelion greens, ginseng, burdock, and black cohosh, to name a few. Just make sure to get all appropriate testing and speak to a professional before giving any herbal remedies to your children.

If low dopamine is the problem, eat foods rich in tyrosine. Almonds, avocados, bananas, lima beans, sesame seeds, and pumpkin seeds can help the body to produce more dopamine naturally. The OCD Recovery Center, offering one of the most scientific, innovative and comprehensive treatment programs in United States, issued a statement that pumpkin seeds have been have been shown to reduce OCD, social anxiety, and depression. They are packed with the amino acid tryptophan, which the brain uses to make neurotransmitters like serotonin.[4]

Also, increase your intake of antioxidants. Dopamine is easy to oxidize, and antioxidants reduce free radical damage to the brain cells that produce dopamine. Exercise and plenty of rest help a great deal, too.

Hypoglycemia

Inflammation in the gut can also trigger insulin resistance, which causes low blood sugar called hypoglycemia and is often aggravated by food sensitivities. So, in addition to all of his other symptoms, Evan had hypoglycemia. I discovered it after reading Kenneth Bock's book, *Healing the New Childhood Epidemics*. Later, testing confirmed what I suspected.

Hypoglycemic symptoms often mimic, amplify, and trigger symptoms of autism spectrum disorders and ADHD. It partially explained his symptoms of insomnia, tendency toward nightmares, excessive night sweats, fatigue, cravings for sweets and starchy foods, and his need for frequent meals and snacks to avoid irritability.

Kenneth Bock, MD, explains in his book that poor cognitive functioning, poor memory, irritability, anxiety, tantrums, poor physical functioning, constipation, "spacy" behavior, physical weakness, confusion, and the inability to communicate can all often be attributed to hypoglycemia. Evan had all of these symptoms.

More extensive testing is usually needed to determine if someone has hypoglycemia. Blood work does not show the milder form of the disorder, so doctors frequently miss the signs altogether.

The good news is that hypoglycemia can be treated naturally. It is recommended to eat healthy, balanced snacks throughout the day, such as an apple with peanut butter to balance the carbohydrates with the protein. Other steps include adding more fiber to your diet, increasing levels of vitamins E and B6, and decreasing consumption of processed foods and refined salts. Raw honey (after the age of one year), cinnamon, curry, ginger, evening primrose oil, black seed oil, and chromium supplements are also helpful.

Low Stomach Acid—Hypochlorhydria

Many children with ADHD and ASD have insufficient stomach acid. Also known as hydrochloric acid, it helps the body to properly digest food, absorb critical nutrients, and metabolize proteins into amino acids. Sufferers of hypochlorhydria often complain of bloating, gas, and indigestion.

Stomach acid is also important for the correct functioning of the immune system. A healthy acid barrier in the stomach easily and quickly kills bacteria and other bugs that enter the body. It also prevents bacteria from the intestines from migrating up and colonizing the stomach.

This condition (more often found in individuals with a type-A blood) is frequently overlooked and may be linked to nutritional deficiencies, constipation, leaky gut, fatigue, high cortisol levels, food allergies, stomach cancer, asthma, gastrointestinal issues (especially inflammatory bowel diseases), GERD, heartburn, and celiac disease. So, if you've made several diet and lifestyle changes and you are still not seeing the results you want, low stomach acid might be to blame.

Here are some ways to increase hydrochloric acid naturally:

- Eat good quality sea salt.

- Increase zinc intake.

- Increase B vitamin intake.

- Eliminate processed foods.

- Eliminate white flour and refined sugars.

- Eat honey; manuka honey produced in Australia and New Zealand is extremely healing.

- Eat cabbage or drink cabbage juice and benefit from its healing enzyme. Also known as vitamin U. Be careful not to drink too much cabbage juice, as it can suppress thyroid activity.

- Consume raw apple cider vinegar.

- Drink ginger tea.

- Limit grain fiber and unfermented soy, which contain phytic acid.

- Drink warm water with lemon before meals.

- Eat dandelion greens with meals or in soups.

- Do not overhydrate or drink ice-cold beverages with meals.

- Eat meat proteins that are well ground up.

- Take quality probiotics and digestive enzymes with DPP IV.

- Take a live-source hydrochloric supplement temporarily in extreme cases, but only after you have discussed this option with a physician. If currently on medication, please ensure that there will not be an adverse reaction to taking it in tandem.

Thyroid Conditions

Another avenue to examine is thyroid functioning. An article published in 2011 in *Autism Research* noted that infants born with low fT4 had an increased risk for autism and that thyroid deficiencies during critical periods of brain development in utero can cause motor delay, deafness, mental retardation, and many neurological ill effects.[5]

And, according to Kenneth Bock, MD, along with allergies and asthma, hypothyroidism is one of the most common physical disorders found in people with ADHD and autism. Hypothyroidism can cause symptoms of cold intolerance, weight gain, depression, constipation, low energy, and impaired cognitive function. Levels are often tested with a blood test, and when they come back "normal," many doctors stop there. However, it is important to dig deeper for a milder form by testing for thyroid antibodies, which may indicate an individual has Hashimoto's (a common autoimmune disease). Elevated thyroid antibodies can cause ADHD-type symptoms. In addition, studies show that a significant percentage of those suffering from celiac or milder gluten sensitivity also have a thyroid problem. Interestingly, research has also shown that when gluten is removed from the diet, thyroid antibodies disappear. This was certainly true for my husband, Steve, who did not want to go on Synthroid. He decided to treat his own hypothyroidism by increasing vitamin D and natural iodine consumption, and by avoiding gluten, raw kale, broccoli and other cruciferous vegetables because of their goitrogenic properties that suppress the function of the thyroid gland by interfering with iodine uptake. Cooking these veggies reduce Goitrogen levels. He was successful.

High Ammonia Levels in the Blood

Physicians have been treating a condition known as hepatic encephalopathy, since the 1960s. Hepatic encephalopathy is a worsening of brain function that occurs when the liver is no longer able to remove toxic substances (such as ammonia) in the blood.

The gut produces ammonia, primarily when protein is digested. Ammonia is a neurotoxin that excites and damages brain cells and the mitochondria (the site of energy production in all cells). As stated in the *Cleveland Clinic Journal of Medicine*, the liver can't detoxify ammonia that well or there is just too much, it can cause neurological damage and "neuropsychiatric dysfunction."[6] It is believed that a buildup of ammonia can sometimes be the root cause of symptoms such as anxiety, OCD, and other neurological conditions.

High ammonia levels can be remedied by clearing out ammonia-producing bacteria in the gut. Suggestions to flush ammonia out of the gut include:

- Eat a protein-reduced diet.

- Improve gut health with probiotics.

- Increase bowel movements with increased fiber intake and other remedies.

- Talk to your healthcare provider about remedies to help restore the liver.

Sleep Issues

Many children on the autism spectrum have trouble sleeping. Here is a quick checklist of possible causes of insomnia, sleep apnea, and restless sleep in children and/or adults that you can investigate in more depth with your health practitioner:

1. Adrenal fatigue and low cortisol

2. Hormone imbalances causing anxiety

3. Asthma

4. Thyroid problems

5. Reflux and other negative food reactions

6. Eating protein too close to bedtime, which keeps the digestive system active

7. Drinking caffeine and taking SSRIs and stimulant medication

8. Drinking alcohol

9. Taking over-the-counter cold medication and blood pressure medication

10. Exercising too late in the day

11. Vitamin B3, B5, B6, and/or B9 deficiency

12. Vitamin D deficiency

13. Amino acid deficiency or imbalance (Look into GABA levels and tryptophan levels)

14. Deficiency of important minerals such as magnesium, zinc, and calcium and iron (check ferritin levels)

15. Hypoglycemia and imbalanced sugar levels

16. Large adenoids and tonsils

17. Habits such as taking naps during the day, watching television, and playing on the computer late at night instead of taking time to wind down in the evening

CHAPTER 21

Identifying Nutritional Deficiencies & Taking Supplements

What Vitamins and Minerals Should My Child Take?

Getting a complete metabolic workup with an integrative physician, naturopath, MAPS doctor (The Medical Academy of Pediatric Special Needs) or DAN "Defeat Autism Now" doctor will paint a complete picture. Make sure to include MTHFR and other gene mutation testing. Minerals, vitamins, and amino acids need to be analyzed. Every child is unique and may require different supplements to create the proper balance in the body, and it can feel like a balancing act. Please refer back to Chapter 12 for a complete listing of vitamins, minerals, and amino acids everyone's body needs.

Remember, too much of a good thing is not always good. While treating Evan with B complex vitamins to help reduce anxiety, the stimulating effect (of too much) actually made him worse, for example. In addition, I can't stress enough about the importance of testing vitamin/mineral levels periodically. For example, too much vitamin A, iron, or potassium can be very dangerous—toxic in fact.

A Deeper Look at Evan's Supplement Treatment Plan

SpectraCell Laboratories is another leader in nutritional testing and vitamin/mineral analysis. The following graphics, created by Spectra-Cell, illustrate the nutrients recommended to prevent and treat ADHD and autism.

RECOMMENDED NUTRIENTS

ADHD

Antioxidant Status: Oxidative imbalance is prevalent in ADHD patients and likely plays a causative role; deficiency of glutathione common in ADHD.

Folate: Low folate status in pregnancy linked to hyperactivity in children; people with the MTHFR (methyl tetrahydra folate reductase) gene are predisposed to folate deficiency and more likely to have ADHD.

Vitamin B6: Evidence suggests high dose supplementation of B6 is as effective as Ritalin for ADHD, probably due to its role in raising serotonin levels.

Magnesium: Deficiency linked to poor function of the neurotransmitters that control emotion, social reactions, hyperactivity and attention; synergistic effect with vitamin B6.

Zinc: Cofactor for dopamine synthesis, which affects mood and concentration in ADHD; Low zinc depresses both melatonin and serotonin production, which affect information processing and behavior in ADHD.

Carnitine: Reduces hyperactivity and improves social behavior in people with ADHD due to its role in fatty acid metabolism; some consider it a safe alternative to stimulant drugs.

Serine: Administration of phosphatidylserine with omega 3 fatty acids improved ADHD symptoms (attention scores) significantly better than omega 3 fatty acids alone, suggesting a synergistic effect; phosphatidylserine increases dopamine levels.

Glutamine: Precursor for the calming neurotransmitter GABA (gamma-aminobutyric acid) that affects mood, focus and hyperactivity; disruption of the glutamine-containing neurotransmission systems may cause ADHD.

Choline: Precursor to neurotransmitter acetylcholine, which regulates memory, focus and muscle control (hyperactivity).

Antioxidant Status: Oxidative imbalance is prevalent in ADHD patients and likely plays a causative role; deficiency of glutathione common in ADHD.

AUTISM

Vitamin D: High dose vitamin D therapy reversed autistic behaviors in severely deficient children; maternal vitamin D deficiency may predispose children to autism.

Vitamin A: One cause of autism may be a defect in a retinoid receptor protein (G-alpha protein), which is critical for language processing, attention and sensory perception; evidence suggests natural vitamin A fixes this protein defect in autistics.

Folate: Oral folate therapy can resolve symptoms of autism in some cases, particularly in autistics with genes that impair folate dependent enzymes.

Glutamine: Blood levels of this amino acid, which acts as a neurotransmitter, are particularly low in autistics. Glutamine also helps prevent leaky gut syndrome, which can exacerbate autistic symptoms.

Vitamin C: Improved symptom severity and sensory motor scores in autistic patients possibly due to interaction with dopamine synthesis; vitamin C also has a strong sparing effect on glutathione.

Glutathione & Cysteine: Commonly deficient in autistic patients, lack of these antioxidants impair detoxification and methylation processes; low levels linked to neurological symptoms in autism, which is often considered an oxidative stress disorder.

Vitamin B1: Deficiency linked to delayed language development; supplementation may benefit autistic patients.

Vitamin B6: Cofactor the neurotransmitters serotonin and dopamine; conversion of B6 to its active form is compromised in many autistics; supplementation trials with B6 resulted in better eye contact, speech and fewer self-stimulatory behavior in autistics; some consider B6 in combination with magnesium to be a breakthrough treatment for autism.

Vitamin B12: Low B12 impairs methylation (detoxification), which causes the neurological damage responsible for many autistic symptoms; deficiency of B12 can cause optic neuropathy and vision loss in autistics; B12 raises cysteine and glutathione levels.

Magnesium: Cofactor for the neurotransmitters that affect social reactions and emotion; Autistics have low levels; improves effectiveness of B6 therapy.

Zinc: Eliminates toxic mercury from brain tissue; zinc/copper ratio is particularly low in autistic kids; low zinc impairs the protein (called metallothionein) that removes heavy metals from the body.

Carnitine: Transports fatty acids into cells; low carnitine (common in autism) impairs the ability to use fatty acids for learning and social development.

Powdered and Liquid Vitamin/Mineral

It was recommended that Evan start taking a high-quality, whole-food powdered multi-vitamin/mineral supplement that can be more easily absorbed. Evan was a good eater, so it was explained to me that when his gut was on the mend I may be able to back off on some of the supplements—except perhaps the ones he needed like B6, B12, methyl-B12, 5-HTP, GABA, magnesium, and zinc, because of his genetic mutations. Nutrient levels would be tested again, and some supplements, such as amino acids, could possibly be eliminated at a later date.

In addition to the daily multi-vitamin/mineral supplement, we added liquid vitamin D drops, magnesium powder, and a complex vitamin B supplement in the form of a spray for easy delivery. Notoriously B vitamins are known to taste awful, but we found a B-complex liquid by Pure Encapsulations that actually tastes pretty good. A few squirts under the tongue in the morning is all it takes. Take in the morning, because B vitamins often have a stimulating effect and can disrupt sleep if given too late in the day.

Vitamin D

Science is beginning to realize that vitamin D is essential for not only skeletal outcomes, but also for the optimal efficiency of our immune system, prevention of cancer, cardiovascular disease, diabetes, and mental disorders including depression and schizophrenia.

Due to Evan's malabsorption issues and his leaky gut, our naturopath tested his amino acid, vitamin, and mineral levels. The results of his tests confirmed that Evan suffered many deficiencies, including vitamin D. His levels were extremely low. This concerned me after learning that reduced levels of vitamin D may contribute to autism and that there was a correlation between vitamin D and autoimmunity.

An article in the *Journal of Neuroinflammation* said, "Aside from the skeletal health effects, vitamin D deficiency has been implicated as a potential environmental factor triggering for some autoimmune disorders. Vitamin D might play a role in the regulation of the production of auto-antibodies."[1]

Another study demonstrated that vitamin D deficiency slowed serotonin production, which may influence social behavior associated with autism spectrum disorder (ASD). The vitamin D hormone activates the gene that makes the enzyme tryptophan hydroxylase 2 (TPH2), which converts the essential amino acid tryptophan to serotonin in the brain. The Children's Hospital Oakland Research Institute (CHORI) showed that serotonin, oxytocin, and vasopressin, three brain hormones that affect social behavior, are all activated by the vitamin D hormone.[2]

Evan's pediatrician had recommended that he begin taking 1,500 IU of vitamin D daily. However, the naturopath disagreed and gave him 5,000 IU (five vitamin D-Mulsion drops per day). High doses of vitamin D regulate the immune system and help stop attacks on the thyroid.

Evan's system was so deficient in vitamin D that our naturopath didn't feel a lower dose would make a dent. She was right. Six months later, he was retested, and his vitamin D level was almost normal. We then tapered down to 3,000–4,000 IU of vitamin D per day.

Researchers believe that vitamin D levels should be routinely measured in everyone because it contributes to so many disease states. It should also become a standard procedure in prenatal care, as well.

Did you know? Many of us may need a supplement because the body cannot make it. We only derive twenty percent of our daily allowance from food sources and need to get the other eighty percent from sunshine. In today's world, we spend less and less time outdoors and use sunscreen, which is important to avoid skin cancer but is also believed to block vitamin D production.

Omega-3

We supplemented Evan with 1.5 teaspoons of OmegAvail Lemon Drop Smoothie (omega 3) as well. Both Evan and Elaina found this fish oil supplement to be extremely tolerable, and I was happy because omega-3 supplementation has been shown to be extremely important for brain health. The American Psychological Association believes those suffering with sensory issues, ADHD, OCD, and depression are often deficient in this essential nutrient.[3]

Evan also started eating sardines, and he loves them. If your kids will eat tuna, try sardines—they are a healthier alternative. They are quite tasty when prepared with organic grape seed oil mayo, chopped celery, and chopped carrots. A child with enough good fats has fewer temper tantrums, sensory issues, and ADHD symptoms. In addition, omega fatty acids enhance sleep and concentration.

DMAE (Dimethylaminoethanol)

Sardines, anchovies, and salmon also contain DMAE, a natural central nervous system stimulant produced by the body. The effect of DMAE is similar to a mild amphetamine and may help memory, mood, and concentration. It may also help to reduce hyperactivity and aggression. If your child will not eat these types of fish, I highly recommend talking to your health practitioner about supplementation. Be aware that this supplement could have a stimulant effect and may not be the best or right treatment for everyone. Starting with a low dose is often best to see how well it works.

When eating fish, remember that smaller fish contain less mercury and wild caught is best. Nutrition experts and doctors highly recommended eating wild salmon rather than farmed. Numerous studies report that farmed salmon contains significantly higher levels of PCBs and other environmental toxins such as dioxins than wild caught. In addition, factory fish are often given many antibiotics to prevent infection and are fed fishmeal most likely containing conventionally grown crops such as soy and corn, containing pesticides, herbicides, and GMOs.

Amino Acid Supplements

Amino acids are responsible for regulating mood by helping the body produce our neurotransmitters such as serotonin and dopamine naturally, so they can be great remedies. That said, it is important to be careful with amino acids, because they can be tricky. It may be better to get appropriate testing before supplementing, because a delicate balance needs to be achieved. Also, if your child takes an SSRI, do not take amino acids without care from a physician because it can be counterproductive and even dangerous. We started Evan on a cocktail of amino acids before getting him tested, and it made his anxiety and behaviors worse. After we got him tested, we discovered that all his amino acid levels were within normal range, except for GABA and 5-HTP, so we started him on those alone and it made all the difference.

B-Complex Vitamins Including Methyl-B12

B-Complex vitamins are often a part of the protocol. Some ADHD and/or autistic children need more or less depending on need. In the case of carrying MTHFR genetic mutations, a child may need to get methyl-B12 shots. Evan only had one of the possible eight MTHFR gene mutations, so a few sprays of complex B vitamins and a sublingual or powered supplement of methyl-B12 was sufficient. Your health practitioner can help you determine what your child needs after genetic testing. Note: Due to their often stimulating effect, it is best to take B vitamins in the morning.

Trimethylglycine (TMG) and Dimethylglycine (DMG)

Trimethylglycine or TMG is a recent and amazing addition to all nutritional-balancing supplement programs and is being used more widely by naturopaths in the treatment of attention-deficit disorder and autism. TMG functions as an antioxidant, anti-inflammatory, energy booster, and methyl donor. As explained in Chapter 19, TMG is given as a supplement to help raise glutathione levels and combat toxic free radicals.

During the metabolic process, TMG leaves behind a compound called dimethylglycine. Dimethylglycine (DMG) is a derivative of the amino acid glycine and has been shown to improve immune and allergy response, neurological function, behavior problems, and speech delays. It can also help assist in the reduction of seizure activity and stimming behaviors.

TMG is made in the body. Unfortunately, some people do not make enough because of inflammation and the presence of certain toxic metals. Some TMG can also be obtained by eating nuts, seeds, meat, and vegetables like broccoli. However, it is often destroyed during the cooking process.

Supplementation is often required. Babies and children need proportionately less TMG than adults depending on their size and weight, so speak to your physician about proper dosing. At age six, Evan was given 500 mg of TMG in a powder form, and because it is very sweet tasting, it was easy to hide in his food. Just remember: elevated glycine levels can cause anxiety, irritability, and other medical problems. Therefore, testing and retesting is very important. It is always a delicate balancing act.

Phosphatidylserine (PS)

We also started Evan on a supplement called "Attentive Child," which included phosphatidylserine. A 2013 study in the *Journal of Human Nutrition and Dietetics* concluded, "Phosphatidylserine significantly improved ADHD symptoms and short-term auditory memory in children. PS supplementation might be a safe and natural nutritional strategy for improving mental performance in young children suffering from ADHD."[4]

This nutrient, normally produced in the brain and found in the inner surface of cell membranes, is often deficient in individuals who are low in B vitamins and essential fatty acids. It's important for proper cell membrane functioning and plays a crucial role in cellular communication and metabolism. Until levels of B vitamins and amino acids maintain stability, it might be helpful to talk to your healthcare provider about supplementing with a product containing phosphatidylserine.[5]

Carnitine

Carnitine in its various forms is often used in the treatment of ADHD. It can help boost the effectiveness of omega-3s, improve memory, and play a role in the synthesis of dopamine. It also reduces toxicity and can improve behavioral problems like aggression and hyperactivity. In addition, many individuals with ADHD have glucose deficiencies that inhibit the uptake of carnitine into the brain.

Hence, supplementing with carnitine is believed to help increase the energy production in the mitochondria.

More About Minerals

We discovered through more extensive testing that Evan needed to take more supplements specifically targeted toward balancing his mineral levels. He was grossly deficient in certain minerals, which could have been hindering his body's ability to detoxify heavy metals and impurities.

We started giving him additional minerals to supply his body with the energy to detox and to also support his thyroid and adrenal glands. These glands are usually stressed by such an unhealthy cycle of events and are among the most affected glands in the body as a result of food sensitivities and allergies.

The hair calcium, magnesium, sodium, and potassium levels indicated that he is a slow oxidizer. This is uncommon for such a young boy (Evan was six years old by this time), as most young children are fast oxidizers. According to Lawrence Wilson, MD, an expert in Nutritional Balancing Science, a slow oxidizer may indicate some degree of adrenal exhaustion and an underactive thyroid.[6]

Evan's calcium/magnesium ratio was slightly higher, indicating that despite his gluten-free diet, he was possibly still overeating simple carbohydrates. His sodium/potassium ratio was only sixty percent of the ideal, possibly indicating some tissue breakdown, infections, gluten intolerances, kidney stress, and liver stress.

His sodium/magnesium ratios were extremely low, which proved to be problematic for him. Both of these minerals are important for carrying an electric charge, for regulating nerve impulses, and for muscle function. Evan's sodium/potassium ratio was also very low, possibly contributing to his chronic sinus infections, eye infections, and bronchial infections. I also learned, through Doctor Lawrence Wilson, that because his calcium/phosphorus levels were extremely low, which could cause more sensitivity to noise and light, frequent colds, allergies, blood that is too acidic, and a tendency toward inflammation.[7]

Evan was given supplements to raise his ratios to support his immunity, stabilize his nervous system, calm his sympathetic nervous system, balance his blood pH, and promote a better night sleep and a better sleep pattern. We also introduced Evan to sea minerals from sources like kelp. We wanted to replenish his body with the minerals he was deficient in, as well as support his thyroid with healthy iodine.

WE EAT WILD PLANET SARDINES!

These sardines are wild caught in the Pacific Ocean and have delicious meaty portions. They are lightly smoked, scale free, and have no BPA in the can lining. If your kids like tuna (without the mercury), they will love these. I make them with grape seed mayonnaise, and Evan and Elaina eat them right out of the can (especially the ones in virgin olive oil).

Nutritional Powerhouse

The nutrients in sardines are many of the same used in the treatment of ADHD, apraxia, and ASD. Ounce for ounce, Wild Planet sardines provide more calcium and phosphorus than milk, more iron than spinach, more potassium than coconut water and bananas, and as much protein as steak. One can contains 313 mg EPA and 688 mg DHA omega-3 and is an ample source of vitamin B12, vitamin D, and selenium. Sardines contain coenzyme Q10 (CoQ10), a nutrient found in the body's cells and believed to have antioxidant and immune system-boosting properties. These sardines are also considered a best choice for sustainability by a consensus of environmental organizations. The company provided the public with periodic press releases, assuring us that their products are vigorously tested for radiation.

Other Supplement Options

Moringa Oleifera Tree—"The Tree of Life"

The Moringa tree is grown in climates such as in India and Thailand. The entire tree is used, including the leaves, roots, and stems, to provide nutrient-rich natural medicine for healing and preventative care.

According to the U.S. National Institutes of Health (NIH), this "food plant has multiple medicinal uses and has been used for centuries by indigenous people to treat and prevent many diseases including malnutrition, allergy abatement, nervous system disorders, digestive disorders, asthma, inflammation, arthritis, hormonal issues, and is an excellent remedy for children with a permeable gut wall, because supplementing your child with Moringa ensures the nutrients are getting more easily absorbed."[8]

One serving of *Moringa oleifera* provides:

- 22% daily value of vitamin C

- 41% daily value of potassium

- 61% daily value of magnesium

- 71% daily value of iron

- 125% daily value of calcium

- 272% daily value of vitamin A

- 92 nutrients

- 46 antioxidants

- 36 anti-inflammatory properties

- 18 amino acids

- 9 essential amino acids

Many moms have contacted me to report tremendous improvement in their children's emotional behaviors at home and at school after taking this supplement. In addition, after researching natural treatments for autism spectrum disorders and Moringa, I found numerous testimonials from mothers who use Moringa to assist in the treatment of autism spectrum symptoms. Parents found the supplement to be particularly helpful in providing essential nutrients for their children who refused to eat nutritious diets due to sensory issues or picky preferences.

Aloe Vera—"The Natural Medicine Plant"

Aloe vera is a very impressive plant that has many healing properties. It contains plant sterols that protect the heart and lowers bad
cholesterol. It contains sugars that can help regulate blood glucose
levels, potent antioxidants to fight free radicals, and vitamins like A,
E, C, B1, B2, B3, and B6. It also contains nine minerals, including iron,
manganese, calcium, and zinc. It can help reduce inflammation in
the body, assist in the healing of autoimmune disorders, reduce high
blood pressure naturally, and can also have an alkalinizing effect on
the body (restoring pH). It may help heal ulcers, irritable bowel
syndrome, Crohn's disease, and other digestive disorders. It also
may help heal and lubricate the intestinal tract, improve constipation, balance electrolytes, and accelerate healing from burns.

However, like other herbal supplements, taking aloe internally can
cause adverse interactions with prescription and over-the-counter
medications. Aloe can also cause adverse side effects and reactions.
Whole-leaf aloe juice/products can potentially cause a skin rash or
diarrhea, because they contain aloe latex (the yellow coating under
the plants skin), which contains anthraquinone, a laxative. There is
also some concern that some of the chemicals found in aloe latex
might cause cancer.

So it is important that if you do purchase aloe for all its amazing
health benefits and nutrient value that you look closely at the ingredient label for it to read "latex-free" or "anthraquinone free."

Sea Vegetables—"The Healing Power of Seaweed"

Sea vegetables from deeper, unpolluted waters are an excellent
source of magnesium, iron, calcium, vitamin A, vitamin C, various B
vitamins, vitamin K, and plant compounds. They also contain one of
the richest sources of natural iodine, which is the mineral responsible
for proper thyroid health, along with various enzymes and dietary
fiber. Seaweed doesn't contain vitamin D, but is contains a substance
that converts D in the body. These amazing vegetables have been
studied extensively and have been documented to help treat diabetes, cancer, heart disease, high blood pressure, high triglycerides,
and thyroid disorders.

Supplement Brands

Many parents have asked me what supplement brand to choose, and I recognize it can be extremely confusing with so many to choose from. The supplement company suggestions I am about to provide are companies that my naturopathic physicians stand behind or a brand that I have personal experience with. Note that I do not promote or endorse any one supplement or product. I recommend discussing all potential treatment options with your naturopath or functional medicine physician before starting any treatments. Every child is unique, and some products may not contain everything your child needs.

Some of the Better Supplement Brands on the Market

Kirkman Labs	Shaklee	Pure Encapsulations
Nordic Naturals	Nature's Way	Spectrum Essentials
Source Naturals	Twinlab	Juice Plus+
Jarrow Formulas	Nature's Plus	Zija
Metabolic Maintenance	Garden of Life	Boiron (Homeopathic)
	Designs for Health	

Your doctor may also order something special from a compounding pharmacy to address a specific need.

Please note: I do not promote any one product. I recommend checking with your healthcare provider before starting any supplement.

I have also received numerous messages and emails from parents who have found it extremely difficult to provide their children with so many different vitamin supplements on a daily basis and have found few products that they love! One product is called SmartMix by Zija made with *Moringa oleifera*. The second product is called Body Balance by Life Force made with aloe vera and nine wild harvested sea vegetables. The third is called Juice Plus+, which provides whole-food-based nutrition from seventeen different fruits, vegetables, and gluten-free grains.

I thought they were important to mention. Note, however, that these products do not contain probiotics, vitamin D, or omega-3 fatty acids, which are often important in treating ADD/ADHD and autism spectrum disorders.

The *Moringa oleifera* in the product Zija is grown on a certified organic farm, and the product doesn't contain any unnatural sweeteners. Moms say, "It has a taste even my picky eaters enjoy." One mom on my blog wrote, "My daughter and I was were on numerous medications before taking these products. I suffered with ADHD and depression, and my daughter son suffered from tremendous allergies, breathing issues and terrible eczema. She was a very picky eater. We all started taking the Zija products, and we were sold. We are no longer on any medication, and I can truly say Moringa oleifera has saved our lives." (Marci Chaney) One dad wrote to me and said, "I refused to put my son on medication, even though he was falling behind in school. The teachers said he wasn't focused. A friend recommended Zija, and we started giving it to him faithfully. Within a few days, my son had more energy, and the teachers started calling. They wanted to know when we started medication." (Michael Stone)

Body Balance is also a certified organic product that has a long nutrient list, which includes vitamins, macro and trace minerals, and plant-based enzymes for digestion, amino acids, fatty acids, and phytonutrients. Although this product does contain aloe, it is latex-free. The aloe affidavit from the company ensures that it only uses organic "inner filet leaf" from mature leaves.

Many moms on my blog also speak very highly of this product and how much it has helped their autistic or ADHD child. One mom writes, "Body Balance has literally rocked our world! My son had an adverse reaction to his MMR vaccine, leaving him with profound sensory processing disorder and low-functioning autism. We altered his diet; gluten, dairy and soy-free; worked at healing his leaky gut and ridding his system of candida; and added Body Balance to our arsenal of tools. We truly feel as though Body Balance was the missing piece in our puzzle that brought everything together. Within days of starting Body Balance, our son began displaying profound changes in regaining vocabulary and verbal skills, fine and gross motor skills, and began to show an understanding of cause and effect. Within one week, his tics, stimming, and flapping were gone, and he began to make beautiful eye contact. Now, only three months later, our son has gone from eight hours of occupational therapy (OT) each week to ninety minutes once a week. His OTs are astounded and so amazed at his continued improvement. He continues to flourish, seeking out and giving signs of affection, interaction, and beautiful social skills." (Erin Schumacher)

Juice Plus+ is made from fresh, high-quality, healthful fruits and vegetables and is carefully tested to ensure that no pesticides or other contaminants affect the natural purity of the product. Made with natural sweeteners and without artificial color/flavor. While oats are present in Juice Plus+ to provide fiber, only the outer shells of the grain is used, not the inner core where gluten resides. Juice Plus+ is available in a capsule or soft chewable form. Many parents have commented to me that this product works. One parent wrote, "I learned about Juice Plus+ by going to an autism seminar. My naturopath concurred it was a worthwhile product. We began using it because of my son's aversion to most food. It has helped transform my son into a healthy and thriving young man. He is free of his meds and his constipation issues are gone. Nature knows how to safely and effectively administer the right amounts of nutrients without the danger of overdosing!"

Why Eat Dark (Non-Dairy) Chocolate?

Studies show that dark (non-dairy) chocolate can improve attention, focus, memory, and motor function, as well as cardiac health. Why flavonols? There is encouraging evidence that foods containing flavonols (a powerful antioxidant) improve cognitive functioning.[9] Recently, the European Food Safety Authority (EFSA), the European regulatory agency similar to the Food and Drug Administration (FDA), issued a positive opinion that flavonols in foods including dark chocolate and cocoa products can help boost "brain" blood flow.

The studies also revealed that flavanols also help control blood sugar, which researchers believe protects the brain from declines associated with insulin resistance. Blood pressure and oxidative stress also decreased in the groups consuming high and intermediate amounts. See the chart below of foods containing flavonols.

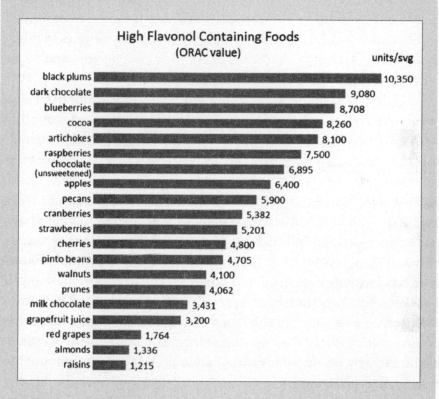

High Flavonol Containing Foods
(ORAC value)

units/svg

black plums	10,350
dark chocolate	9,080
blueberries	8,708
cocoa	8,260
artichokes	8,100
raspberries	7,500
chocolate (unsweetened)	6,895
apples	6,400
pecans	5,900
cranberries	5,382
strawberries	5,201
cherries	4,800
pinto beans	4,705
walnuts	4,100
prunes	4,062
milk chocolate	3,431
grapefruit juice	3,200
red grapes	1,764
almonds	1,336
raisins	1,215

This chart demonstrates ORAC (Oxygen Radical Absorbance Capacity), a measure of antioxidant capacity.

CHAPTER 22

Eastern Medicine & Body Work Practices

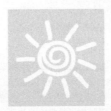

Craniosacral and Osteopathic Treatment

As discussed earlier, in addition to motor-functioning issues, Evan suffered from torticollis and a flat head as an infant. Evan was restricted by his umbilical cord, had a transverse lie in the womb, and was lying on his back in an incubator for quite some time, all which potentially explained his condition.

We found Tamara Kichar-Barry, OTR/L, founder of The Body's Wisdom, an alternative health and wellness therapy center. Tammy is a phenomenal licensed occupational therapist, who practices craniosacral therapy. She used a gentle hands-on body work approach to release the soft connective tissue in his neck and reshape his flat head. We continued with treatments even after those two situations resolved, and she continued to work on his body to release any residual birth trauma and help him heal from his frequent ear infections and illnesses.

I also learned that for children with ADD/ADHD and other similar issues, craniosacral therapy can be very helpful when used in concert with other treatments. It's important to note that the earlier the restrictions are released, the better the chance for significant progress.

It was on Tammy's table that Evan rolled for the first time, and I continued to see many improvements in him after each session. He saw Tammy for craniosacral work on and off for years.

Evan also saw a well-respected doctor of osteopathic medicine, Michael Burruano, DO, with more than thirty years of experience. Doctors of osteopathy attend osteopathic medical school and obtain graduate medical education through internships, residencies, and fellowships. They gain a specialty in the musculoskeletal system and often practice functional medicine. Although they are considered more "alternative," just like MDs they are fully qualified and considered equal in terms of their authority to diagnose and treat various health conditions.

Cranial osteopathic treatment differs from craniosacral treatment in that it does not only treat the membranes; it addresses the entire musculoskeletal system, the bones, the cartilage, and the fluid. It seeks the health within the system and enhances that "health" to bring about clinical improvement. By so doing, the cranial restrictions can be alleviated. As stated in *Alternative Therapies in Health and Medicine*, by author Jim Jealous, DO, "Once these restrictions are released, the brain has an opportunity to grow in its intended fashion."[1]

Evan had many restrictions. He was diagnosed with acute cervical derangement; spasm of the neck and back, plagiocephaly (head flattening), and neuro-developmental delays. Dr. Burruano believed that Evan had some birth trauma from his emergency delivery and from being restricted by his umbilical cord in utero. Apparently, a newborn's head is like a floating balloon, and any jarring to the head or disruption to its body can cause many of these symptoms. He said that a C-section baby is more prone to derangements because in a normal birth, the birth canal acts as a chiropractic adjustment and properly aligns the spine.

Evan was treated by Dr. Burruano every three weeks for approximately four months. He worked to gently release restrictions in Evan's neck, brain, and body to enable the normal movement of spinal fluid and vital nutrients in and out of the brain. We believe that this treatment helped Evan on many levels by allowing the spinal fluid to feed the brain with all of the essential nutrients it needed to function well.

There are reports within osteopathic literature dating back to the 1930s of cranial distortion contributing to altered cerebral function and of osteopathic treatment restoring children to normal or to markedly improve functioning.[2]

After Evan's initial treatments, his behaviors worsened at first because the treatment takes time to process. However, after the fourth treatment or so, he became a calmer and less irritable little boy. He was also more coordinated and slept a bit better. Once the restrictions were relieved, Evan began to demonstrate a marked increase in eye contact, initiation of social interaction, and improved speech.

In a 2006 article titled "Osteopathic Medicine and Autism," this osteopathic cranial strain pattern is not the cause of autism spectrum disorders, but if there is a cranial strain pattern and other causes, the brain is more susceptible to outside adverse influences such as vaccines, toxins, etc.[3]

While there are published reports and discussions in books on osteopathic medicine and cranial osteopathy that describe the relationship between cranial distortions and autism spectrum disorders, they have largely been ignored by mainstream medical practices.

There have been studies on the effects of different environmental factors and cranial osteopathic treatments. The majority of children in one particular study demonstrated a characteristic common cranial distortion and responded well to a highly integrated therapy treatment plan.[4]

Studies showed that cranial osteopathic treatment has a clear positive impact on cognitive, behavioral, and neurotransmitter function.[5]

The treated children improved significantly in spatial awareness, coordination, attention, social communication, and speech skills.[6]

The results showed gross improvement in the areas of communicating sentences, initiating social contact, and demonstrating spontaneous imaginative play. In addition, those treated to reverse the effects of the vaccines showed improvement in cognitive function and socialization.

I don't believe that cranial osteopathy is the only or complete cure, but I believe it brought us one step closer to healing Evan. Again, this treatment only removes restrictions. In addition to the brain, the entire system must then be rehabilitated with any number of reasonable and appropriate interventions, including homeopathy, vitamin supplementation, allergy elimination, detoxification, behavior modification, sensory integration, and extensive occupational therapy, physical therapy, and speech rehabilitation.

For more information, read "Effect of Osteopathic Medical Management on Neurologic Development in Children" in the *Journal of the American Osteopathic Association.*[7]

Chiropractic Care—Another Drug-Free Solution

We had originally not gone down the route of chiropractic care to treat Evan, only because we had so many other treatments on board and felt it similar to cranial osteopathic care. However, after reading studies and a lot of positive feedback from moms and professionals online saying that chiropractic care works, we tried it.

Like cranial release work, the chiropractor triggers the neurotransmitters to assist in the treatment of autism spectrum disorders. From a chiropractor's point of view, spinal movement problems, typically at the top of the neck, contribute to distorted nerve function in the central nervous system.

Like a powerful computer, the brain controls and monitors all bodily functions. Brain messages move in a vast network of connections, our nervous system, which allows the brain to communicate with every part of the body. Manipulations by the chiropractor correct head/neck misalignment, release the nerve and energy blockages to allow the body to come back into balance, and reactivate brain communication to the areas affected by misalignment. As soon as the correction is made, muscles begin to relax, blood and oxygen circulation increases, the immune system gains strength and vitality, and the body's natural, self-healing process begins.

Upper cervical techniques were used on a nine-year-old boy with Tourette's, ADHD, depression, asthma, and headaches to review the effectiveness of chiropractic care on children with these disorders. The case report published by the Chiropractors Association declared that after six weeks of care, all conditions were no longer present. He stopped numerous medications including Albuterol, Depakote, and Adderall, and he was still without symptoms five months later at the conclusion of his case.[8]

Reiki, Massage, and Reflexology— Restoring the Energy Balance in the Body

Reiki is an ancient Japanese method of healing, promoting the body to heal itself. It is a "laying on of hands" approach. The practitioner channels an unseen "life force energy" and helps balance the client's body and mind. Reiki is used to heal a person's physical health, as well as maintain harmony and systemic balance in the brain and nervous system without side effects. As a Reiki practitioner myself, I use reiki as a part of my psychotherapy practice, as well as giving Evan frequent reiki treatments while he sleeps. It is amazing how well my clients, as well as my family, respond to treatment. In fact, when the kids are having a bad day or when they feel a tummy ache or headache coming on, they will ask for reiki.

Therapeutic massage is widely and effectively used in treatment of autism spectrum disorders (ASDs) to address sensory issues, motor problems, and touch receptivity. Some autistic individuals who are withdrawn or dissociated from their environments may respond defensively to being touched and tend to respond negatively to certain textures. Massage offers a safe and nurturing approach to improving the improper or incomplete maturation of the tactile system.

Reflexology is another nontraditional practice that may help to relieve many conditions associated with autism spectrum disorders. Reflexology is the application of appropriate pressure to specific points and areas on the feet, hands, or ears. Reflexologists believe that these areas and reflex points correspond to different body organs and systems, and that pressing them has a beneficial effect on the organs and person's general health. For example, reflexology holds that a specific spot on the "big toe" corresponds to the brain. When a reflexology practitioner uses thumbs or fingers to apply appropriate pressure to this area, it affects brain functioning. Some of the issues treated with reflexology include ADHD, insomnia, obsessive compulsive disorder, asthma, sinus issues, liver and kidney issues, irritable bowel syndrome, and other digestive disorders, to name a few.

Therapeutic Massage and Bodywork for Autism Spectrum Disorders: A Guide for Parents and Caregivers by Virginia Cowen is a wonderful resource for those who would like to further explore the benefits of message and other body work practices.

Acupuncture—A 2,000-Year-Old Healing Method

Acupuncture has been used in the treatment and prevention of illnesses, including autoimmune and digestive disorders, for more than two thousand years. Scientific studies are showing us that the ancient Chinese practice of acupuncture improves certain functions and symptoms in autistic children.[9] There are no negative side effects, and the needles are extremely small and thin, causing little to no pain.

The basic theory of acupuncture starts with the meridian system and flow of energy (called qi, pronounced "chee") between organs and the blood. Acupuncture is used to regulate the functions of organs via the flow of energy and blood through the meridian system. The needles can balance the blood flow between the right and left frontal lobes of the brain.

Numerous clinical trials on autistic individuals have tested the validity of such treatment. While the design and control of the studies were not perfect, there were marked statistical improvements in behavior and/or development in children with autism.

The studies have shown that when a comparison group was used, acupuncture-treated groups experienced superior improvement over behavioral therapy-treated groups. When acupuncture was used in conjunction with other modalities such as Chinese herbal treatments, massage, and music therapy, the outcome was even better than with acupuncture alone.

The reported improvements among the studies include better language communication function and/or social interaction, reduction of repetitive behaviors, improvements in fine motor, self-care, and/or cognitive function. As reported by the *Evidence Based Complementary Alternative Medicine Jounal*, the rates of improvement were more than eighty percent in the acupuncture-treated groups versus more than fifty percent in the comparison groups.[10] Findings were inconsistent, however. While many children showed dramatic improvements, others showed little to no improvement. It reminds us that there is no perfect fix and that what works for one child may not work for another.

Still, I remain hopeful that when you find the right combination of treatments that fit your child's unique profile, real healing can take place.

NAET—Nambudripad's Allergy Elimination Technique

We were originally told by Evan's naturopath that he may not need to be on a restrictive diet forever, which was a relief. I agreed that a whole-food diet restricting dyes and other harmful ingredients was a good practice anyway, but I wanted to believe that we could give Evan a slice of whole-wheat bread or a scrambled egg at some future date.

The protocol was to keep Evan away from all offending foods for about two years to allow his gut to make a full recovery. I was skeptical and afraid that his symptoms could return when we reintroduced the foods, and my fears were not dampened after reading blogs and talking with other moms. It seemed that there was a strong possibility that Evan's body would start fighting the foods again.

New hope arrived when my husband and I attended the fortieth birthday party of a friend we had not seen in years. I met a speech language pathologist there named Fran. We spoke about the endless therapy appointments and numerous treatments to address Evan's PDD, ADHD, food sensitivities, and apraxia. Fran asked me if I had ever heard of NAET (Nambudripad's Allergy Elimination Techniques).

NAET is a combination of knowledge and techniques already known from Western medicine, chiropractic, muscle testing/kinesiology, and acupressure/acupuncture (Eastern medicine). I did some research and found that NAET has been used to treat autism and allergies. A noninvasive procedure that uses muscle testing (applied kinesiology) and acupressure to diagnose and reverse the allergy or sensitivity, the technique does not require any blood draws, scratch tests, or shots. If the child is small, an adult becomes the energy conduit.

In the book *Say Good-bye to Allergy-related Autism*, Devi Nambudripad discusses how this approach dramatically reduces allergies and sensitivities in a large percentage of the children. When these allergies are aggressively treated, the children often gradually come off their very restricted diet and the variety of food intake improves dramatically.[11]

And in a 2011 study published in the *Journal of Integrative Medicine*, "autism spectrum children have been studied following aggressive allergy elimination treatment (NAET) with quite remarkable success. . . . NAET treatment provides an effective treatment modality for children with autism to decrease autistic traits and improve their speech, language, communication skills, social interactions, sensory and cognitive awareness, and overall physical health and behavior."[12] In addition, the Department of Medical Laboratory Sciences at Weber State University in Utah reports that NAET has also been used to treat severe peanut allergies with success.[13]

I also read that going through allergy elimination treatments for foods, amino acids, vitamins, and other substances could allow sensitive children to do much better and be more receptive to other interventions.

Evan was muscle-tested, and he tested positive for the same foods that showed up on his blood test. I asked why this would happen a year after we had eliminated all of those irritating foods. The NAET practitioner explained to me that Evan's body was still programmed energetically to believe that those particular foods were harmful to him. Her testing also showed that Evan had many sensitivities the blood work didn't pick up, such as issues with amino acids, vaccines, food dyes, vitamin B, anesthesia, magnesium, and phenols/salicylates, to name a few.

I learned that all children have their unique sets of sensitivities. For example, children with a seizure disorder, often have energy blocks to B vitamins and sugar imbalances. I also discovered that a child who appears more symptomatic than Evan may only have one or two big issues. For example, one nonverbal little boy with severe autism was tested by my NAET practitioner, and his biggest issues were with heavy metals. Within a few treatments, he showed improvements.

Devi Nambudripad further says, "NAET techniques reverse 'the switch' by eliminating energy blockages (allergies) permanently and restore the body to a healthy state. During the NAET treatment, the brain creates a new friendly memory for the allergen. After the completion of the NAET treatment, the irritant or allergen becomes a non-irritant and a non-allergen in the energy field."[14] Removing these blockages allow our children to receive the right supply of nutrients to the brain because the body is no longer pushing them away.

Evan's treatment with the NAET practitioner tested and treated the basic twelve sensitivities first. For Evan, that included chicken/egg, milk/calcium mix, B complex mix, sugar mix, mineral mix, corn, grain mix, and yeast. Later, he was tested and treated for many others, including magnesium, digestive enzymes, sugar, adrenal gland and liver detox, metals, and amino acids. The goal was to continue the process of returning his body to homeostatic balance. It was remarkable that after the sessions, Evan gained color in his face, his eyes appeared clearer, and his behavior improved. Within a few weeks after the B treatments, he appeared more coordinated and clearer in his thinking.

One of the treatments was to address sugar imbalances and his inability to process sugar correctly. The NAET practitioner gave him a vial of sugar while doing acupressure. His face turned bright red, he got hives, and he began jumping around her office in a hyper state. She had him hold the vial in his sock for ten to fifteen minutes. Evan left the office extremely fatigued and a little irritable. We had to keep all sugars and carbohydrates away from him for twenty-six hours so that his body could "reset." Within days, we noticed a calmer and less hyper child.

Evan was also treated for amino acids and fatty acids. His body was blocking some essential and nonessential amino acids and essential fatty acids (omega-3).

Finally, after testing the basic allergens and heavy metals, she tested him for some of the other 78 different allergens in the autism kit. A few of the other tests in this kit included vaccines, artificial food coloring, neurotransmitters, and different parts of the brain that control specific functions. When she had him hold the vial that corresponded to his temporal lobe, his body became very weak. The temporal lobe involves auditory perception, memory, emotional responses, language, and visual perception.

To find a NAET practitioner near you, visit http://naet.com/sub scribers/drnamerica.html.

BioSET

Another allergy elimination technique used in the treatment of allergy-related autism spectrum disorders is called BioSET. It is similar to NAET in that it utilizes acupressure, enzyme therapy, and the laws of quantum physics to redirect and reprogram a body's immune responses to ordinarily benign substances like food. However, it uses different protocols and instruments.

To find a BioSET practitioner near you, visit the creator's website at www.drellencutler.com/pages/practitioners/.

Essential Oils

During our path of healing, I was introduced to the benefits of essential oils for the treatment of ADHD and autistic-related conditions. I recognized that many of the treatment oils were made up of healing herbs, municipal flowers, and healing foods that mimic the same principles as homeopathy.

One drop of cinnamon essential oil, for example, reaps the health benefit of ingesting a whole stick of cinnamon. Experts agree that smelling cinnamon can help boost cognitive functioning and increase mental alertness and concentration. (Cinnamon is also an excellent remedy for anxiety, poor memory, inflammation, digestive issues, yeast overgrowth, and regulating glucose levels in cases of diabetes and hypoglycemia.)

Primrose oil high in gamma-linoleic acid (omega-6) when coupled with omega-3 also boosts the immune system, aids nerve health, and helps to maintain healthy glucose levels, as well. In fact, one study in Australia revealed that taking a combination of fish oil and evening primrose oil capsules along with a multivitamin/mineral reduced symptoms of ADHD by as much as fifty percent. There were improvements in attention span and memory, and reduced restlessness, hyperactivity, and impulsivity.[15]

Julie Behling-Hovdal, author of *The Essential Survival Guide to Medical Preparedness*, wrote about the effectiveness of essential oils on brain health. "Essential oils work by oxygenating and enlivening the body's cells, including those in the brain. They can help to clear the cell membranes of toxic chemicals that may be interfering with proper neurotransmitter and hormone balance. They can help to literally heal emotional traumas and clear emotional baggage that may be keeping children from thriving. It has even been postulated that certain essential oils may help to heal issues on the level of the DNA!"[16]

Terry Friedmann, MD, the cofounder of the American Holistic Medical Association, conducted a study to determine the healthful effects of essential oils on children who had ADHD. Each group was pretested using a baseline evaluation with real time EEG and the T.O.V.A. Scale. An electroencephalogram (EEG) is a test to measure the electrical activity of the brain, and the T.O.V.A. Scale is a neurological assessment tool (using a simple computer game) that measures a person's attention while screening for attention deficit hyperactivity disorder. Generally, the test takes approximately 21 minutes to administer. It measures a number of variables involving the test takers' response to either a visual or auditory stimulus.

The essential oils chosen for the case study were lavender, vetiver, cedarwood and Brain Power (a blend of frankincense, sandalwood, melissa, cedarwood, blue cypress, lavender and helichrysum). The oils were administered in this fashion: one of the oils were administered by inhalation three times a day for thirty days. The inhalation of the oils proved to settle the brainwaves back into normal patterns and improved the children's scholastic performance and behavioral patterns. The results indicated that essential oils were highly effective in treating hyperactivity and inattention. Lavender increased performance by fifty-three percent, cedarwood increased performance by eighty-three percent, and vetiver increased performance by a hundred percent.[17]

Testimonials from numerous moms report that these oils have made a huge difference in the autistic symptoms of some kids and have helped, in some cases, to reverse the diagnosis so that children could stop taking medication. Bear in mind, however, that some of these oils are extremely potent remedies.

SOME ESSENTIAL OIL REMEDIES

Symptom	Remedy
Adrenal Fatigue	Clove, Coriander, Cyprus, Geranium, Rosemary
Attention—Promotes mental clarity, memory, and focus	Brain Power, Basil, Bergamot, Cedarwood, Cinnamon, Clarity, Cyprus, Geranium, Frankincense, Lavender, Peppermint, Rose, Sandlewood, Vetiver, Evening Primrose
Anger, Irritability, and Stimming Behaviors	Vetiver, Purification, Grounding
Anxiety, Stress, and OCD	Angelica, Bergamot, Chamomile, Frankincense, Geranium, Lavender, Nutmeg, Peace & Calming, Sandlewood, Release
Allergies/Sensitivities	Lavender, Chamomile, Harmony, Valor
Autism	Basil, Bergamot, Cedarwood, Clary Sage, Eucalyptus, Frankincense, Geranium, Lavender, Melissa, Peppermint, Rosemary, Sandlewood, Vetiver
Boredom	Grounding
Brain Balance	Frankincense, Evening Primrose
Candida/Yeast	Lemongrass, Clove
Constipation	Fennel, Ginger, Juniper, Lemon, Marjoram, Orange, Patchouli, Peppermint, Rose, Rosemary, Sandlewood, Tangerine, Tarragon

Symptom	Remedy
Diarrhea	Fennel, Geranium, Ginger, Lemon. Melissa, Myrrh, Orange and Sandlewood, Peppermint, Cinnamon, Clove, Nutmeg
Poor Digestion	Bergamot, Cinnamon, Clary Sage, Cyprus, Dill, Frankincense, Lavender, Myrrh, Orange, Patchouli, Sage, Peppermint, Tangerine, Black Seed, Di-Gize
Frustration and Depressed Mood	Joy, Lemon
Heavy Metal and General Toxicity	Coriander, JuvaFlex, Peppermint, Ginger, Tangerine, Tarragon
Hyperactivity	Peace & Calming, Grounding
Hypoglycemia	Lavender, Thieves, EndoFlex, Cinnamon, Cumin, Clove, Thyme, Coriander, Lemon, Dill, Evening Primrose
Immune System Support	Immunpro, Eucalyptus, Black Seed, Evening Primrose
Night-Time Fears	Lavender, White Angelica, Valor, Sacred Mountain
Lack of Self-Esteem, Courage & Confidence	Jasmine, Frankincense, Valor, Joy
Sleep Difficulties	Angelica, Bergamot, Eucalyptus, Frankincense, Peace & Calming, Lavender, Vetiver, Valor, Roman Chamomile, Clary Sage, Citrus Fresh, Sandlewood, Orange, Valerian, Ylang ylang

Applying Oils

Pure essential oils can be diffused in your home, misted from a water bottle, ingested, or rubbed onto the body in a massage. Carrier oil such as almond oil, coconut oil, or vegetable oil can be used to spread the essential oil and dilute it slightly. The oil can be rubbed on the bottoms of your child's feet (especially on the big toe, which is an acupressure point that affects the brain), and then rubbed upward toward the very top of the spine or shoulders.

- Oils like Joy can be rubbed on the chest over the heart for depression.

- Oils like cedarwood, vetiver, Brain Power, Clarity, lavender, and Common Sense can be mixed with a carrier oil and applied to the back of the neck before school for help with focus and attention.

- Oils for the adrenal glands should be applied topically over the kidney area, which is the lower back on each side of the spine. A warm compress should then be placed over the area for approximately 3 minutes.

- Oils for digestion can be dropped and consumed in a large glass of water.

The two essential oil companies I most recommend are Young Living and dōTERRA. Both of these companies are committed to producing therapeutic-grade oil you can trust. Before using essential oils, I highly recommend purchasing an essential oil book to learn how to muscle test and properly apply the oils to get the best results. Muscle testing will determine whether or not your child is sensitive to a particular oil. This is important to prevent a negative reaction. One great resource is *Releasing Emotional Patterns with Essential Oils* by Carolyn L. Mein.[18]

The Healing Benefits of Herbal Teas

As I am not a fan of most juice drinks like Kool-Aid, sports drinks, or even drinking too much fruit juice, I often turn to decaffeinated herbal tea. I make iced tea and keep it in the refrigerator. When my kids want to feel grown-up, we sip warm herbal tea together.

Making homemade brewed tea is a good alternative to other kids' beverages. It is an excellent way to keep kids hydrated, and decaffeinated teas have plenty of natural flavor and many health benefits. Sugar, honey, or nectars can be added when the tea is still hot, or add a splash of juice, such as lemon, orange, pineapple, or cranberry at any time to sweeten the tea.

I buy only organic teas since reading the horrifying truth about

many of the commercial teas being sold in malls all across America. I
learned from reading a blog from Vani Hari of *Food Babe*, "Many of
today's expensive tea brands are operating under the guise of providing health benefits and promoting clean living, but are actually
laden with pesticides, toxins, artificial ingredients, added flavors,
and GMOs."[19]

HERBAL TEAS FOR SPECIFIC AILMENTS

Ailment	Tea for Health
Anxiety and Mood Disorders	Chamomile, oat straw, passionflower (for children over 4), peppermint, holy basil (Tulsi), lavender, lemon balm, catnip, rosemary
Colic	Fennel, chamomile, peppermint A breastfeeding mother can drink the tea (1 cup three times per day), or the tea can be diluted and given to the infant with a medicine dropper (1 diluted teaspoon three times per day).
Constipation	Flaxseed tea added to oatmeal or fruit juice, Senna (a proprietary blend senna leaf), licorice root, bitter fennel fruit, organic sweet orange peel, organic cinnamon bark, organic coriander seed, organic ginger rhizome, orange peel oil
Indigestion and Stomachache	Ginger, peppermint, chamomile, lemon balm, lavender, catnip, rosemary
Healing the Gut	Licorice, slippery elm, marshmallow root, black cherry, turmeric, echinacea Proprietary blend: calendula, chamomile, peppermint, fennel, malva, Canadian fleabane, estafiate, plantain
Immune System	Peppermint, hibiscus flower (sorrel), rosehip, echinacea, chamomile, dandelion
Mental Clarity and Focus	Acai berry, ginseng, blueberries, cinnamon

Ailment	Tea for Health
Sleep Aid	Peppermint, chamomile, mint, catnip, lemon balm, black cherry, valerian

If on medicine, it is best to consult with your doctor before consuming any herbs. For example, chamomile interacts with drugs such as aspirin, platelet inhibitors, anticoagulants, antidepressants, propranolol (beta-blocker), and others.

Please consider the possible risks, as well as the benefits, of these traditional medicinal plants. Consult your healthcare provider or a trained herbalist before giving herbs to young children.

CHAPTER 23

Other Healing Practices and Therapy Treatments

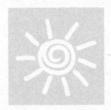

As mentioned throughout this book, speech and language therapy, as well as physical/occupational therapy, is extremely helpful in enhancing and/or restoring a person's functioning so that they achieve independence in all areas of their life. Speech therapy focuses on communication skills and improved intelligibility. Physical therapy focuses on gross motor skills, such as walking and running, and occupational therapy primarily focuses on more fine motor skills, such as dressing, playing, and eating. These therapies are often a vital part of treatment for children with ADHD, apraxia, sensory processing disorder, and autism and helps them improve cognitive, physical, and motor skills, while, at the same time, enhances self-esteem and interpersonal relationships. Next, I will provide an overview of many other treatment methods for ADHD and autism spectrum disorders.

Brain Balancing Therapy

Brain Balance Achievement Centers were created by Dr. Robert Melillo to help kids with ADD/ADHD, dyslexia, and ASD reach their physical, social/behavioral health, and academic potential. This therapy has been clinically proven to be extremely effective for use with children with ADD/ADHD.[1]

Dr. Robert Melillo is an internationally known lecturer, author, educator, researcher, and clinician in the areas of neurology, rehabilitation, neuropsychology, and neurobehavioral disorders in children. He's also an expert in nutrition with more than twenty years of clinical experience.

In his book *Disconnected Kids*, Melillo states, "In order for the brain to function normally, the activities in the right and left hemisphere must work in harmony, much like a concert orchestra."[2] He goes on to explain that a slow-developing left brain causes problems with reading and staying on task, while a child with a slower developing right brain may have more difficulty with social interaction and reading social cues.

A child's brain is very changeable, and with specific therapies, it can rewire itself to enable fully balanced functioning. Dr. Melillo believes that brain balancing therapy, in conjunction with dietary modifications and the correction of nutritional imbalances, can reverse spectrum disorders and its many features such as sensory-related issues. His approach includes vision therapy, sensory-motor exercises, light stimulation, musical brain balance activities, Brain Gym®, vestibular training, proprioceptive exercises, and core stability exercises. His book provides many at-home exercises and other Brain Gym ideas to bring to your physical and occupational therapist. Brain Gym began with Paul Dennison, a teacher and reading specialist. In 1975, he received his PhD and alongside his wife Gail, co-founded and co-created Educational Kinesiology and the Brain Gym activities. These 26 activities are aimed at helping children foster eye teaming, spatial awareness, listening skills, hand-eye coordination, and flexibility in order to enhance learning capabilities.

I never wanted Evan to give up on himself or on school, and luckily, we were blessed with an amazing educational team at our town's elementary school. They completely "got it" when it came to the importance of Brain Gym activities for Evan. Amazingly, they integrate the above activities with all of the children at the school, whether they are neurologically typical or not. They firmly believe that these exercises help students to learn better in general, read better, achieve a higher level of functioning and a gain a greater level of inner stability.

Transitioning from a birth-to-three program, Evan started a half-day special education program on his third birthday. His half day was followed by a couple of hours of support services, including speech and language, occupational therapy, and physical therapy. The entire therapy team at the school worked with Evan by doing core strength exercises and cross-crawl exercises to work on motor planning and help "balance" his brain.

All of the children at his school learned specific movements prior to learning new skills to improve their stability, mobility, flexibility, and eye-hand and/or sensory motor coordination. Doing these activities definitely helped to activate Evan's brain for optimal retrieval of information.

Evan loved his highly structured multisensory approach to learning. He eagerly approached each and every day and was excited about going to school where he would perform his best in his teacher's presence. Evan's teachers and therapists adored his sweet, gentle, and hard-working disposition.

Integrative Reflex Therapy:
Targeting Underlying Neurosensorimotor Pathways

Motor reflexes are a set of automatic movements that begin in the womb. The reflexes are vitally important for the proper development of the brain, nervous system, and the sensory systems. There are many reasons that the reflex movements are underdeveloped or incomplete. When this occurs, it causes challenges from mild to severe in learning, motor development, sensory integration, emotions, and behavior.

The primitive reflexes are important for our survival. The Moro reflex (startle reflex) allows us to react to danger. Walking reflexes allow us to start the pattern of walking from infancy. The rooting reflex allows the baby to turn toward his/her food source such as a bottle or breast. The palmer grasp and planter are the reflexes that close the fingers and curl the toes. The galant reflex allows the baby to twist when you put a little pressure on the spine.

Infant stress, toxins, and illness are just a few of the causes that can prevent a child's reflexes from integrating properly. Enzyme deficiency is another potential cause that prevents the necessary chemicals in the brain from becoming activated. These insults, along with nutrient deficiencies, interfere with the proper development of the nervous system.

Another interesting correlation is described in a book titled *Fight Autism and Win: Biomedical Treatments That Work.* Underdeveloped primitive reflexes leave the baby more susceptible to nutritional deficiencies, poor immune responses, allergies, and the negative effects of food additives.[3]

The Moro reflex (startle reflex) directly affects adrenaline and cortisol, and imbalances can lead to aggressive and oppositional behavior. The child is constantly in a state of "fight or flight." Sudden surges of cortisol can also lead to blood sugar imbalances. The proper functioning of the Moro reflex is important for the ability to focus and track, pay attention, and block out background noise.

The asymmetrical tonic neck reflex is initiated when the head turns right and left on a horizontal plane, and it is responsible for eye-hand coordination and essential for the normal maturation of the link between the two halves of the brain. When this reflex is underdeveloped, children prefer right brain activity and are better at seeing the whole picture rather than finer details. They use intuition rather than problem-solving to find solutions. A right-brained child could exhibit more learning difficulties, emotional upsets, impatience, and impulsivity.

Many of the symptoms of ADD/ADHD and apraxia/dyspraxia can be caused by the retention of these important reflexes. Integrative therapy can help target underlying neurosensorimotor pathways to improve or even restore function.

For more information or to find a provider, visit http://masgutova method.com. For read more about Integrative Reflex Therapy or to find a provider, please visit the Svetlana Masgutova Educational Institute® *The Masgutova Neurosensorimotor Reflex Integration—MNRI® Method:* http://masgutovamethod.com.

Also a great book of interest is *Reflexes, Learning and Behavior: A Window into the Child's Mind: A Non-Invasive Approach to Solving Learning & Behavior Problems* by Sally Goddard.[4]

Aquatic Therapy

Physical and occupational therapy conducted in an aquatic environment has been extremely helpful for Evan. Research supports that water is an excellent medium to exercise and rehabilitate the body, especially if the water temperature is maintained between ninety-three and ninety-six degrees to relax muscles. Besides learning the necessary life skill of swimming, aquatic therapy helps children with ASD to improve motor skills, elongate the muscles, improve flexibility, improve core strength, overcome sensory issues, enhance their learning potential, and practice interpersonal skills (when the therapy is conducted in a group setting). If you are interested in aquatic therapy, find a qualified facility that specifically works with special needs individuals. Angelfish Therapy is one such innovative pediatric company. Angelfish has been helping children with a variety of special needs, sensory issues, and motor coordination difficulties reach their full potential through fun and challenging aquatic therapy sessions and swim lessons, in camp, individual, and group settings. Also, Angelfish educates therapists, swim instructors, care givers, and parents how to use the water to improve a child's motor skills and overcome sensory issues to learn how to swim. To purchase a training DVD titled *Swim Whisperers* or to learn more, visit them at http://campangelfish.com.

Equine Therapy

Horse-assisted therapy for special needs children can be extremely beneficial. Kids and animals is a very natural combination. Equine therapy (Hippotherapy) can help children with a very wide range of disabilities, including autism, developmental disorders, cerebral palsy, seizure disorders, sensory processing issues, learning disabilities, and behavioral/emotional problems. Equine therapy provides opportunities for physical as well as emotional therapy. Riding horses improves strength, muscle tone, and helps with balance, posture, flexibility, motor coordination, and concentration. At the same time, confidence and self-esteem improve. It not only focuses on the therapeutic riding skills but also the development of a relationship between horse and the rider. Equine therapy provides a nurturing and non-judgmental environment in which a child with special needs can flourish. To read research articles and success stories or find a provider near you, please go to www.americanhippotherapyassociation.org, www.pathintl.org, and www.frdi.net.

Hyperbaric Oxygen Therapy

Hyperbaric oxygen therapy offers a treatment option for people with cerebral palsy and autism spectrum disorders. A child climbs into a safe and noninvasive chamber with slight pressure and oxygen as not to upset their fragile bodies. The oxygen helps to reduce inflammation of the brain and the gut therapeutically. Breathing one hundred percent oxygen would not accomplish the same thing because the atmospheric pressure does not reach all areas of the body the way the oxygen can travel in the hyperbaric chamber. This therapy has been well proven, and there are numerous studies in *BMC Pediatrics* and the *Lancet* pointing to its efficacy.[5]

This treatment can be very costly, but many believe that it has helped their child tremendously. This therapy is offered in some autism treatment facilities, and portable hyperbaric chambers are available for sale or rent.

Neurotherapy: Neurofeedback and Auditory Integration Training (AIT)—Retraining a Dysregulated Brain

Also known as EEG biofeedback, neurofeedback offers an additional treatment option for people with a variety of disorders such as anxiety, depression, tics, seizures, ADHD, and autism spectrum disorders. It was introduced in the 1960s, and although it has not met scientific standards for efficacy, it is believed by many to be very effective in conjunction with traditional psychotherapy.

The brain is an intricate system of chemical and electrical activity that is designed to work like a well-oiled machine and function well all the time. However, for a variety of reasons which I have mentioned throughout this book, the brain becomes dysregulated and does not function the way it was originally designed.

Neurofeedback works to put the "train back on the tracks," so to speak. It is an operant conditioning tool that simply retrains the brain to behave "normally," arousing when appropriate and calming when appropriate. It's a noninvasive treatment that does not shock or manipulate the brain in any way. The client sits in front of a computer monitor, and electrodes are attached to the scalp. The clinician sits behind another to read the EEG data. The client plays computer games, and when the brain waves behave similar to the waves the computer wants, the client hears a beep and receives visual reinforcement on the screen.

Neurofeedback can be expensive, however, costing $2,000–$5,000. Nevertheless, consistent evidence for improvements in ADHD symptoms after EEG-neurofeedback training in children with ADHD have been provided by several studies. One such study was conducted by Vincent Monastra, PhD, founder of the FPI Attention Disorders Clinic in New York. He conducted a year-long, uncontrolled study with 100 children who were on medication and also receiving neurofeedback. Monastra's results indicated some patients were able to reduce medication dosage by about fifty percent after treatment and that the benefits seemed to remain after the treatment had ended."EEG biofeedback was determined to be 'probably efficacious' for the treatment of ADHD."[6]

Auditory Integration Training (AIT) was pioneered in France by Guy Bérard, MD, who promoted it as a cure for clinical depression and suicidal tendencies, along with what he said were very positive results for dyslexia and autism. Although there has been very little empirical evidence regarding this notion, there have been many anecdotal studies that point to this therapy as being highly effective.

AIT typically consists of twenty half-hour sessions over ten days that involve listening to specially filtered and modulated music. It was used in the early 1990s as a treatment for autism, and it has been promoted as a treatment for ADHD, depression, and a wide variety of other disorders.

One particular study in *Procedia—Social and Behavioral Sciences* provides support for the use of neurofeedback and AIT as helpful components of effective intervention in children with ASD.[7]

Results from the study presented in the article indicated a substantial decline in autistic behavior and considerable improvements in socialization, vocalization, self-stimulating behaviors, flexibility, sucking, and assertiveness. The frequency of repetitive stereotyped behaviors was reduced, and there was improvement in speech and language indexes and subscales of language competency.

To learn more, visit these links: www.aboutneurofeedback.com, www.neurofeedbackfoundation.org, and www.aitinstitute.org/.

Vision Therapy

Although we haven't gone down the route of prism glasses or formal vision therapy yet, I felt it extremely important to talk about it. Evan has seen a behavioral optometrist a few times and was prescribed glasses for nearsightedness. He performs eye exercises at home to strengthen his ability to focus, and we believe it has helped. For example, Evan plays with a zigzag marble track made of wood. When he rolls a marble down the track, he can follow it with his eyes. He also does eye exercises by tracking a marble as it moves around a tin pie plate.

There are many easy exercises like these that can be done at home when time or resources are limited.

Unfortunately, vision is the area that often gets ignored in ADHD and autistic children. It can be overlooked by teachers, educators, and pediatricians, because they associate behavioral problems and clumsiness with motor-planning issues, apraxia, sensory issues, and learning disabilities. It's believed that for some of our kids with sensory-related issues, vision therapy helps tremendously and may need to be addressed before occupational and physical therapy can take hold.

We were lucky to have teachers and therapists at our public elementary school who recognized Evan's vision and tracking issues. They incorporated exercises in the classroom and taught us exercises to do at home. We saw many positive changes with Evan's balance and spatial orientation as a result of the vision work, and that helped his progress in other therapies.

Prism glasses can help to correct the positioning of the eye or eyes so that a person no longer sees double (diplopia) and no longer has tracking problems. Double vision is when a viewer sees two individual images using both eyes, instead of the one that most people see. Some people with diplopia see one image, but it's blurred. Others only see images on one plane and can't see in three dimensions.

A quick and easy test to screen your child for focus problems is to hold a pencil at the tip of his or her nose. Your child should be able to tell you that he or she can only see one pencil. If your child sees two pencils, focusing is probably a problem.

Vision therapy has been around for a long time. In the 1970s, it was a widely popular therapy. My brother, Paul, and I went for intense eye therapy at a vision center. We were asked to track blinking lights on a large circular board. I remember the words jumped all over the page. I experienced double vision before I began therapy, and after about four months, Paul and I were reading better and performing better in school.

While vision therapy does not cure ADHD or autism alone, it can significantly improve academic and sports performance, and it can enhance the child's quality of life by allowing him or her to participate in more typical, age-appropriate activities.

If you see an eye doctor, make sure it is a behavioral optometrist who can diagnose correctable vision problems. The College of Optometrists in Vision Development (COVD) is a certifying body for doctors in the optometric specialty called Behavioral/Developmental/Rehabilitative Optometry. Some offer services right in their office or clinic, while others assign specific eye focus exercises your child can do at home.

Even a lazy eye can be treated with the proper eye exercises. So, before surgery is presented as an option, make sure to seek help from a good behavioral optometrist. I've heard stories of moms who were being talked into surgery before they realized there was therapy that could correct the problem. The surgery corrects muscle problems, but lazy eye is often a brain problem, not a muscle problem at all.

Traditional Psychotherapy:
CBT, Social Skills Groups, and ABA

In my psychotherapy practice, I treat many people who come to me with the diagnoses of ADHD, OCD, and depression. Even without medication, I have observed dramatic improvements within a few months of treatment when I use cognitive and behavioral therapies. Clients report a reduction of impulsivity, hyperactivity, disorganization, procrastination, perfectionistic thinking, depression, and anxiety. They also feel improvements in their self-esteem, interpersonal relationships, and organizational habits. I find combining strength-based approaches (focusing on a person's special gifts) with coaching and psychotherapy produces the best overall results.

Although I am not currently running any social skills groups, I often encourage clients to seek them out. Social skills groups are facilitated primarily by licensed clinicians such as licensed social workers, mental health counselors, marriage and family therapists, and licensed professional counselors. At times these groups are also run in speech, occupational, and physical therapy offices as an essential component to treatment.

Cognitive behavioral therapy (CBT) is a problem-focused approach to helping people identify and change the dysfunctional beliefs, thoughts, and patterns of behavior that contribute to their problems. Its underlying principle is that thoughts affect emotions, which then influence behaviors. CBT combines two very effective kinds of psychotherapy: cognitive therapy and behavioral therapy.

Cognitive therapy concentrates on thoughts, assumptions, and core beliefs. With cognitive therapy, people are encouraged to recognize and to change faulty or maladaptive thinking patterns. Cognitive therapy is a way to gain control over inappropriate repetitive thoughts that often feed or trigger various presenting problems. For instance, if a person continuously tells themselves that they are "stupid," the therapist would ask them to practice reframing their statement to reflect a more accurate one. Such as, "That test was difficult, but I am typically a good student."

Behavioral therapy concentrates on specific actions and environments that either change or maintain behaviors. For instance, when someone is trying to stop a negative behavior, the person is encouraged to replace the behavior with a more appropriate one to help change behaviors, particularly when the new behavior is reinforced.

The combination of cognitive therapy and behavioral therapy is highly beneficial and changes are seen quite rapidly if the client is engaged. It is extremely goal orientated and action focused, so results are quite measurable. In my practice, parents often report that CBT and other forms of therapy are more helpful than medication alone.

Social skills groups are supportive and nurturing peer group environments that help to foster healthy peer relationships, and the skills taught relate to real-world experiences and relationships. Clients learn communication skills. They learn how to listen, make a friend, read nonverbal social cues, and how to network, which are essential for the maintenance of all relationships. Ultimately, these life skills lead to increased happiness and a healthier life.

Applied behavior analysis (ABA), previously known as behavior modification, is a behavior-modification-type approach to learning based on the work of Dr. B. F. Skinner; the application of operant and classical conditioning that modifies human behaviors, especially as part of a learning or treatment process. ABA is a highly researched and effective behavioral therapy technique used by many therapists and school systems to treat autism related behavioral issues, while at the same time improving communication, play, self-care, and living skills in children. Since its induction in the early 1960s, a variety of practices have evolved from it. Basically, therapists and teachers use an antecedents-behavior-consequences model to improve cognitive and language abilities. This therapy manages the consequences of behavior by rewarding positive behavior and, to deter certain behaviors, will apply consequences for poorer behavior when appropriate. Goals are often tailored and choices are often provided to reduce the likelihood of problem behavior. Then, the skills are taught to allow individuals to be more successful and less reliant on problem behavior to meet their needs.

Psychodrama and Family Constellations

Two experiential methods most frequently used in psychotherapy and educational settings have offered help for children and adults with ADHD and autism spectrum disorders. They are recognized as more effective than traditional talk therapy. One is psychodrama, which is an action method that uses spontaneous dramatization, role playing, and other interactive structures to gain a better understanding of the roles that we play and how to connect with others in our world.

Developed by J. L. Moreno, MD, who died in 1974, and continued for decades by his widow, Zerka Moreno, it is a therapeutic modality for children, as well as adults, to improve social relationships, self-acceptance, self-esteem, attentiveness, impulsivity, and other behavioral concerns.

The psychodrama practitioner may use games, fairytales, puppets and other props, music, or movement to create a safe place where feelings can be contained, expressed, and witnessed in individual, group, and family settings. When used by a skilled practitioner, psychodrama is highly engaging, helping people express their truths in an accepting environment and practice new roles and behaviors.

In psychodrama, the client is invited to act out life scenes relating to inner conflicts, past hurts, unfinished situations, personal dramas, fantasies, and dreams, with the help of group members or the practitioner and sometimes trained helpers. The child or adult may replay a wished-for scene to gain a corrective re-experience. For instance, it might be standing up to a childhood bully rather than fleeing. The role playing may involve practicing social skills that will eventually transfer to greater comfort in real-life situations.

Another modality is called Family Constellations, sometimes known as Systemic Constellations, created by Bert Hellinger, a German psychotherapist. This phenomenological method is used to uncover the source of chronic conditions, illnesses, and emotional difficulties that may have roots in the intergenerational family system, rather than the individual, and may sometimes be connected to a key stress event. This moving and powerful work in the family's energetic field has been used to examine the emotional factors connected to conditions such as illness, allergies, alcoholism, ADHD, and autism. Some parents of autistic children have experienced profound transformations as a result of this work for themselves, as well as for their families.

Martial Arts Training

Kids on the autism spectrum often respond well to martial arts training. This vigorous exercise allows a child to expend anxious energy and get endorphins going. Numerous studies show and parents concur that this highly structured and vigorous sport can drastically improve strength, balance, attention, motor coordination, social skills, eye contact, as well as confidence and self-esteem to defend themselves. One such study conducted by the University of Isfahan in Iran also found that repetitive behaviors decreased as the student with autism continued to train.[8]

CHAPTER 24

Preconception and Prenatal Safety Checklist

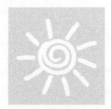

I've heard from many moms who are afraid they will have a child with autism, or they are afraid to have a second child if their first was affected. I've also wondered what I could have done differently to protect Evan from developing ADHD and autism.

As advanced as we are as a society, I believe we miss the mark when it comes to prenatal care. We all know that a healthy pregnancy leads to a healthier baby, but are we doing enough? We are living in a toxic world, so there is certainly more we can do to prepare our bodies before conception. What follows are suggestions that I believe you should discuss with your doctor and address before conceiving your next baby.

Get Tested for the MTHFR Mutation Gene

A simple blood test can determine if you carry the MTHFR gene mutation. This will let you know if you need to be supplemented with more than the recommended dose of methyl-B12 and folate. Folic acid is the synthetic form of folate and often the prescribed supplement. Some agree that taking folate supplements is the better choice. This simple test could help you avoid having a miscarriage and could prevent your baby from developing birth defects, neurological problems, and other medical issues.

According to an article in the *Journal of the American Medical Asso-*

ciation on February 13, 2013, "Women taking folate before pregnancy were 40 percent less likely to have a baby later diagnosed with autism, according to a new study."[1]

On October 12, 2011, the same journal stated, "The use of folic acid/folate supplements in early pregnancy was associated with a reduced risk of severe language delay in children at age 3 years."[2]

Get Tested for Pyrrole Disorder

Symptoms of pyrrole disorder include anxiety, mood swings, aggression/bad temper, poor tolerance of stress, and hypersensitivity to light, sounds, tastes, and/or touch. A simple urine test can detect this problem. If zinc and vitamin B6 are being dumped into your urine, it means these nutrients aren't being correctly metabolized in your body. Both are essential for a healthy pregnancy and a healthy baby.

Resolve Infections

Get yourself checked to see if you have any chronic inflammations, yeast infections, urinary tract infections, or low-grade chronic infections. If you do have any infections, consider avoiding prescription medications, and try to have the issues treated naturally.

Check Thyroid Functioning

As discussed in Chapter 20, checking for low thyroid functioning and elevated thyroid antibodies is very important before and during your pregnancy. Experts believe that getting enough iodine and treating thyroid conditions can help safeguard against ADHD and autism.

Take Probiotics and Prebiotics

Rebuild your gut with human-strain probiotics and feed the probiotics with plenty of dietary fiber. A healthy gut is essential to your health and your child's health.

Also, take digestive enzymes—and chew your food well—to ensure you're digesting and absorbing nutrients properly.

Drink Water

Drink lots and lots of mineralized water. Try to get water that is stored in BPA-free bottles, and have your tap water tested for heavy metals, helpful mineral levels, pH, and bacteria.

Eat Healthy

Eat carefully, and increase your intake of healthy protein and mineral-rich foods such as kelp, small fish, and organic root vegetables.

There are a variety of ways to ensure a healthy diet. The following strategies are among the most important:

Avoid Toxic Foods

Avoid processed and chemical-laced foods. Our mainstream food supply is so processed and refined that many vitamins and minerals essential to health are stripped away, while chemicals and preservatives that are bad for you are added.

Avoid tuna, marlin, swordfish, tilefish, grouper, bluefish, Chilean sea bass, shark, king mackerel, and other large fish known to contain high levels of mercury, which is poisonous. Fish containing the least amount of mercury include anchovies, sardines, flounder, haddock, herring, wild-caught salmon, sole, squid, shrimp, scallops, and clams.

Increase Levels of Glutathione

Eat sulfur-rich foods such as broccoli, cauliflower, Brussels sprouts, and cabbage. Eat foods high in selenium, such as Brazil nuts, sunflower seeds, shellfish, meat, poultry, eggs, mushrooms, and onions, and herbs such as cinnamon and cardamom that have compounds that can restore healthy levels of glutathione.

Talk to your physician about N-acetylcysteine (N-AC) injections or supplements. Liposome capsule supplements are best because they protect the glutathione from the digestive process and allow it to be absorbed into the body.

Go Organic

Whenever possible, buy organic foods. In a comparative study between organic and conventional tomatoes, "A farming experiment at the University of California, Davis, has found that organically grown tomatoes are 70–97% richer in certain kinds of flavonoids than conventionally grown tomatoes. The increased flavonoid levels could stem from the difference in how organic and conventional tomatoes are fertilized."[3] Plants grown without fertilizers and pesticides react to the environment by building their own defenses. The result means higher levels of antioxidants, benefiting the tomato and the consumer. These powerful antioxidants increase detoxifying enzymes in the body.

In a 1994 study in the *Journal of Clinical Nutrition*, food labeled "organic" and selected randomly from Chicago food markets had an average of twice the mineral content of standard supermarket food. That makes sense because in modern mainstream farming, one crop is grown over and over on the same piece of land, depleting the soil and its nutrients. Also, toxic sprays damage microorganisms that help the plants absorb minerals from the soil.

Don't forget that primitive man consumed five to eleven times the amount of the essential minerals most of us get from mainstream food. When food is low in essential minerals, the body absorbs and makes use of more toxic metals.

Vitamins and minerals are essential for boosting your energy and keeping you feeling your best. In contrast, chemicals add toxins to your system that may remain in your body for decades and lead to a variety of illnesses.

Another reason to eat organic is that conventional foods contain a lot of synthetic pesticides, which are considered neurotoxins. Our main exposure to these chemicals comes through our diets. According to *Rodale News*, pesticides in food are linked to ADHD in kids, and Phil Landrigan, MD, Professor and Chair of the Department of Community and Preventative Medicine at Mount Sinai School of

Medicine in New York City, agrees. "People who switch to an organic diet knock down the levels of pesticide by-products in their urine by 85–90 percent."[4]

Warning: Mike Adams of Natural News says to steer clear of organic foods, herbs, and supplements from China, which is one of the most polluted nations on Earth with high levels of toxins, including lead, cadmium, and arsenic routinely appearing in its foods.[5] Look for the USDA "certified organic" logo to ensure you're buying genuine organic food.

Avoid Extreme Diets

Any diet that is without balance has the potential to cause health problems. For example, don't live on protein drinks, as they lack many vital minerals. Even a strict vegetarian diet is typically deficient in zinc and other essential nutrients that help detoxify the body. Such a diet can also be deficient in vitamin B12 and amino acids, which are essential for your baby's brain health. If you're committed to a vegetarian diet, you must take extra special care to ensure you're getting all of the nutrients you and your baby need through vitamin supplements and foods that address these potential deficiencies.

Get Enough Zinc

Zinc is critical for many bodily functions, including fertility, maintaining the right hormone levels, and cell division. It's also a powerful antioxidant and may help prevent cancer.

According to a 2007 article in the *American Journal of Clinical Nutrition,* zinc deficiency may be a hidden cause of genetic defects: "Genetic birth defects may be caused by faulty DNA or by faulty gene expression. Even if one's DNA is perfect, the synthesis of proteins from that DNA can be faulty. For example, zinc is required for a key enzyme in gene expression, RNA transferase."[6]

Get Enough Omega-3

Omega-3 fatty acids provide numerous health benefits, including reducing blood pressure, reducing inflammation, improving joint and bone health, improving skin, and improving mental health.

Top sources for omega-3 include small fish such as sardines and/or quality small fish supplements free of pesticides. Other sources are ground flaxseeds and flaxseed oil, walnuts, pumpkin seeds, sesame seeds, ground chia seeds, primrose, borage, grape seeds, coconut oil, walnuts, kidney beans, black beans, and canola oil. Just be cautious about canola oil, due to possible GMO.

Take Vitamin and Mineral Supplements

Bioavailable, whole-food prenatal vitamins with adequate amounts of minerals will help both you and your baby.

Cleanse Your System

Detoxify your organs, glands, and tissues of heavy metals, estrogen-mimicking chemicals, and other toxins. Virtually all of us have toxins built up in our systems, and eliminating them is very important. These toxins can lead to birth defects, miscarriages, or illnesses in our children. Some experts advise starting a detox regimen two years before conception.

Warning: Don't perform any detoxification regimens once you become pregnant, because toxins that you release from your body could transfer to your baby. Detoxifying *before* you become pregnant is very highly recommended, but not after.

Cut Toxins Out of Your Life

As a first step, cut out any lifestyle habits that put toxins into your body. Avoid:

- Smoking.

- Alcoholic beverages.

- Harmful drugs.

- Environmental toxins you may be exposed to regularly at work or home—including secondhand smoke and industrial chemicals. Avoid contaminated air, such as industrial fumes, as much as possible. Use air filters in your home and office to trap toxic airborne chemicals.

- Skin care and beauty products that contain toxic ingredients can seep in through your skin or scalp. Don't put anything on your skin that you don't want absorbed into your system.

- Toxic cleaning products and air fresheners. Use natural products instead.

- Over-the-counter medications, such as antacids, that contain high levels of aluminum and other harmful ingredients.

- Unnecessary prescription medications. Educate yourself so that you can weigh the costs versus benefits of medications and vaccinations for you and your baby.

Flush Toxic Metals

You can help remove toxic metals from your body by consuming foods and supplements that contain sulfur, such as cabbage, beans, and garlic. You can also take hot clay and sea salt baths, as mentioned in Chapter 19. Make the water as hot as you can stand, and add essential oils such as rosemary (10 drops), lavender (10 drops), or a tiny bit of tea tree oil (2 drops). Then, soak for forty-five minutes.

Exercise Regularly

If you exercise and sweat at least thirty minutes a day, it will help sweat toxins out of your system.

Get Enough Sleep

When you get eight to nine hours of sleep daily, you're giving your body the opportunity to detoxify, heal, and rebuild. This is critical to achieve optimal health.

Avoid Stress

Take good care of yourself so that your pregnancy can be as stress-free as possible. Natural therapies such as body work, chiropractic work, and energy work can greatly facilitate digestion and alleviate stress.

CHAPTER 25

What to Feed Your Infant

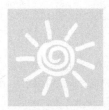

I frequently hear from mothers who are worried about the best ways to feed their babies and toddlers. This chapter explains how to improve your young child's nutritional health.

Breastfeeding Tips

I'm often asked whether breastfeeding is still considered the best way to feed one's baby. Typically, it is. Breastfeeding creates a wonderful bonding experience between mother and baby, and it's healthy for both mom and child . . . most of the time.

The caveat is that for your baby to get the most benefit from your milk, you need to be in the healthiest state possible. You can achieve this by reading and following the advice in the previous chapter. Virtually everything described in Chapter 24 also applies after you give birth.

That said, I recommend paying extra attention to cleansing and to your immune system health. Any toxins in your system may be passed on to your baby through your breast milk, and the same goes for your good or bad gut flora.

You should, therefore, take care to continue eating well, drinking water often, and taking your prenatal supplements, including probiotics. Remember, human milk does contain casein. So if you are breastfeeding a baby with a milk allergy or sensitivity, you should avoid milk products and make sure you are taking the correct dose of vitamin D and calcium supplements.

Finding the Right Formula

Many very wonderful, caring, and dedicated moms have no choice but to bottle feed their baby because they have a difficult time latching. Some moms do not produce enough breast milk, acquire an infection or need to return to work. So finding the right formula is key—especially if the baby has a sensitivity to cow's milk.

A report in *Environmental Health Perspectives* estimated that eighteen to twenty-five percent of babies in the U.S. are found to have an intolerance to cow's milk and are put on formula by their pediatricians.[1]

In these cases, pediatricians typically recommend a soy-based formula for full-term infants. Currently, soy formula consists of up to twenty-five percent of the infant formula market. Soy was first thought to be a healthy alternative to breast milk and milk-based formula, but there are now concerns about soy impairing iodine absorption in infants, which can interfere with thyroid function and overall development. Soy can also partially block mineral absorption because of its high phytic acid level. This can lead to deficiencies in calcium, magnesium, iron, and zinc, all of which are necessary for the proper functioning of the central nervous system and immune system. As mentioned earlier, ninety percent of soybeans grown in the U.S. are estimated to be genetically modified.

Soy formula contains more aluminium than human milk. Per serving, human milk is believed to contain 4–65 mg of aluminium, while soy-based formula is believed to contain 600–1,300 mg. The American Academy of Pediatrics does not recommend soy-based formula for preterm infants. Studies comparing cow's milk formula to soy-based formula demonstrated that some babies who received soy-based formula had problems with bone growth. In addition, high levels of aluminium could be toxic.

Most baby formulas try to mimic the nutrients found in breast milk. However, many versions are made with other genetically engineered crops, such as corn (for corn syrup) and canola. On top of that, they are largely composed of sugar (via corn syrup, cane sugar, and/or sucrose).

To avoid toxic pesticides like cupric sulfate or genetically engineered ingredients, one may want to use organic infant formula, which is usually made with complex carbohydrates like brown rice and provides essential digestive enzymes and probiotics. These formulas also leave out the toxins, chemicals, and unhealthy sugars included in most conventional formulas.

If you find an organic formula you like that doesn't include probiotics, buy quality infant probiotics, and add that into the formula yourself before feedings.

Organic formula carries a few caveats: Make sure that whatever brand you consider doesn't include synthetic forms of DHA (from algae) and ARA omega-6 (from soil fungus). These are extracted using petroleum-derived hexane solvent and other unhealthy substances, and they are approved as organic due to a faulty FDA interpretation of organic regulations.

One study out of Dartmouth College found that organic products containing "brown rice syrup" contained high levels of arsenic. The testing included seventeen infant formulas. In March 2013, Nature's One, one of the organic formula manufacturers, released a statement that claims they are using compliant technology to filter and remove arsenic from their organic brown rice syrup.

Also, watch out for organic formula that contains palm oil. It has been added to the formula to try to mimic fatty acids in human milk—only human infants do not absorb it well; it reacts with calcium and can cause "soaps" in the baby's gut. As reported in the *American Academy of Pediatrics* journal, this can negatively affect a baby's intestinal tract. All organic formulas from PBM Nutritionals, including Earth's Best, contains palm oil.

Lastly, watch out for carrageenan. A review by the University of Iowa Carver College of Medicine warns us about its harmful effects. It is a food additive in many conventional and organic foods that plays a potential role in the development of inflammatory bowel disease and gastrointestinal malignancy.[2] It has been banned from all infant formula in Europe (conventional and organic), but here in the United States, it can be spotted in some organic formulas, including Earth's Best and Similac Organic Ready to Feed.

If your baby has allergies, turn to elemental formulas such as Neocate and Elecare. These contain vitamins, minerals, and individual amino acids without the food proteins to which allergic babies may react. The main ingredient is corn, but it is non-GMO and doesn't contain any corn protein, so it is generally safe even for children with corn allergies. These formulas are lifesavers. You can try a few and see which works best for your baby.

Alternatively, you can choose to create formula yourself. There are many recipes in books and online for homemade formulas. If you go this route, be sure that your formula contains the correct levels of nutrients and consult with your doctor or nutritionist.

Some parents create the foundation of their homemade formula using a powdered supplement called UltraCare from Metagenics, which is made with rice protein powder. Other parents prefer to use coconut milk, raw cow's milk, or raw goat's milk. Remember: coconut milk is low in protein and calcium; goat's milk is deficient in vitamin D, B12, iron, and folate; and raw milk can harbor dangerous bacteria, such as salmonella, E. coli, and listeria.

CHAPTER 26

Instilling Healthy Practices Including Getting Your Child to Eat Better

When Your Child Is a Picky Eater and Craves the Wrong Things

While part of being a parent is encouraging good eating habits in your child, it also means paying attention when your child is exhibiting unusual eating choices. For example, Evan has always loved to eat, but from an early age, he was a picky eater when it came to certain foods. Surprisingly, foods he didn't want to eat included those other kids are crazy about such as macaroni and cheese and the cheese on pizza (which he pulls off before eating a slice).

My pediatrician told me it was just a phase. Later on, Evan's therapists told me his sensory issues were causing him to be averse to certain food tastes, textures, and consistencies.

After reading the book *Cure Your Child with Food* by Kelly Dorfman,[1] I realized that Evan has a genuine sensitivity to certain kinds of foods—including dairy—and is intuitively pushing them away.

In other words, sometimes picky eating is a kid just refusing to try something new or is simply about taste or texture. Other times, however, picky eating is a sign that certain foods are irritating your child and actually damaging his/her health.

I know what some of you are thinking: "But my kids won't eat anything but macaroni and cheese or pizza. If I change their diet, they'll starve!" Many parents with kids on the autism spectrum would agree that their kids do not eat well and that their diets are limited.

Unfortunately, limited diets without fruit, vegetables, and healthy protein limit the nutrients the body needs to function well. And the foods our kids crave like cheese, yogurt, and bread often contribute to the symptoms our children exhibit. So what do you do? The proceeding section will outline some very important tips on getting your child to eat healthier. Just remember to investigate all possible underlying issues. It could be due to sensory integration issues, but commonly could also be tied to digestive woes, nutritional deficiencies, food sensitivities, and sometimes even side effects from medication.

It can require a certain amount of detective work to figure out which is which. Reading books such as Dorfman's (mentioned earlier) and/or working with a knowledgeable naturopathic doctor or dietician can help enormously.

Another great resource is Karen Le Billon's book, *French Kids Eat Everything*. It contains recipes, practical tips, and easy-to-follow steps on how to end picky eating and raise happy and healthy children. She writes, "French parents think about healthy eating habits the way North American parents think about toilet training, or reading. If your children consistently refused to read, or even learn the alphabet, would you give up trying to teach them? Would you be content to wait for your children to toilet train by themselves, assuming that they'd eventually "grow out of it" or "figure it out"?"

Persuading Your Child to Eat Fruits and Veggies

While supplements arc important, the most bioavailable forms of nutrients still come from everyday foods. Nutrition remains the best medicine. A lot of kids aren't thrilled at first about consuming vegetables and fruits, so here are some tips to steer your child to lifelong healthy eating habits.

Stop Serving "Kids Meals" and Be Persistent

Too many households serve the adults one dinner and give the kids mac and cheese and processed chicken nuggets. Food is food. Start serving healthy food when your children are young. Persistence. Even if your child turns down a particular vegetable the first few times you offer it, don't give up. It may take around ten tries, but your child may well grow to like what you're selling. Persistence often wins the day.

Homemade Fruit Popsicles

These treats are a great source of calcium, potassium, fiber, iron, vitamin A, vitamin B6, and antioxidants. Here's the recipe:

1 cup coconut water or coconut milk   1 pitted date   Fruit (as desired)

Blend the ingredients together at high speed until milky (if too thick, add a little water). Add blueberries, cherries, or mango pieces. Pour into a Popsicle mold, and place in the freezer until frozen.

Encourage Participation in Meal-Making

Take your children with you when you shop for organic food. Then, when you get home, take them into the kitchen to help you prepare what you've purchased. The latter needn't be any more challenging than what your kids can manage; even just washing the fruits and vegetables is a genuinely useful contribution.

If you care to take this a step further, create your own vegetable garden, and have your children help you maintain it. Few things are as desirable and taste as wonderful as what you've grown yourself.

When you involve your children in the process that goes into making lunch or dinner, they're much more likely to happily eat everything you put on their plates.

Make Veggies and Fruits Fun

Sometimes, kids don't object to a food across the board but just to its texture or the way it looks. In these cases, preparation and presentation can make a world of difference.

For example, at first I had trouble getting Evan to eat broiled asparagus. Then, I decided to make it a special treat instead of an obligation. I now give Evan a pastry brush for painting the asparagus with olive oil, and I let him sprinkle the stalks with sea salt to his taste. When he's done, I bake the asparagus at 400 degrees until the stalks are crunchy. Evan loves these green treats and tells me they taste better than French fries.

I use the same approach to make baked cauliflower taste like fresh popcorn. I especially like doing this with purple cauliflower, which is even more delicious and contains more minerals, vitamins, antioxidants, and fiber than the white variety.

As for any fruit that Evan isn't drawn to, I have him cut it up with a cookie cutter into shapes that tickle him, or I put slices of the fruit on a skewer. Making the food visually appealing somehow makes it tastier.

If you're similarly creative in making veggies and fruit fun for your children, you're much more likely to get them to love eating what's good for them.

Enforce a "No Thank You Bite" Rule

If there is a healthy food your child refuses to eat, wait until he/she is hungry before offering it. Your child can refuse to eat the whole serving, but the rule is that he/she is required to take at least one bite to know what he/she will be missing. If your kid still refuses the food after the first bite, simply say, "Too bad! It's good for you."

Use Fruit and Veggies as Snacks, Decorations, and Treats

We need to be sneaky feeders. When your child wants a snack, offer an organic fruit. If that doesn't fly, offer organic dried fruit, which contains more sugar and tastes more like candy.

Another way is to purée the veggies or fruits, and sneak them into everyday foods like pasta sauce, soups, or breads like pumpkin or zucchini, using gluten-free flour.

When your child wants a treat, allow him/her to dip fruit into coconut yogurt. Other good snacks are apple slices and veggies dipped in organic peanut butter.

When you make smoothies, sneak in some kale or spinach when your kid isn't looking, and decorate the glass with fruit. This way, your child will not only eat more fruit but will start to think of it as extra special.

There is a wonderful recipe book to help you make the most

delicious smoothies titled *Salad Under Cover: Smoothies for Superhero Kids*, by Kristen Taylor of Beegreenfoods.com.

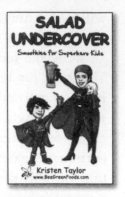

Whole-food enthusiast Kristen Taylor offers fantastic and creative solutions for the "picky eater." She, too, was a "mama lioness" with a fierce commitment to heal her son on the autism spectrum. She agrees that diet modifications and eating nutrient-rich foods turned their lives around.

Kristen's Blueberry Monster Milk

2 cups almond milk or coconut milk	2 tbs of hemp seeds
	1 cup blueberries
1 tbs coconut oil	2–3 tbs chia seeds

Buzz all ingredients together in a high-powered blender. Drink and enjoy!

Persuading Your Child to Play Outside

Both exercise and sunshine help a child to produce more dopamine and other neurotransmitters such as serotonin. Exercise increases blood calcium, which stimulates the production and uptake of dopamine in the brain. Jumping rope, walking, running, and swimming at least fifteen to thirty minutes a day make a dramatic difference in mood and energy levels. School systems need to make sure not to discount the importance of recess and fun play.

School recess plays an important role in school success for children. There is a connection between recess/physical activity and attention/academic performance. A study released in *Pediatrics* in 2013 demonstrates that minimizing or eliminating recess may be counterproductive to academic achievement, as a growing body of evidence suggests that recess promotes not only physical health and social development but also cognitive performance.[2] Dr. David L. Katz, MD, an authority on nutrition says, "We need to treat ADHD with recess not Ritalin." He created a program called ABC for Fitness (Activity Bursts in the Classroom.) When the program was studied, "it showed a reduction in medication use for asthma and ADHD."[3] The ABC for Fitness program shows schools how to restructure physical activity into multiple, brief episodes of activity into classrooms throughout the day without taking away valuable time for classroom instruction. Exercise encourages your brain to work at optimum capacity. Research in pediatric literature has demonstrated that the more physically active schoolchildren are, the better they do academically.[4] Yet, many schools in the U.S. are removing rather than improving their physical education programs.

There is also a positive correlation between spending time in nature, serotonin synthesis, and the hours spent in the sunshine. A series of studies published in the June 2010 issue of *Journal of Environmental Psychology* infer that children who regularly play outside are healthier and are happier than those who do not. It is time to instill practices that allow children more exercise and more sunshine. Educators should be encouraging more outdoor activities and parents should be pushing their children out the door and away from the computer, phone, television, and video games.

Persuading Your Child to Relinquish the iPad and Get Enough Sleep

Having a structured bed routine and getting at least eight to ten hours of sleep are critical. Routinely getting enough sleep helps the body recover from the day and allows a child's neurotransmitters to build up naturally while they sleep. Chronic fatigue means that they are less likely to perform well. Neurons do not fire optimally, muscles are not rested, and the whole system is not synchronized.

Studies from the Division of Sleep Medicine at Harvard Medical School imply that sleep plays a critical role in mood, metabolism, focus, memory, learning, and immune functioning.[5] Turning off the television, computer, iPad, and iPhone at least one hour before bedtime signals the brain to release the necessary melatonin to allow the mind and body to fall asleep more easily.

EXPERT RECOMMENDATIONS FOR CHILDREN'S SLEEP (per night)			
Age 1–3	12–14 hours	Age 5–11	10–11 hours
Age 3–5	11–13 hours	Age 11+	8.5–9.5 hours

Persuading Your Child to Drink More Water

Today's kids are loading up on sugary drinks that contain harmful chemicals and artificial flavors. Soda and sports drinks are too often a substitute for water. Drinking eight to ten cups of water a day helps maintain the balance of body fluids, aids normal bowel function, improves digestion, helps the body burn stored fat, helps flush away toxins, enables muscles to become stronger and work harder, reduces fatigue, increases cognitive function, helps supply ample oxygen to the brain, and supports nerve function. Water also ensures that electrolyte levels remain high enough to allow the nerves to relay messages to and from the brain.

For some people who lack sufficient levels of stomach acid and digestive enzymes, drinking water with meals causes bloating. Some experts believe these people should not consume water during mealtime because the water could dilute the necessary enzymes and stomach acid needed for proper digestion. For some of our gut-sensitive kids, limiting liquids during mealtime may be a good idea. Some are underweight and need to eat more and drink less.

How to Get Your Child to Drink More Water

- Offer water throughout the day.
- Serve more fruits and vegetables.
- Make their favorite non-BPA cup or water bottle more available, and remind them to take at least five sips.
- Add ice. Many kids like water better when it's cold, although warmer water is better for digestion.
- Let your child drink water through a straw to make it more fun.
- Mix a splash of 100% fruit juice into water to give it a little flavor.

- Add a drop of lemon or fresh orange.

- Foster independence by leaving a spouted pitcher or water dispenser on the counter or low shelf in the refrigerator, and allow kids to get water themselves.

- Limit other options.

- Make natural lemonade with raw honey, and get loads of benefits. Lemon juice activates the salivary glands and helps the digestive system break down essential minerals in the food for better absorption, boosts the immune system, cleans the liver, and alkalizes the body. It also contains calcium, magnesium, vitamin C, bioflavonoids, and pectin, which promote immunity and fight infection. It even helps us lose weight. Raw honey heals the gut, reduces allergies, and helps us sleep better by balancing out blood sugar. Get rid of artificial substitutes that often contain high fructose corn syrup, refined sugar, and food dyes.

Homemade Lemonade

Juice of 4–6 lemons $3/4$ cup honey* (warmed to liquefy)

Combine the ingredients in a pitcher with 6 cups water and ice, and enjoy!

*WARNING: Honey is not safe for children under one year of age.

Persuading Your Child to Take Vitamins

Getting a young child to take vitamins or other supplements can be tricky. Some kids respond well to rules, visual schedule reminders, a reward system, and simply being told the vitamins are good for them. But if your child is picky, has motor/sensory issues, has a strong gag reflex, or for any other reason has difficulty swallowing pills, convincing him/her to take pills on a daily basis can be challenging.

- Kids tend to be more accepting of chewable or gummy vitamins, so if you can find such forms that don't contain the harmful additives listed in this book, they might be your best choice.

- If you must use supplements that come only in capsule or tablet form, pull the capsules apart or grind the tablets so that they can be dissolved in water or juice.

- Along similar lines, if your child flat-out refuses to take vitamins and other supplements, hide the powered form in their drinks and/or food. I put Evan's supplements in natural apple sauce or throw them into organic sunflower seed butter that I spread on celery stalks and apple slices. If a supplement tastes especially awful, I hide the taste with organic chocolate dairy-free syrup.

Certain supplements, such as high quality omega-3 fish oil in liquid form, are easily added to a smoothie. For example, OmegAvail Lemon Drop Smoothie is delicious and contains 1,820 mg of EPA and DHA fatty acids per serving.

Talk to your health provider about other bioavailable liquid multivitamins that may be easier to administer. As mentioned before, SmartMix by Zija or Body Balance by Life Force may be an option.

Many other supplements mix well in a fruit or veggie smoothie. The mortar and pestle are now my friends. I find the finer the powder, the more dissolvable it is in liquid, and the less gritty it tastes.

To help the smoothies go down even smoother, Evan and I make up silly names for different varieties. Here's our recipe for "Olivia the Orange."

Olivia the Orange Dairy-Free Creamsicle Smoothie

16 ounces frozen orange juice or cold orange juice

Ice

3/4 cup coconut milk

3 tablespoons raw honey*

2 teaspoons pure vanilla extract

2 teaspoons probiotic powder

3,000 IU vitamin D3 drops

Add more supplements, if desired, adjusting for taste

Blend all ingredients to desired consistency. YUM!

*WARNING: Honey is not safe for children under one year of age.

CHAPTER 27

Opening the World of Improvements

There have been remarkable improvements in Evan's health, and many of his autistic symptoms have disappeared. After putting the alternative treatments into practice and addressing underlying nutritional deficiencies, Evan's progress catapulted. His teachers and therapists report huge advancements in his academic, social, and emotional well-being. In addition, his work habits improved since the introduction of alternative and homeopathic treatments one year ago.

Evan has always demonstrated a positive attitude toward learning that is reflected by his enthusiasm and willingness to try. I strongly believe that his school and therapy sessions have provided a safe, patient, and positive environment for him. I also believe that the speech, occupational, and physical therapy has helped Evan improve in many areas by providing him with tools and promoting the development of new brain pathways.

After a year of treating Evan naturally and biomedically, he stays on task and is less careless. He has less difficulty listening and following directions, and he isn't as distracted by background noise. He listens to his teachers and responds appropriately when asked a question. He's able to retain information and speaks more clearly to convey his ideas.

When he was tested at age five-and-a-half, his level of development was only that of a three-and-a-half-year-old. Developmentally, he was two years behind his peers. A year later, after implementing the alternative treatments, Evan's testing demonstrated a huge improvement in all areas of development. At six-and-a-half, his level of development was that of a five-and-a-half-year-old. Now, he was only one year behind his peers.

There is a tremendous jump in Evan's expressive language and speech articulation; it's more complex and conversational. His comprehension skills are also much better. He is able to formulate a thought and carry out his plans. He is now forming new ideas and trying them out on others.

Evan's true personality started to emerge, and it was discovered that he has a very dry sense of humor. One day, while Evan's grandma was cooking a new stew recipe that included cinnamon as her "special ingredient," she hit her wooded spoon against the pot, causing a piece of the spoon to fly off. She warned us all to watch out for it because she had no idea where it flew. After dinner, grandma asked if anyone could taste what the special ingredient was. Without hesitation, Evan said, "Spoon."

He is less anxious and no longer grunts and screams when he is upset. He is coping better with changes in routine and with frustrating situations. He no longer throws himself into fits of uncontrollable rage, throwing his toys, hitting others, or displaying sudden mood swings. In addition, his sensory issues are lessening greatly. Loud noises and uncomfortable clothing no longer bother him as much.

Evan's pre-kindergarten treatment plan included a communication device to help him write and communicate. There is no need for this device anymore. His fine motor skills have significantly improved, and he is able to write his letters as well as many of his peers. We now see a confident little boy who is eager to join in group activities.

His motor-planning difficulties have jumped from extremely disordered to barely noticeable. We notice an increase in imaginative play, and there is greater independence in daily activities of living.

Socially, Evan is also doing much better. He makes eye contact more often and now greets his friends at the playground. He no longer enters into a trance-like state or detaches himself from the world. Evan talks to strangers in waiting rooms and has whole conversations with people. He is able to assert himself and tell people what he likes and doesn't like and what he wants and doesn't want.

On Evan's seventh birthday, his grandfather joked with him by saying, "Mmm . . . your cake looks so good; I think I'm going to eat your piece." In the same breath, Evan replied, "That's okay, Grandpa; I'll just eat yours." Demonstrating a marked improvement in social ability, increased self-esteem, and tremendous growth on so many levels, he got the joke, stood up for himself, responded with sharp wit, and delivered it in a loving and nonaggressive way. We are so proud of him.

We have noticed that Evan's sweet cravings have lessened, and he's no longer overly thirsty. The dark bluish circles under his eyes have disappeared. His eczema and fungal infections have cleared. He no longer suffers from sinus infections, respiratory infections, or eye infections. His constipation issues continue to improve. He's no longer straining, and his bowels are less sluggish. He doesn't suffer from nightly head sweats anymore, and the quality of his sleep has improved. His immune system seems stronger. In fact, he has only missed a few days of school since starting his treatment.

Teachers, therapists, his swimming instructor, and family members have all commented on how well Evan is doing. They say, "I don't know what you're doing, but we see a huge difference in Evan. Keep it up." Just this past summer, I enrolled him in a typical art camp with his sister Elaina for a week. I told the teachers about my book and all the ways that I have been trying to help Evan. They looked at me and said, "Evan is on the spectrum? I would never have guessed that in a million years." That was certainly music to my ears.

Evan is now eight years old and progressing well. When I recently asked him, "What do you think helped you more—all of the intense therapy or your diet changes and vitamins?" He looked at me with the biggest smile and with huge inflection in his voice and said, "Mom, they helped each other work better."

So, we continue appointments with the naturopathic physician to address any emerging health concerns or imbalances. We continue his dietary modifications, and we continue his therapies so that we can optimize his health as much as possible. We still have rough days from time to time, but then again who doesn't—it's all part of the fun.

CHAPTER 28

Natural Remedies
Often Scrutinized

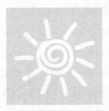

It is important to realize that not all naturopathic physicians are created equal. Some use homeopathic remedies, some use mineral therapy, some use herbal remedies, some create serums to address food allergies, and some use NAET and other allergy elimination techniques. Some treat with numerous supplements, and some don't. Some believe in energy healing, some believe in essential oils, some believe in acupuncture, and some believe in chiropractors, osteopaths, and craniosacral care. Unfortunately, the lack of consistency of practice causes many science-minded individuals to become skeptical and even cynical. In spite of the inconsistencies, I encourage you to keep an open mind.

Homeopathy is a system of alternative medicine originated in 1796 by Samuel Hahnemann, and alternative methods like it have been used for centuries. Before it was coined "homeopathy," Native American Indians practiced many forms of natural healing.

I believe that homeopathy and other functional medicine practices have the ability to reach deep into the body and trigger change in a way nothing else can. Alternative medicine methods also known as "complementary" or "functional" medicine seek to address the entire person, not just a set of symptoms.

These methods are steeped in tradition. In numerous other countries, the practices are considered mainstream. Homeopathic remedies are available at nearly all pharmacies throughout Europe and

many other parts of the world. Believe it or not, our ancestors imple-
mented many of these natural practices in our country for a long
time before pharmaceuticals were introduced to the public in the late
1900s. Slowly, these early holistic practices were abandoned to make
way for new advancements in medicine. Newer often forgets the
older and wiser, leaving behind the tried and true. Modern interventions and modern medicines often save lives. Yet seeking to quickly
suppress symptoms by using artificial chemicals that carry potential
adverse effects—seems fundamentally irrational. We should use current technology to identify disease origins, and couple laboratory
findings with good old-fashioned doctoring.

I was amazed when I ironically came across *The Household Physician—A 20th Century Medica* in the basement while cleaning out
Steve's great grandfather's belongings. This twelve-volume text dating back to 1918 includes "the latest discoveries in medicine and the
most approved methods of treatment." There is a section on "Diseases of the Brain" that specifically targets stress, convulsions, and
illness of the mother during gestation, excessive use of mercury, and
issues of the bowels and digestive tract. The text then discusses treatments such as sea baths and the importance of minerals, necessary
treatment of constipation "when the bowels are bound," the use of
"magnesia" (magnesium), and tonics for debility (herbal treatments
such as chamomile and cinnamon). Many of the homeopathic remedies my naturopath prescribed were in the book as well. Those
included calcarea carbonica, nux vomica, pulsatilla, and sulfur for
"cradle cap, eczema in allergic persons, yeast management, distress
in the stomach, digestive tract and constipation."

The book talks about the importance of eliminating sugar, tomatoes, and all stimulants. It recommends a wholesome diet of fats
and protein, as well as the need to drink plenty of alkaline mineral
water for health.

CHAPTER 29

A Call to Action:
Shifting Current Practices

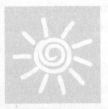

We cannot live in this world without the advances of modern medicine. There are new treatments every day for many debilitating illnesses and diseases, and new medications are developed that save lives or dramatically raise the quality of a person's life. However, according to Beth Lambert and Victoria Kobliner's book, *A Compromised Generation*, "One of the fundamental flaws of our existing medical paradigm is the tendency to approach health and sickness only through a disease-based or organ-focused lens. Most branches of medical specialties are almost exclusively dedicated to specific organs, organ groups, or diseases. Physicians are some of the most intelligent, hardworking, and highly trained professionals in our society, but few are trained to use a 'systems biology' approach to manage the health of their patients."[1]

We need to begin looking at health care from a broader vantage point. We need to learn to respect each other's disciplines and recognize that there is a need for collaboration between traditional Western medicine and Eastern holistic treatments. We need multidisciplinary teams in the areas of education, research, and clinical care that can work in tandem to address our illnesses.

I find it funny that we call our original medicine humans have been using for thousands of years "alternative" when modern medicine was only discovered about 100 years ago!

I recognize that alternative medicine can't set a broken bone or perform a much-needed operation. In an emergency, I also recognize that it may be necessary to medicate our kids for a time as we dig deeper to find possible underlying causes and implement psychotherapy and more natural remedies. In many cases, we should look at psychiatric medications as a rescue remedy or a bridge, not a long-term solution.

We need an "integrative medicine" approach. A healing-oriented medicine that takes the whole person (body, mind, and spirit) into account, including all aspects of lifestyle. We need to emphasize the therapeutic relationship and make use of all appropriate therapies, both conventional and alternative. We need a medical system that neither rejects conventional medicine nor accepts alternative therapies uncritically. Good medicine should be based on good science, be inquiry-driven, and be open to new paradigms. We need to use natural, effective, and less-invasive interventions whenever possible. We need a system that promotes prevention of illness as well as the treatment of disease.

Although many parents claim that psychotropic medication has completely changed their child's life for the better, we must not forget that giving a six-year-old medication does nothing to change the conditions that derail their development in the first place. Yet, those conditions are not currently receiving any attention. Policymakers are so convinced that these children have an organic disease that they have all but called off the search for a better understanding of the conditions. It isn't enough to simply be alive. The quality of life is also important. A cancer patient, for example, could benefit tremendously from treatments that could improve the quality of life during radiation and chemotherapy. In my opinion, it's essential that we begin to include chiropractors, massage therapists, naturopaths, acupuncturists, osteopathic physicians, Oriental medicine practitioners, and others in our treatment plans. We need more organizations to enable its members to understand and collaborate with one another and relate their messages to conventional biomedicine, insurance, and government agencies with a unified voice. By including preventive care, we decrease disease and reduce the overall cost of health care.

If there had been a team of alternative doctors alongside traditional doctors in the NICU coming up with a specific protocol to treat Evan's immature digestive system and gut flora issues, might he never have suffered so much? Is it possible that if some of my health issues were addressed holistically, as well as medically, before conception and during pregnancy that Evan's health would have greatly benefited? I believe so.

Could the elimination of unnecessary vaccines be accomplished so that tiny babies are not getting their first hepatitis B vaccine before they leave the hospital? Could we administer these vaccines in adolescence or when they are at a higher risk? Could measles, mumps, and rubella combination shots be causing problems? Would it perhaps be better if they were split up and spread out so that babies didn't receive so many in one visit? Could vaccines be produced without all of the harmful ingredients and preservatives? Could we have blood work before a second MMR shot is administered to determine if a second shot is necessary? Many times, antibodies are present after only one vaccination.

Some of the vaccines are absolutely necessary due to potential risks. Are they all necessary? In the early 1980s, there were seven vaccines administered (23 doses), and today there are sixteen vaccines (69 doses). Perhaps we need to think about our personal risk factors before deciding if we want or need to vaccinate. We may want to accept some vaccinations and refuse others, or we may want to alter our vaccine schedule.

According to the Centers for Disease Control and Prevention, "In the U.S., no federal vaccination laws exist, but all 50 states require certain vaccinations for children entering public schools. Depending on the state, children must be vaccinated against some or all of the following diseases: mumps, measles, rubella, diphtheria, pertussis, tetanus, and polio."[2] However, as stated in Chapter 10, vaccines are medical interventions. Parents can deny vaccinations because of allergic reactions or other medical reasons, and in 48 states exemptions for non-medical reasons are also acceptable.

It is also important to remember that a vaccination decision does not have to be black and white. You can accept some vaccines and reject others. It is important to learn about vaccine benefits as well as their potential risks. Pro-vaccine information is readily accessible through the American Academy of Pediatrics, the CDC, and health-care and government-sponsored organizations.

If you would like to review medical and scientific literature sur-rounding vaccination risks as well as hear personal stories from those whose lives have been touched by vaccine-related injuries, Markus Heinze has written a book titled *VACCeptable Injuries: Increasing Childhood Diseases & Developmental Disorders*.[3]

If you would like to learn more about how to legally avoid vac-cines, a doctor of osteopathic medicine, Sherri Tenpenny has written a book titled *Saying No to Vaccines*."[4]

If you would like to learn how to protect your child from infec-tious diseases and find homeopathic alternatives to vaccination, Kate Birch, RS Hom (NA), and Cilla Whatcott, HD (RHom), CCH, have written a book titled *The Solution: Homeoprophylaxis: The Vaccine Alternative*.[5]

Treating and Preventing Disease Naturally Meets Resistance

Why is there so much resistance to treating and preventing disease with nutrition and natural methods? Why is medication always the first line of defense? Unfortunately, many people are unaware that there are healthier and more natural solutions available. And some are resistant to change and are looking for a quick fix. A doctor may recommend exercise and dietary changes for weight loss or for improved health. Yet, we resist, often looking for the easier and/or cheaper way out. We must remember, a healthy diet may be cheaper than our medical bills in the long run. We need to take time out of our busy lives and start investing in our health. We are worth it!

Another issue is that disease equals big money! Pharmaceutical companies have set out to discredit alternative medicine—especially in those areas of greatest drug profits, such as cancer, heart disease, psychiatric disorders, and allergies. These companies aren't only in the business of saving lives. They're also in the business of inflating the profit margins on their drugs as much as possible. According to research firms, these drug companies use the term "scientific evidence" as a political definition to control the FDA and National Institutes of Health. They buy investigative journalists with their advertising. They pay doctors and psychiatrists to speak on their behalf and offer up expensive trips and steep payments. They block financial contributions by using terms like "unproven treatments," and many "charitable organizations" are completely controlled along with Congress. These are only some of the practices of the large pharmaceutical companies that spend millions of dollars to implement carefully designed plans. R. Webster Kehr of the Independent Cancer Research Foundation says, "The FDA, NIH, NCI, ACS and medical schools are their puppets."[6]

I personally know this to be true. Six years ago, before I started my own private practice as a psychotherapist, I worked for a group of psychiatrists. As clinicians, we were invited by these pharmaceutical companies to attend lavish monthly dinner parties at posh restaurants and were provided with lunches at least one or two days per week. Many of our office supplies were also paid for by these companies.

The doctors received large sums of money to give five-minute speeches on the importance of certain drugs over others, and they would change their tune the next week to sing the praises of a different drug. It all depended on who was paying for the meal. I remember laughing with other therapists about certain drugs being the "one of choice" for the month. For example, it appeared as though everyone had bipolar disorder and everyone would be on the same medication after that particular company came in to speak to us.

If the therapists wanted to introduce "alternative" therapy treatments or modalities to treat our patients who suffered from ADHD, anxiety, or depression, the doctors wouldn't encourage us or support us.

Wikipedia even mentions how the medical community refers to alternative medicine as "folk knowledge" and homeopathy as "quackery." It seems clear that there are some self-serving reasons for those labels. For example, pharmaceutical companies are even going as far as packaging products that come naturally like fish oil and acidophilus and charging our insurance companies exorbitant amounts of money for what we can buy over-the-counter for one-tenth the price.

Changing American Consciousness

Big change can only come from the collective consciousness of its people. The issues are systemic. All of the pollutants, including chemicals, dyes, artificial ingredients, and heavy metals are what our American culture is now built upon. These pollutants are integrated into every aspect of our lives from the toxins in our atmosphere, to the foods we eat to the medications we take to the clothes we wear to the cosmetics we use. We are poisoning ourselves, and the consequences are starting to show with the incredible rise of diseases like cancer, asthma, diabetes, and countless autoimmune disorders like autism.

Interesting anecdote: My neighbor Judy, an elementary school nurse for 24 years stated, "In 1984, all I did was put Band-Aids on kids. I had no idea what autism was. There were no allergies, no EpiPens, zero inhalers and one kid on Ritalin. By the time I retired in 2010 in my one school alone, I took care of 45 kids on inhalers, 14 kids that needed EpiPens, there were over 25 kids on meds for ADHD and at least 18 diagnosed with moderate to severe autism. There were many others that were undiagnosed, but clearly somewhere on the spectrum."

Our soils are now contaminated and lacking naturally occurring vitamins, minerals, and nutrients. A simple and cheap solution would be to start replacing the minerals we have lost in our soil with sea minerals, which are plentiful. We can also use our resources to create indoor ecosystems to grow our food using hydroponic technology and organic fertilizers and plant nutrients, rather than using genetically engineered technology to create genetically altered food.

But you can bet that pharmaceutical, oil, food, and insurance companies have no interest in changing current practices no matter how sick they're making all of us. Currently, these companies are adhering to FDA guidelines and are not violating any federal laws, so we need to start changing those laws. It would mean fighting big lobbyist groups and big companies that generate trillions of dollars. Therefore, it's time for us to take our power back and put health before wealth in this country.

It's going to take grassroots change. "We the people" need to start a movement. We need to insist on cleaner fuel, we need to refuse to buy anything with artificial dyes and chemicals and only buy products made from organic and all natural ingredients. We need to buy whole food that is minimally processed and join local farming co-ops in our communities. We need to start cooking on a regular basis instead of relying on "convenience" meals. We need to stop serving poison in our lunchrooms. We must start treating our diseases naturally and not relying so heavily on pharmaceuticals. This would force the large companies to turn their practices around in order to continue making a profit.

To begin, there is a free smartphone app that I mentioned in a previous chapter called Buycott. You scan a barcode of a product, and the app tells you the name of the "mother" manufacturing corporation. It helps you avoid supporting companies that do not support our health. For example, it will alert you if the product contains GMOs or if the company does not support GMO labelling.

We must demand changes. Many countries have already banned many processed food ingredients that are making us sick. GMOs have been banned in a number of countries, but the U.S. has even refused to demand labelling of GMO products and produce. In fact, food companies are making healthier versions of their products for other countries because of the bans. For example, Nutri-Grain bars in Europe are made without high fructose corn syrup and are made instead with beet juice, annatto, and paprika extract for color instead of artificial dyes.

Why aren't they making a higher quality product for us in the United States? According to Mike Adams of *Natural News*, "Health insurance companies and pharmaceutical companies invest billions in fast food chains and crappy synthetic vitamin companies."[7] It's all to keep us as customers. So what can we do? We can all check our investment portfolios and make sure we aren't funding this craziness. We should be investing in green companies and companies that support our health instead.

What else needs to change? All insurance companies need to get on board and pay for natural treatments that work. They should be covering homeopathic remedies, naturopathic physicians, and many of the therapies currently considered alternative or complementary, such as chiropractors, craniosacral therapy, and massage therapy. Again, money is the reason they don't. The more services they exclude from coverage while still selling policies to patients, the better for their businesses. To change this, we and the companies we work for must start refusing to buy policies without this essential coverage.

In reality, many of the alternative remedies and nutritional supplements cost less in comparison to medications and expensive trips to specialists, and they are often very effective if taken as recommended by your physician. If all of the insurance companies got on board, tons of money would be saved in the long run. They would help us prevent illness and disease by making these treatments easily accessible, and it would benefit them by reducing the number of claims, ultimately protecting and increasing their profit margins.

We simply need to wake up and make a stand for real change. We can no longer put a price tag on our physical and mental health. The amount of pain we are creating for our families and our children is a high price to pay for the way we conduct our business.

APPENDIX A

Questions & Answers

Who should I contact if I want to start treating my child naturally?

I recommend finding a naturopath, Defeat Autism Now (DAN) doctor, a Medical Academy of Special Needs (MAPS) doctor, or a homeopath to do the first line of testing. I would find one in your area who specializes in autism. I've learned through this experience that even in the field of alternative medicine, there are differences. I needed to find a team to treat Evan. Our first naturopath performed many of the appropriate tests, addressed gut issues, and treated Evan with homeopathy, which was her specialty.

As I dug deeper in the research, I sought out a Defeat Autism Now (DAN) doctor who specialized in autism. Although not as well versed in homeopathy, Dr. Skowron discovered Evan's various gene mutations, treated his neurotransmitter imbalances, adrenal fatigue, and hypoglycemic issues.

Therefore, a combination of practitioners may be the best choice.

To find a provider, please visit the following websites:

- www.dandoctorlist.org

- www.naturopathic.org

- www.icimed.com

- www.holisticmedicine.org

- www.ahha.org

- www.mapdr.com

- www.naet.com

- www.drellencutler.com/pages/practitioners

- www.biobalance.org

- www.generationrescue.org/resources/find-a-physician

- www.sharedabilities.com/resources-links

- www.nationalcenterforhomeopathy.org

I tried the gluten free/dairy free diet, and it didn't work.

Again, I highly recommend going to a knowledgeable practitioner who knows how to test, interpret, and treat all of the underlying conditions. A complete metabolic workup and treatment is recommended to make a fuller recovery. Unfortunately, only addressing one piece of the puzzle will yield a less positive outcome for some children.

What particular tests should I ask the doctor about?

I recommend making a complete checklist of all of your questions and concerns, and provide your doctor with a list of specific tests you would like performed. I also learned throughout this process that these tests are not routinely performed by the mainstream medical community, and it took steady perseverance to find the right team of professionals to address all of my concerns.

A holistic doctor will most likely start with a metabolic and nutritional profile such as an Organic Acid Test (OAT) and food sensitivity testing. When it comes to sensitivity testing, some practitioners prefer the ALCAT over IgG and IgE testing. These tests can sometimes produce false positives causing patients to unnecessarily cut foods out of their diet. The ALCAT studies the reaction of your white blood cells, rather than testing for antibodies. To learn more, you can locate them at www.greatplainslaboratory.com and www.alcat.com.

The chart on the following page lists some of the tests you might want to include.

COMPLETE METABOLIC WORKUP

Gut Analysis	Good/bad bacteria (Candida)	Genova Test
	Lactulose/Mannitol	Leaky Gut
	Fecal or Urine	Parasites
Food Sensitivities	Blood Testing IgG and IgE Food Panel or ALCAT panel, which tests ones response to foods, medicinal herbs, food dyes and additives, environmental chemicals, and mold	
Heavy Metal Testing	Hair Sampling or Blood	
Neurotransmitter Testing	Neurobalance Profile—Urine	
Adrenal Fatigue/Cortisol	Blood or Urine	
Amino Acid Testing	Urine or Blood	
Vitamin Testing	Blood	
Mineral Testing	Hair Sampling or Blood	
MTHFR, COMT & MAO Gene Mutations	Blood or Saliva (23andme.com)	
Pyrrole/Pyroluria Gene Mutation	Urine	
Histadelia	Blood Test for Histamine Levels	

Another test that often indicates nutritional deficiencies is the RBC. This tests the child's red blood cell count. Lower than normal numbers of RBCs could indicate malnutrition and specific nutritional deficiencies that need to be addressed, such as low iron causing anemia, as well as low levels of copper, folate, vitamin B6, and vitamin B12. If results show low levels (even just marginally), I recommend insisting on deeper testing to find out exactly why.

Iron deficiency may require a battery of tests. By the time the hemoglobin (protein that carries oxygen to the body) and the hematocrit (percentage of red blood cells) levels are low, a person is in later-stage iron deficiency anemia. Other tests a doctor can order include serum ferritin (the storage form of iron in the body) and transferrin saturation (the transportation form of iron in the blood).

Does insurance pay for visits with a naturopath?
How much does all this testing cost?

The answer to these questions depends on your particular insurance policy. Some policies cover naturopathic doctors, and others do not. Everyone's policy is unique. My insurance did not cover NDs. However, the cost of all lab work was covered under the normal medical portion of our policy. In some cases, insurance companies will pay for one test and not the other. I had one client whose doctor's visits were covered, but he needed to pay out of pocket for certain lab work because it wasn't covered. Finding an integrative physician or other medical doctor (MD) who specializes in metabolic issues and nutrition may be a safe bet, and one that many insurance policies would cover. When you find the right provider, they may be willing to work with you in regard to price and payment options. If not, going to your regular pediatrician or family doctor first with the list of tests you want done may be one idea. Just know, that physician may not know how to interpret the testing or know how to treat, but it's a great first step.

In addition, there are numerous laboratories you can find online that will assist you with testing and with locating a physician. Some labs require a doctor's order, but others do not. A traditional lab may charge you a much higher rate, which your insurance company may deny. Therefore, shopping around for the best price is important. A few laboratories that conduct the proper testing include Great Plains Laboratory, SpectraCell Laboratories, US Biotek Laboratories, and Genova Diagnostics (Diagnostic Insight—Australia).

What do you think of the GAP, Specific Carbohydrate, or Feingold Diet?

We never followed a specific diet. We simply got the test results and followed the protocol designed by our two naturopathic physicians. I read many books and researched various available autoimmune diets. There are many different "diets" out there all claiming to be the best. These include the GAP diet, Candida-free diet, the Feingold Diet, the Gluten/Casein-Free diet, the Specific Carbohydrate diet, the Immune Quieting diet, and others. Most of these focus on the need to reduce inflammation in the gut and eliminate offending foods such as dairy, wheat, eggs, and sugar, along with processed foods, etc. Many recommend staying away from artificial colors, flavors, and preservatives such as BHT and TBQH. They also want us to avoid artificial sweeteners and artificial fragrances.

I believe that all of these different protocols are like different makes of cars with the goal of going to the same place. Some of these diets are highly regimented with long lists of foods and ingredients to avoid. The problem is that you still may not be avoiding the ones that are actually causing your child's trouble. I wish there was a cookie-cutter approach to healing our kids, but every child is unique. For example, Evan was sensitive to mustard.

I highly recommend getting the food allergy and sensitivity testing by a naturopath or integrative physician, so that you're addressing all of the correct offenders. I also recommend seeking out an NAET or other allergy-elimination practitioner to test for some of the more obscure substances like amino acids and digestive enzymes. Sometimes, it's the amino acids in the foods, not the foods themselves, that are the problem. An allergy-elimination technique professional can address such issues.

To learn more, please visit the following websites:

- www.gaps.me
- www.feingold.org
- www.breakingtheviciouscycle.info
- www.thecandidadiet.com
- www.bodyecology.com

What is an elimination diet?

A procedure used to identify foods that may be causing an adverse effect in a person, in which all suspected foods are excluded from the diet and then reintroduced one at a time.

What is a rotation diet?

Once definite food sensitivities have been identified, doctors or allergists may recommend following a rotation diet. This plan requires that you eat different foods throughout the day in a four-day period to decrease the likelihood of developing new allergies or sensitivities. I do this with Evan. He has a very slight sensitivity to peanuts and almonds so I make sure not to give it to him too often. People with mild food intolerances may find that if they follow the rotation diet, they can eventually tolerate certain foods better. However, rein-troducing these foods should be done very carefully.

What about products like Focus Formula & Bright Spark?

Focus Formula is an herbal remedy approach to help people main-tain concentration and improve their attention span. Many parents report success with such products. I would, however, warn about herbal supplements for children without proper consultation with a doctor or practitioner. Herbs can mimic medications and have simi-lar side effects. My naturopath has given Evan herbs to correct cer-tain imbalances, monitoring it very carefully and then removing them when imbalances were corrected. Here is one mom's testimo-nial: "After reading reviews, I had really high hopes for this product for my 8 year old daughter with ADHD. I decided to put her on it. I started noticing slight changes in her for the better, but my MD was concerned about liver function so she ordered a blood test. My daugh-ter's liver enzymes came back elevated. I searched on the internet for a cause of elevated liver enzymes and found out that the herb skullcap can affect the liver. Now we need follow-up blood work."

Just remember natural does not always mean safe. Herbs can be harmful, especially in supplement form. Please do your research and speak with your physician.

What about the use of caffeine to treat ADD/ADHD?

I get asked this question a lot. I agree it does help. Unfortunately, once again like with any other drug, it only really "helps" the symp-toms and can cause other ill effects.

Teachers and parents are often frustrated when dealing with chil-dren with inattention, hyperactivity, impulsivity, and behavioral problems. Many parents feel pressured to either medicate or try a "natural" alternative stimulant like caffeine, which appears to be the safer choice because even though it's a stimulant, it's a less objec-tionable one. Millions use caffeine daily in the form of coffee, energy drinks, and caffeinated soda to provide a quick jolt. They feel that caffeine helps them stay awake and concentrate.

So, why wouldn't caffeine be a good choice for managing

ADHD? Although my response may not be a popular one with many of you who feel that caffeine has helped your child immensely, we must remember that caffeine (although naturally produced in plants) is still considered a drug. It comes with numerous side effects and also only addresses symptoms, not causes. Side effects of caffeine include agitation, tremors, insomnia, dependency, and withdrawal. Caffeine also interferes with the way the amino acid GABA binds to its receptors to cause a calming effect.

Many would advise against giving caffeine to children because it can trigger many of the same symptoms as prescribed stimulants, including loss of appetite, digestive problems, and malnutrition.

Coffee especially has many negative health effects in gut-damaged people who suffer from leaky gut, irritable bowel syndrome, Crohn's disease, colitis, and ulcers. Coffee can harm the stomach and intestines by irritating it lining, and it depletes hydrochloric acid, which is needed to assist in digestion. Coffee also contributes to acid reflux, invites bacteria to thrive, prevents the gut from healing because of its acidic nature, acts as a laxative, and blocks the absorption of important minerals.

What about the use of cannabis oil to treat autism, seizures (epilepsy), insomnia, anxiety, irritability, and rage?

While no double-blind study has been done on the effect of medicinal marijuana and autism, anecdotal evidence begins to mount. Many suggest that the active ingredient in cannabis oil, called CBD (Cannabidiol), can help reduce many symptoms of ADHD and autism, including seizures, anxiety, insomnia, and self-injurious/aggressive behavior. CBD is a non-psychoactive cannabinoid that is considered a supplement by the FDA, and although not approved as a medicine, it is available for purchase. According to the Epilepsy Foundation in Colorado, "A number of people with epilepsy report beneficial effects from using marijuana/cannabinoid, including a decrease in seizure activity. Those who promote the medical use of marijuana often include treatment of epilepsy in the long list of disorders for which marijuana is supposed to be helpful. In fact, multiple states now have laws allowing the prescription of marijuana for the treatment of epilepsy."[1] Medicinal marijuana is also being used to treat persons with HIV, Parkinson's disease, Alzheimer's, and even cancer.

Doctors at the Center for Autism Research and Treatment at the UC Irvine Center in California believe that there is a genetic mutation preventing the brain's pathways from functioning properly. They believe that cannabis oil may help assist the body's endocannabinoid system to work more effectively. "American and European scientists have found that increasing natural marijuana-like chemicals in the brain can help correct behavioral issues related to fragile X syndrome."[2] While the autism community continues to debate the subject about the possible benefits of marijuana, more and more parents are willing to explore other options and alternative treatments to help their child. Some parents report that marijuana/hemp oil or hemp seeds containing cannabinoid compounds have helped in the treatment of their child. So, eating crushed hemp seeds loaded with protein and other healthy nutrients may also serve another important purpose.

What should I do if I want my child to get off of his/her medication?

It is important to realize that there are specific tapering strategies when going off of psychotropic medication. You should never stop taking a particular medication without the assistance of your physician.

It is recommended that there is ample communication between the patient's prescribing physician, such as the family doctor or psychiatrist, and the clinician proposing the tapering plan. The plan should involve stopping one drug at a time and should only be done with patients who are medically stable. The plan needs to be very gradual and methodical to reduce the possibility of side effects, withdrawal, and destabilization.

Some of the possible side effects if the patient does not taper off a psychiatric drug slowly include tremors, restlessness, anxiety, flu-like symptoms, headaches, abdominal pain, nightmares, nausea, weakness, and dizziness.

For more information on tapering off of medication properly and safely, please refer to Townsend Letter, The Examiner of Alternative Medication, February/March 2013, *What to Do When Patients Wish to Discontinue Psychotropic Medications?* At www.townsendletter.com/FebMarch2013/whattodo0213.html.

Do you have any other suggestions for epilepsy and seizures? My child takes Depakote and Lamictal, and she is having many side effects even though it hasn't made much of a difference. Are there natural remedies?

I recommend doing some research into the ketogenic diet. This high-fat, adequate-protein, low-carbohydrate diet has helped many children who suffer from epilepsy. I recommend reading *Treating Epilepsy Naturally: A Guide to Alternative and Adjunct Therapies* by Patricia A. Murphy.[3] Then, I suggest that you find a naturopath or integrative physician. Unfortunately, medications often mask symptoms and do a lousy job of it most of the time.

Find an NAET practitioner as well who can work on reversing sensitivities to foods and other environmental triggers. Seizures can be triggered by numerous things, including sugar imbalances and blocks to vitamin B. Some kids are also "allergic" to fluorescent lights, among other strange things. NAET is recommended by many in the treatment of seizure disorders.

I also recommend watching a wonderful movie released in 1997 called *First, Do No Harm*. It was based on a true story of a mother who went against medical advice and sought biomedical treatments after her son was getting worse on medication.

Visit www.jacobteitelbaum.com/natural_cures/epilepsy.html and www.epilepsyfoundation.org/aboutepilepsy/treatment/ketogenic diet/for more information.

Are there any diagnostic tools that a parent can purchase to determine whether or not their child has ADHD, apraxia, or autism?

It's important to get professional testing, but the inventories listed here are extremely helpful in giving you an idea as to whether or not you need to seek professional help.

The Child Development Inventory for age twelve months to four years is a series of three screening tests that that can be used as an early detection tool to help identify autism by determining the child's developmental needs. Visit www.childdevrev.com.

Ages and Stages Questionnaire for ages four months to five years is a questionnaire that focuses on communication, motor skills, social skills, and problem solving. Visit www.brookespublishing.com/store/books/squires-asq/system.htm.

Social Communication Questionnaire is appropriate for most age groups and focuses on language development and social interaction. It has been used to identify autism. Visit www.testagency.com/?/test/show/64/.

When should I seek professional testing and services?

I believe it's important for you to follow your gut instincts. You are your children's most informed caretaker, and you know them best. If you feel something is wrong, it probably is. I remember how easy it would have been to stick my head in the sand and follow the recommendations of others. I'm glad I didn't.

Get your child evaluated as soon as you suspect a problem. Most states have an early intervention program. If your child qualifies for services, the state can help provide your child with services such as occupational, physical, and speech therapy. It is really important to get therapies as early as possible; this is one key element to successful treatment in all cases.

In Evan's case, he qualified for all services except for speech until he was close to age three, although he was completely unintelligible. The therapists assured me not to panic or assume that all children develop at the same pace. They felt that once his gross and fine motor skills emerged, the speech would eventually come.

Side Note: After talking with numerous speech language pathologists (SLPs) and after personal experience, it's important to note here, that Evan would have benefited by earlier intervention and that it's essential to get speech therapy on board right away. According to Esther Thelen, the author of a book about human development, "It takes 70 muscles and 8 different body parts to utter a single l-syllable word."[4]

Should I get my child tested by the school system for early intervention?

In my experience, it's a good idea. The brain is continuously growing and developing from birth. It's imperative to help create new pathways in the brain from a young age. The expectations for kindergarteners these days are nothing like we remember. They are expected to interact socially with peers, read level one and two books, and write complete sentences in their journals. They are asked to sit quietly in their seats and use expressive and receptive communication skills appropriately. They are even expected to tell and recite stories.

I remember our goal for Evan was to "be ready for kindergarten." Although early intervention does not guarantee a trouble-free school experience, I can tell you that getting him all of the appropriate services beforehand paved the way for a more successful year.

Are there any services available from age three until the entrance into kindergarten besides private therapy and private schools?

Yes, there are. Many towns have special education preschool programs funded by the town. At three years old, Evan was enrolled in a special education preschool program at our town's elementary school.

Why do our kids have such difficulty with potty training?

Many children on the autism spectrum have difficulty with motor planning—i.e., getting their bodies to do what's needed to complete a task. Evan had trouble knowing when he had an urge, and when he did, he had trouble figuring out what he needed his muscles to do in order to address it.

I read an article, "Autism and Toilet Training," by Danica Mamlet, who explains the difficulties autistic children have when potty training.[5] They all fit Evan.

Difficulty with comprehending language and logic can inhibit the ability to understand toilet procedures, too. Autism can also create resistance to a change in routine. Plus, the bathroom can be an overly stimulating environment with its bright lights, noise coming from running water, and the change in temperature when removing clothes.

Most children with autism have gastrointestinal problems that make a regular toilet training schedule a challenge. GI problems such as abdominal pain, bloating, gaseousness, constipation, and/or diarrhea are more prevalent in children with autism.

I remember feeling embarrassed that my son was almost four and not showing any signs of potty training readiness. I became more and more frustrated at Evan, and it was difficult to find size-seven diapers. So, I hired a "potty training specialist" to help me train him.

It's my belief now that if we had addressed all of his gastrointestinal problems long before his fourth birthday, I may not have needed to hire anyone.

My son scored low on his IQ test; is that a true indication of his potential?

Although many children on the spectrum are quite brilliant, some children with apraxia or autism spectrum disorders have some cognitive impairment. Most are milder cases. At age six, Evan's IQ test scored low, but I needed to remember to take the results with a grain of salt. It can be tremendously difficult to ascertain capability from a less compliant child. In addition, since language deficits are part of the triad, the verbal portion can be expected to be lower than more typical peers. There are some nonverbal IQ tests that can be administered in the place of others, but even with those, I needed to remember that Evan's behavior and intelligence outside the testing arena demonstrated more competency than his IQ scores showed.

A reminder: Due to the speech and language motor planning component, children with apraxia often exhibit signs of learning disabilities that include problems with reading and writing.

Should I hold my child back from entering kindergarten?

It was very heartbreaking to keep Evan back from entering kindergarten at age five-and-a-half. I cried as he walked back into the preschool classroom for the third straight year. I was upset by how much taller my son looked than the other children in his class. I noticed that in a classroom of twelve children, Evan was only one of two boys, which was very unusual for a special education classroom. I worried that he might not have any good friends by the time of his birthday party. I wondered if I had made a terrible mistake and immediately sought parents and educators who could reassure me that I was doing the right thing. In their experience, they had never heard of a case where a parent regretted holding their child back. More often, they heard of an upset parent who pushed a child ahead when they weren't ready. For me, allowing Evan an extra year to mature and master his basic skills was a blessing and the right decision. He started kindergarten at age six-and-a-half, and it was the best thing we could have done.

Childhood Developmental Guidelines

Each child develops at his/her own particular pace; it's impossible to tell exactly when your child will master a given skill. The developmental milestones listed here will give you a general idea of the changes you can expect as your child gets older, but don't be alarmed if he/she takes a slightly different course. Act early and alert your pediatrician if your child displays a possible developmental delay. The following are milestones—what most babies can do at the ages shown.

1 MONTH OF AGE

Social/Emotional Development

Focuses 8 to 12 inches (20.3 to 30.4 cm) away

Eyes wander and occasionally cross

Prefers black-and-white or high-contrast patterns

Language/Communication

Prefers the human face to all other patterns

Hearing is fully mature

Recognizes some sounds

May turn toward familiar sounds and voices

Movement/Physical Development

Makes jerky, quivering arm thrusts

Brings hands within range of eyes and mouth

Moves head from side to side while lying on stomach

Head flops backward if unsupported

Keeps hands in tight fists

Strong reflex movements

2 MONTHS OF AGE

Social/Emotional Development

Begins to smile at people in the family

Can briefly calm himself or herself

May bring hands to mouth and suck on hand

Tries to look at parent

Language/Communication

Coos, makes gurgling sounds

Turns head toward sounds

Cognitive (Learning, Thinking, Problem-solving)

Pays attention to faces

Begins to follow things with eyes

Begins to act bored (cries, fussy) if activity doesn't change

Movement/Physical Development

Can hold head up and begins to push up when lying
on tummy

Makes smoother movements with arms and legs

4 MONTHS OF AGE

Social/Emotional

Smiles spontaneously, especially at people

Likes to play with people and might cry when playing stops

Copies some movements and facial expressions, like smiling or frowning

Language/Communication

Begins to babble

Babbles with expression and begins to copy sounds heard

Cries in different ways to show hunger, pain, or being tired

Cognitive (Learning, Thinking, Problem-solving)

Lets you know if she/he is happy or sad

Responds to affection

Reaches for toy with one hand

Uses hands and eyes together, such as seeing a toy and reaching for it

Follows moving things with eyes from side to side

Watches faces closely

Recognizes familiar people and things at a distance

Movement/Physical Development

Holds head steady, unsupported

Pushes down on legs when feet are on a hard surface for short periods

May be able to roll over from tummy to back

Can hold a toy and shake it and swing at dangling toys

Brings hands to mouth

When lying on stomach, pushes up to elbows

6 MONTHS OF AGE

Social/Emotional

Knows familiar faces and begins to know if someone is
a stranger

Likes to play with others, especially parents

Responds to other people's emotions and often seems happy

Likes to look at self in a mirror

Language/Communication

Responds to sounds by making sounds

Strings vowels together when babbling ("ah," "eh," "oh")
and likes taking turns when parents make sounds

Responds to own name

Makes sounds to show joy and displeasure

Begins to say consonant sounds (jabbering with "m," "b")

Cognitive (Learning, Thinking, Problem-solving)

Looks around at things nearby

Brings things to mouth

Shows curiosity about things and tries to get things that are
out of reach

Begins to pass things from one hand to the other

Movement/Physical Development

Rolls over in both directions (front to back, back to front)

Begins to sit without support in tripod position

When standing, supports weight on legs and might bounce

Rocks back and forth, early for crawling, some crawl backward
first

9 MONTHS OF AGE

Social/Emotional

May be afraid of strangers

May be clingy with familiar adults

Has favorite toys

Language/Communication

Understands "no"

Makes a lot of different sounds by combining consonants like "mabada"

Copies sounds and gestures of others

Uses fingers to point at things

Cognitive (Learning, Thinking, Problem-solving)

Watches the path of something as it falls

Looks for things he sees you hide

Plays "peek-a-boo"

Puts things in his/her mouth

Moves things smoothly from one hand to the other

Picks up things like cereal o's between thumb and index finger

Movement/Physical Development

Stands, holding on

Can get into sitting position

Sits without support

Pulls to stand

Crawls

12 MONTHS OF AGE—AT THE FIRST BIRTHDAY

Social/Emotional

Is shy or nervous with strangers

Cries when Mom or Dad leaves

May become fearful in certain situations

Tests parental responses

Has favorite things and people

Shows fear in some situations

Hands you a book when he wants to hear a story

Repeats sounds or actions to get attention

Puts out arm or leg to help with dressing

Plays games such as "peek-a-boo" and "patty cake"

Language/Communication

Responds to simple spoken requests

Uses simple gestures, like shaking head "no" or waving "bye-bye"

Makes sounds with changes in tone (sounds more like speech)

Says "mama" and "dada" and exclamations like "uh-oh!"

Babbles with reflection

Tries to imitate words

Responds to "no"

Cognitive (Learning, Thinking, Problem-solving)

Explores objects in many different ways (shaking, banging, throwing, dropping)

Finds hidden things easily

Looks at the right picture or thing when it's named

Copies gestures

Starts to use things correctly; for example, drinks from a cup, brushes hair

Bangs two things together

Puts things in a container, takes things out of a container

Pokes with index (pointer) finger

Uses pincer grasp and starts feeding self

Begins to use objects correctly (drinking from cup, brushing hair, dialing phone, listening to receiver)

Follows simple directions like "pick up the toy"

Movement/Physical Development

Gets to a sitting position without assistance

Crawls forward on belly by pulling with arms and pushing with legs

Gets from sitting to crawling or prone (lying on stomach) position

Pulls up to stand, walks holding on to furniture ("cruising")

May stand alone

May take 1 to 3 steps without assistance

18 MONTHS OF AGE

Social/Emotional

Likes to hand things to others as play

May have temper tantrums

May be afraid of strangers

Shows affection to familiar people

Plays simple pretend, such as feeding a doll

May cling to caregivers in new situations

Points to show others something interesting

Explores alone but with parent close by

Language/Communication

Says at least 10 single words (articulation not important)

Says and shakes head "no"

Points to show someone what she/he wants

Cognitive (Learning, Thinking, Problem-solving)

Knows what ordinary things are for; for example, telephone, brush, or spoon

Points to get the attention of others

Shows interest in a doll or stuffed animal by pretending to feed it

Points to one body part

Scribbles on his/her own

Can follow 1-step verbal commands without any gestures; for example, will sit when asked to

Movement/Physical Development

Walks alone or while pushing a toy

Can help undress himself/herself

Drinks from a cup

Eats with a spoon

2 YEARS OF AGE

Social/Emotional

Copies others, especially adults and older children

Gets excited when with other children

Shows more and more independence

Shows defiant behaviors

Plays mainly beside other children; however, starting to include them. May engage them with a game of chase

Language/Communication

Says minimum of 50 words

Points to things when they are named

Knows names of familiar people and body parts

Says 2–3-word sentences

Follows simple instructions

Repeats words overheard in a conversation

Points to things in a book

Cognitive (Learning, Thinking, Problem-solving)

Finds things covered even under 2 or 3 covers

Begins to sort shapes and colors

Completes sentences and rhymes in familiar books

Plays simple make-believe games

Builds towers of 4 or more blocks

Might use one hand more than the other

Follows 2-step directions like pick up your shoes and put them in the closet

Names pictures in a book such as cat and dog

Movement/Physical Development

Walks alone and pulls toys from behind

Stands on tiptoe

Kicks a ball

Begins to run

Climbs onto and down from furniture without help

Walks up and down stairs with support

Scribbles spontaneously

Makes or copies straight lines

3 YEARS OF AGE

Social/Emotional

Copies adults and friends

Shows affection for friends without prompting

Takes turns in games

Shows concern for a crying friend

Understands the idea of "mine" and "his" or "hers"

Shows a wide range of emotions

Separates easily from Mom and Dad, if temperament allows

May get upset with major changes in routine

Dresses and undresses self with help

Language/Communication

Follows instructions with 2- or 3-step directions

Can name most familiar things

Understands words like "in," "on," and "under"

Says first name, age, and sex

Names a friend

Says words like "I," "me," "we," and "you" and some plurals (cars, dogs, cats)

Talks well enough for strangers to understand most of the time

Carries on a conversation using 2 to 3 sentences

Cognitive (Learning, Thinking, Problem-solving)

Can work toys with buttons, levers, and moving parts

Plays make-believe with dolls, animals, and people

Works puzzles with 3 or 4 pieces

Understands what "two" means

Copies a circle with pencil or crayon

Turns book pages one at a time

Builds towers of more than 6 blocks

Screws and unscrews jar lids or turns door handles

Movement/Physical Development

Climbs

Runs more easily

Kicks a ball forward with intention

Pedals a tricycle (3-wheel bike)

Walks up and down stairs, one foot on each step

4 YEARS OF AGE

Social/Emotional

Enjoys doing new things

Plays "Mom" and "Dad"

Is more and more creative with make-believe play

Would rather play with other children than alone

Cooperates with other children

Often can't tell what's real and what make-believe is

Talks about what he/she likes and what he/she is interested in

Language/Communication

Knows some basic rules of grammar, such as correctly using "he" and "she"

Sings a song or says a poem from memory such as the "Itsy Bitsy Spider" or "Wheels on the Bus"

Tells stories

Can say first and last name

Cognitive (Learning, Thinking, Problem-solving)

Names some colors and some numbers

Understands the idea of counting

Starts to understand time

Remembers parts of a story

Understands the idea of "same" and "different"

Draws a person with 2 to 4 body parts

Names four colors

Plays board or card games

Follows three-part commands

Tells you what he/she thinks is going to happen next in a book

Movement/Physical Development

Hops and stands on one foot up to 2 seconds

Throws ball overhead

Catches a bounced ball most of the time

Moves forward and backward with agility

Pours, cuts with supervision, and mashes own food

Draws circles and squares

Begins copying or writing some capital letters

Uses scissors

5 YEARS OF AGE

Social/Emotional

Wants to please friends

Wants to be like friends

More likely to agree with rules

Likes to sing, dance, and act

Is aware of gender

Can tell what's real and what make-believe is

Shows more independence (for example, may visit a next-door neighbor by himself/herself; adult supervision is still needed)

Is sometimes demanding and sometimes very cooperative

Language/Communication

Speaks very clearly

Tells a simple story using full sentences

Uses future tense; for example, "Grandma will be here."

Says name and address

Cognitive (Learning, Thinking, Problem-solving)

Counts 10 or more things

Can draw a person with at least 6 body parts

Can print some letters or numbers

Copies a triangle and other geometric shapes

Knows about things used every day, like money and food

Movement/Physical Development

Stands on one foot for 10 seconds or longer

Hops; may be able to skip

Can do a somersault

Uses a fork and spoon and sometimes a table knife

Can use the toilet on his/her own

Swings and climbs

Adapted from the Centers for Disease Control and Prevention (CDC) *Developmental Milestones,* www.cdc.gov/NCBDDD/ACTEARLY/milestones/; *Bright Futures: Guidelines for Health Supervision of Infants, Children, and Adolescents,* Third Edition, edited by Joseph Hagan, Jr., Judith S. Shaw, and Paula M. Duncan, 2008, Elk Grove Village, IL.: American Academy of Pediatrics; The Child Mind Institute, New York, NY, www.childmind.org

APPENDIX C

Autism Research Institute Parent Rating of Behavioral Effects of Biomedical Interventions

Adapted from Autism Research Institute, ARI Publication 34/March 2009.

The parents of autistic children represent a vast and important reservoir of information on the benefits—and adverse effects—of the large variety of drugs and other interventions that have been tried with their children.

The following data have been collected from the more than 27,000 parents who have completed our questionnaires designed to collect such information. For the purposes of the present table, the parents responses on a six-point scale have been combined into three categories: "made worse" (ratings 1 and 2), "no effect" (ratings 3 and 4), and "made better" (ratings 5 and 6). The "Better:Worse" column gives the number of children who "Got Better" for each one who "Got Worse."

DRUGS	Got Worse[A]	No Effect	Got Better	Better: Worse	No. of Cases[B]
Actos	19%	60%	21%	1.1:1	140
Aderall	43%	26%	31%	0.7:1	894
Amphetamine	47%	28%	25%	0.5:1	1355
Anafranil	32%	39%	29%	1.1:1	440
Antibiotics	33%	50%	18%	0.5:1	2507
Antifungals[C]					
Diflucan	5%	34%	62%	13:1	1214
Nystatin	5%	43%	52%	11:1	1969
Atarax	26%	53%	21%	0.8:1	543
Benadryl	24%	50%	26%	1.1:1	3230
Beta Blocker	18%	51%	31%	1.7:1	306
Buspar	29%	42%	28%	1.0:1	431
Chloral Hydrate	42%	39%	19%	0.5:1	498
Clonidine	22%	32%	46%	2.1:1	1658
Clozapine	38%	43%	19%	0.5:1	170
Cogentin	20%	53%	27%	1.4:1	198
Cylert	45%	35%	19%	0.4:1	634
Depakene[D]					
Behavior	25%	44%	31%	1.2:1	1146
Seizures	12%	33%	55%	4.6:1	761
Desipramine	34%	35%	32%	0.9:1	95

DRUGS	Got Worse[A]	No Effect	Got Better	Better: Worse	No. of Cases[B]
Dilantin[D]					
Behavior	28%	49%	23%	0.8:1	1127
Seizures	16%	37%	47%	3.0:1	454
Fenfluramine	21%	52%	27%	1.3:1	483
Haldol	38%	28%	34%	0.9:1	1222
IVIG	7%	39%	54%	7.6:1	142
Klonapin[D]					
Behavior	31%	40%	29%	0.9:1	270
Seizures	29%	55%	16%	0.6:1	86
Lithium	22%	48%	31%	1.4:1	515
Luvox	31%	37%	32%	1.0:1	251
Mellaril	29%	38%	33%	1.2:1	2108
Mysoline[D]					
Behavior	41%	46%	13%	0.3:1	156
Seizures	21%	55%	24%	1.1:1	85
Naltrexone	18%	49%	33%	1.8:1	350
Low Dose Naltrexone	11%	52%	38%	4.0:1	190
Paxil	34%	32%	35%	1.0:1	471
Phenobarb.[D]					
Behavior	48%	37%	16%	0.3:1	1125
Seizures	18%	44%	38%	2.2:1	543

DRUGS	Got Worse[A]	No Effect	Got Better	Better: Worse	No. of Cases[B]
Prolixin	30%	41%	28%	0.9:1	109
Prozac	33%	32%	35%	1.1:1	1391
Risperidal	21%	26%	54%	2.6:1	1216
Ritalin	45%	26%	29%	0.6:1	4256
Secretin					
Intravenous	7%	50%	43%	6.4:1	597
Transderm.	9%	56%	35%	3.9:1	257
Stelazine	29%	45%	26%	0.9:1	437
Steroids	34%	30%	36%	1.1:1	204
Tegretol[D]					
Behavior	25%	45%	30%	1.2:1	1556
Seizures	14%	33%	53%	3.8:1	872
Thorazine	36%	40%	24%	0.7:1	945
Tofranil	30%	38%	32%	1.1:1	785
Valium	35%	42%	24%	0.7:1	895
Valtrex	8%	42%	50%	6.7:1	238
Zarontin[D]					
Behavior	34%	48%	18%	0.5:1	164
Seizures	20%	55%	25%	1.2:1	125
Zoloft	35%	33%	31%	0.9:1	579

A. "Worse" refers only to worse behavior. Drugs, but not nutrients, typically also cause physical problems if used long-term.

B. No. of cases is cumulative over several decades, so does not reflect current usage levels (e.g., Haldol is now seldom used).

C. Antifungal drugs and chelation are used selectively, where evidence indicates they are needed.

D. Seizure drugs: top line behavior effects, bottom line effects on seizures.

E. Calcium effects are not due to dairy-free diet; statistics are similar for milk drinkers and non-milk drinkers.

BIOMEDICAL/ NON-DRUG/ SUPPLEMENTS	Got Worse[A]	No Effect	Got Better	Better: Worse	No. of Cases[B]
Calcium[E]	3%	60%	36%	11:1	2832
Cod Liver Oil	4%	41%	55%	14:1	2550
Cod Liver Oil with Bethanecol	11%	53%	36%	3.4:1	203
Colostrum	6%	56%	38%	6.8:1	851
Detox. (Chelation)[C]	3%	23%	74%	24:1	1382
Digestive Enzymes	3%	35%	62%	19:1	2350
DMG	8%	50%	42%	5.3:1	6363
Fatty Acids	2%	39%	59%	31:1	1680
5 HTP	11%	42%	47%	4.2:1	644
Folic Acid	5%	50%	45%	10:1	2505
Food Allergy Trtmnt	2%	31%	67%	27:1	1294
Hyperbaric Oxygen Therapy	5%	30%	65%	12:1	219
Magnesium	6%	65%	29%	4.6:1	301
Melatonin	8%	26%	66%	8.3:1	1687
Methyl B12 (nasal)	10%	45%	44%	4.2:1	240
Methyl B12 (subcut.)	6%	22%	72%	12:1	899
MT Promoter	8%	47%	44%	5.5:1	99
P5P (Vit. B6)	11%	40%	48%	4.3:1	920
Pepcid	11%	57%	32%	2.9:1	220
SAMe	16%	62%	23%	1.4:1	244
St. Johns Wort	19%	64%	18%	0.9:1	217
TMG	16%	43%	41%	2.6:1	1132

BIOMEDICAL/ NON-DRUG/ SUPPLEMENTS	Got Worse[A]	No Effect	Got Better	Better: Worse	No. of Cases[B]
Transfer Factor	8%	47%	45%	5.9:1	274
Vitamin A	3%	54%	44%	16:1	1535
Vitamin B3	4%	51%	45%	10:1	1192
Vit. B6/Mag.	4%	46%	49%	11:1	7256
Vitamin C	2%	52%	46%	20:1	3077
Zinc	2%	44%	54%	24:1	2738
SPECIAL DIETS					
Candida Diet	3%	39%	58%	21:1	1141
Feingold Diet	2%	40%	58%	26:1	1041
Gluten-/Casein-Free Diet	3%	28%	69%	24:1	3593
Low Oxalate Diet	7%	43%	50%	6.8:1	164
Removed Chocolate	2%	46%	52%	28:1	2264
Removed Eggs	2%	53%	45%	20:1	1658
Removed Milk Products/Dairy	2%	44%	55%	32:1	6950
Removed Sugar	2%	46%	52%	27:1	4589
Removed Wheat	2%	43%	55%	30:1	4340
Rotation Diet	2%	43%	55%	23:1	1097
Specific Carbohydrate Diet	7%	22%	71%	10:1	537

Additional Resources

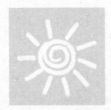

Shared Abilities is an online community for sharing information about special needs and celebrating all we are able to accomplish! This website contains current news and information, more than 100 discussion groups, and a provider directory. To take advantage of this wonderful resource, please visit www.sharedabilities.com.

Apps for Children with Special Needs provides a valuable resource to the special needs community. It assists families of children with special needs and the wider community of educators and therapists who support them by producing videos that demonstrate how educational smart apps work and provides information and advice about how the different apps can assist a child's development. For more info, visit www.a4cwsn.com.

Social Thinking Groups are helpful, as they teach individuals how their own social minds work and why they and others react and respond the way they do; how their behaviors affect the way others perceive and respond to them; and how this affects their own emotions, and responses to relationships with others across different social contexts. "Think Social" is one such social thinking curriculum used for school-age students. Visit www.socialthinking.com.

Psychodrama in Practice: I have the privilege of knowing Karen Carnabucci, MSS, LCSW, LISW-S, TEP, a facilitator and author of such therapeutic practices. She has cowritten two astounding books, one with Ronald Anderson titled *Integrating Psychodrama and Systemic Constellation Work: New Directions for Action Methods, Body-Mind Therapies and Energy Healing*, and the other with Linda Ciotola titled *Healing Eating Disorders with Psychodrama and Other Action Methods: Beyond the Silence and the Fury*.

DyeDiet provides a wonderful website, created by a chemist, that offers food reviews, health risks, and nutritional values based on the analysis of food additives and artificial dyes. Creator of the Health Risk and Nutrition Calculator: www.dyediet.com/calculator/

- Eliminates need to understand meanings of food additives
- Eliminates confusion over which foods to avoid
- Eliminates confusion over which foods to consume
- Educates consumers about which foods are safe and which are not
- Offers links to detailed information about foods or food additives of interest.

In terms of **Health Risk** values, the Dye Diet Calculator indicates which food additives and products are better to *avoid* for prevention of health issues, especially with regard to the long-term effects and chronic intoxication. In terms of **Nutritional Values,** it shows which food products are nutritious and *safe* to consume *in moderation.*

CONTACT INFORMATION

If you liked this book and would like to learn more and/or if you have a question you'd like to share with me and other readers, please visit my website www.healingwithouthurting.com, on Facebook at Healing ADHD & Asperger's Without Hurting (www.facebook.com/onyourpathtohealing), or on Twitter @ADHDNoHarmMeds. If you have private comments about this book or if you'd like to consider using my services, please don't hesitate to contact me at onyourpathtohealing@gmail.com.

Glossary

Acid Reflux—*see Gastroesophageal Reflux Disease.*

Acupuncture—A traditional Chinese practice of inserting fine needles through the skin at specific points, especially to cure disease or relieve pain. With children, needles are often replaced with other tools. *See also Acupressure.*

Acupressure—The application of pressure (as with the thumbs or fingertips) to the same discrete points on the body stimulated in acupuncture that is used for its therapeutic effects (as the relief of tension or pain).

Adrenals—A pair of complex endocrine organs near the anterior medial border of the kidney, consisting of a mesodermal cortex that produces glucocorticoid, mineralocorticoid, and androgenic hormones, and an ectodermal medulla that produces epinephrine and norepinephrine.

Adrenal Fatigue—A term used in alternative medicine to describe the unproven theory that the adrenal glands are exhausted and unable to produce adequate quantities of hormones, primarily the glucocorticoid cortisol. The term "adrenal fatigue" may be applied to a collection of mostly nonspecific symptoms such as "tiredness, trouble falling asleep at night or waking up in the morning, salt and sugar cravings, and needing stimulants like caffeine to get through the day." There is no scientific evidence supporting the concept of adrenal fatigue, and it is not recognized as an actual diagnosis by the medical community.

Allergy—An exaggerated or pathological immunological reaction by the body to substances, foods, situations, or physical states. A food allergy requires the presence of Immunoglobin E (IgE) antibodies against the food. Symptoms may include sneezing, difficulty breathing, itching, or skin rashes.

Amino Acid—A molecule that is the basic ingredient necessary to create a protein. Amino acids link together in chains to form proteins. Some amino acids are created by the body, but others can only be obtained by eating foods that contain them, such as meat, dairy products, or beans. Amino acids are used both as the basic building blocks of proteins and as an alternative source of energy in cells. They are necessary for all cells in all known living things.

Inadequate intake of amino acids (and/or protein) can have extremely serious health consequences. Amino acids naturally assist the body to make the brain's neurotransmitters without the use of medication. Eating enough foods containing amino acids completes a very important biological process.

Applied Behavior Analysis (ABA)—Previously known as behavior modification, ABA is the application of operant and classical conditioning that modifies human behaviors, especially as part of a learning or treatment process. Behavior analysts focus on the observable relationship of behavior to the environment, including antecedents and consequences, without resorting to "hypothetical constructs." By functionally assessing the relationship between a targeted behavior and the environment, the methods of ABA can be used to change that behavior.

Applied Kinesiology—An alternative healing diagnostic tool that allows you to ask your body "yes or no" questions. It works with the idea that a positive association or "yes" strengthens the muscles, while a negative association or "no" weakens them. Bypassing conscious thought, muscle testing accesses your intuitive and energetic systems. It is not a replacement for conventional medical diagnostics but can be very useful when a blood test is not available.

Apraxia—Apraxia is a disorder that can stand alone or coexist with other conditions. Apraxia is a neurologically based motor-planning disorder that impacts speech and often affects gross motor skills (crawling, walking, and jumping) and fine motor sequencing (writing, dressing, and brushing teeth). Confusion about this condition is reflected by the number of terms used to define it, including childhood apraxia of speech, developmental apraxia, developmental dyspraxia, and speech dyspraxia.

Asperger's Syndrome—A subtype of autism that is categorized as a condition by which a person has relative preservation of linguistic and cognitive development. However, the person has issues with some basic skills, most notably with nonverbal communication—e.g., problems with eye contact and facial expressions. Asperger's children may also have problems socializing with others, feeling empathy for others, and using imagination. These children often have limited interests and exhibit eccentric repetitive movements. They have trouble making friends because of their lack of social skills. At times, these children do not respond to their names when called and act like others around them do not exist. Characteristically, these children appear awkward and have many problems maintaining reciprocal relationships. Children with ASD may engage with adults long enough to get their needs met, but may virtually ignore that same adult afterward. These children may often get stuck in an obsessive thought pattern in their heads with little room for much of anything else.

Note: The American Psychiatric Association (APA) announced the publication in May 2013 of their new diagnostic manual, in which Asperger's Syndrome was removed as an independently listed condition (as well as Pervasive Development Disorder—Not Otherwise Specified) and instead replaced it with a sole diagnosis of Autistic Spectrum Disorder (ASD).

Attention Deficit Disorder (ADD)—A syndrome of disordered learning and disruptive behavior that is characterized primarily by symptoms of inattentiveness and distractibility.

Attention Deficit Hyperactivity Disorder (ADHD)—A syndrome of disordered learning and disruptive behavior that is characterized primarily by symptoms of inattentiveness or primarily by symptoms of hyperactivity and impulsive behavior (such as speaking out of turn).

Auditory Integration Training (AIT)—Auditory integration training (AIT) is one specific type of music/auditory therapy based upon the work of French otolaryngologists Dr. Alfred Tomatis and Dr. Guy Berard. The premise upon which most auditory integration programs are based is that distortion in how things are heard contributes to commonly seen behavioral or learning disorders in children. Some of these disorders include attention deficit/hyperactive disorder (ADHD), autism, dyslexia, and central auditory processing disorders (CAPD). Training the patient to listen can stimulate central and cortical brain organization.

Autism Spectrum Disorder (ASD)—A set of complex neurodevelopment disorders that cause individuals to display mild to severe persistent impairments in social interaction and communication along with restricted, repetitive, and stereotyped patterns of behaviors, interests, and activities. Children with the disorder have marked difficulties with social interaction and display problems with verbal and nonverbal communication. They often exhibit ritualistic behavior ("stimming," which is short for self-stimulating behavior) like hand flapping or rocking. Thoughts are often obsessive, and behaviors are compulsive. Severity is based on social communication impairments and restricted repetitive patterns of behavior.

Autoimmune Disorder/Disease—Any of a large group of diseases that arise from an inappropriate immune response of the body against substances and tissues normally present in the body (autoimmunity).

Biofilm—A usually thin and resistant layer of microorganisms (such as bacteria) that form on and coat various surfaces. In a healthy gut filled with beneficial microflora, the biofilm remains thin so that the nutrients can pass through the intestinal wall and actually assist in the moistening of the intestinal tract, protecting from infection, inflammation, and toxins that are ingested. If the gut is unhealthy, the film remains thicker and becomes a source of inflamma-tion. Unhealthy biofilm houses toxins like heavy metals and promotes more bacteria, parasites, and yeast overgrowth. In addition, because nutrients can-not be properly absorbed, the thicker biofilm causes nutritional deficiency.

Biomedicine—The branch of medical science that deals with the ability of humans to tolerate environmental stresses and variations. The application of the principles of the natural sciences, especially biology and physiology, to clinical medicine.

Biomedical Protocol—With regard to ADHD and autism spectrum disorders, it is a systemic evaluation and treatment of the entire child. It is the combi-nation of mainstream and alternative modalities working in harmony to heal the child. The protocol includes close examination of the gastrointestinal sys-tem, immune system, metabolic and underlying conditions, along with nutri-ent therapy. Although biomedical treatment is considered alternative by the American Academy of Pediatrics, there is no denying that biomedical treat-ments often help to treat these disorders successfully.

BioSET—An allergy elimination technique created by Dr. Ellen Cutler. It is being used in the treatment of allergy-related ADHD and autism spectrum disorders, along with many other ailments. It uses applied kinesiology, acupressure, enzyme therapy, and the laws of quantum physics to redirect and reprogram a body's immune responses to ordinary benign substances like food.

Candida—A genus of yeast-like fungi that are commonly part of the normal flora of the mouth, skin, intestinal tract, and vagina, but which can overgrow and cause a variety of infections. Thrush is found on the tongue of children. Candida/yeast infections lead to a variety of illnesses and symptoms, both medically and emotionally. The holistic community believes it to be one of the underlying causes of autoimmune disorders.

Casein—The protein commonly found in mammalian milk, making up eighty percent of the proteins in cow's milk and between twenty and forty-five per-cent of the proteins in human milk. Many people have an intolerance to milk protein. This is not the same thing as lactose intolerance. *See lactose.*

Celiac Disease—An autoimmune disorder in the small intestine to the protein gluten, found in wheat, rye, barley, and sometimes oats. This inflammation damages the tissues and results in impaired ability to absorb nutrients from foods. It is also called sprue, nontropical sprue, gluten sensitive enteropathy, celiac sprue, and adult celiac disease. It may be discovered at any age.

Childhood Disintegrative Disorder—Also known as Heller's syndrome, this disorder marks a regression in at least two areas of development, including language, potty training, social skills, and motor skills. The child begins losing important developmental milestones. The onset of CDD is between age two and ten years.

Chiropractic—A healthcare profession that focuses on disorders of the musculoskeletal system and the nervous system and the effects of these disorders on general health. Chiropractic care is used most often to treat neuromusculoskeletal complaints, including but not limited to back pain, neck pain, joint pain of the arms or legs, and headaches. Doctors of chiropractic are often referred to as chiropractors or chiropractic physicians. However, they are not licensed to prescribe medication. They practice a drug-free, hands-on approach to health care that includes patient examination, diagnosis, and treatment. Chiropractors have broad diagnostic skills and are also trained to recommend therapeutic and rehabilitative exercises, as well as to provide nutritional, dietary, and lifestyle counseling.

Congenital Disorder of Glycosylation Type Ia (CDG)—One of several rare inborn errors of metabolism in which glycosylation of a variety of tissue proteins and/or lipids is deficient or defective. Congenital disorders of glycosylation are sometimes known as CDG syndromes. They often cause serious, sometimes fatal, malfunctions of several different organ systems (especially the nervous system, muscles, and intestines) in affected infants. This disorder can have varying degrees of severity. The disorder was previously called carbohydrate-deficient glycoprotein syndrome.

Cortisol—A steroid hormone, more specifically a glucocorticoid, produced by the zona fasciculata of the adrenal cortex. It is released in response to stress and a low level of blood glucocorticoids. Its primary functions are to increase blood sugar through gluconeogenesis; suppress the immune system; and aid in fat, protein, and carbohydrate metabolism. It also decreases bone formation. Low cortisol levels can be very dangerous and can result in muscle weakness, muscle pain, joint pain, fatigue, loss of appetite, weight loss, cravings for salt, low blood pressure, low energy, low blood sugar, darkening of skin, changes in mood, sleep disturbances, depression, and irritability.

Cradle Cap—A yellowish, patchy, greasy, scaly, and crusty skin rash that occurs on the scalp of recently born babies. It is usually not itchy and does not bother the baby. Cradle cap most commonly begins sometime in the first three months of life. Similar symptoms in older children are more likely to be dandruff than cradle cap. The rash is often prominent around the ear, the eyebrows, or the eyelids. It may appear in other locations as well, where it is called seborrheic dermatitis rather than cradle cap.

Cranial Distortion—A condition characterized by an asymmetrical distortion (flattening of one side) of the skull. It is characterized by a flat spot on the back or one side of the head. Often, there is also facial asymmetry.

Craniosacral Therapy—A form of bodywork or alternative therapy focused primarily on the concept of "primary respiration" and regulating the flow of cerebrospinal fluid by using therapeutic touch to manipulate the synarthrodial joints of the cranium. Craniosacral therapy was developed by Dr. John Upledger in the 1970s, and is loosely based on osteopathy in the cranial field (OCF), which was developed in the 1930s by William Garner Sutherland. In the United States, OCF, or cranial osteopathy, as it is more commonly known, can only be practiced by fully licensed occupational therapists and physicians (DOs, MDs), and, in some states, licensed naturopathic physicians (NDs).

DAN (Defeat Autism Now) Doctor—An MD or naturopathic physician who uses biomedical techniques to treat children with autism. A project of the Autism Research Institute, founded in the 1960s by Dr. Bernard Rimland, DAN Doctors are trained in the "DAN Protocol," an approach to autism treatment that starts with the idea that autism is a biomedical disorder. Specifically, these doctors feel that autism is a disorder caused by a combination of lowered immune response, external toxins from vaccines and other sources, and problems caused by certain foods.

Depression—A state of sadness and unhappiness; a disorder showing symptoms such as persistent feelings of hopelessness, dejection, poor concentration, lack of energy, inability to sleep, and, sometimes, suicidal tendencies.

Dopamine—A pleasure-producing neurotransmitter (messenger) in the brain. It is classified as a catecholamine (a class of molecules that serve as neurotransmitters and hormones). At correct levels, it helps a person feel happy and is important for cognition, motor movement, and cognitive stability. Elevated dopamine can contribute to OCD, impulsivity, and pleasure-seeking and repetitive behaviors such as the compulsion to play video games or an obsession with violence. Reduced levels can contribute to fatigue, irritability, and the inability to carry out simple tasks.

Dyslexia—A learning disorder marked by a severe difficulty in recognizing and understanding written language, leading to spelling and writing problems. It is not caused by low intelligence or brain damage.

Dyspraxia—*see Apraxia.*

Eczema (aka Atopic Dermatitis)—An inflammatory skin condition characterized by reddening and itching and the formation of scaly or crusty patches that may leak fluid.

Elimination Diet—Procedure used to identify foods that may be causing an adverse effect in a person, in which all suspected foods are excluded from the diet and then reintroduced one at a time.

Epinephrine—Also called adrenaline. A hormone secreted by the adrenal medulla upon stimulation by the central nervous system in response to stress, such as anger or fear, and acting to increase heart rate, blood pressure, cardiac output, and carbohydrate metabolism. Our "fight or flight" response. Too much epinephrine can create severe anxiety and heart palpitations.

Essential Oils—Any of a class of volatile oils obtained from plants, possessing the odor and other characteristic properties of the plant, used chiefly in the manufacturing of perfumes, flavors, and pharmaceuticals.

Equine Therapy—Also known as hippotherapy, equine therapy is the use of horses in a form of therapeutic riding in order to achieve goals that enhance physical, emotional, social, cognitive, behavioral, and educational skills for people who have disabilities. It not only focuses on the therapeutic riding skills but also on the development of a relationship between horse and rider. It uses a team approach in order to provide treatment for the individual with the guidance of a riding instructor.

Feingold Diet—A food elimination program developed by Ben F. Feingold, MD, to treat hyperactivity. It eliminates a number of artificial colors and artificial flavors, aspartame, three petroleum-based preservatives, and (at least initially) certain salicylates. There has been much debate about the efficacy of this program. The mainstream medical establishment dismissed it as an "outmoded approach" lacking evidence and efficacy, but some medical practitioners, as well as many people living with ADHD and parents of children with ADHD, claim that it is effective in the management of ADHD and a number of other behavioral, physical, and neurological conditions, including salicylate sensitivity. The debate has continued for more than thirty years, involving not only consumers and physicians, but scientists, politicians, and the pharmaceutical and food industries.

Fermented Soy—The breaking down of the organic raw soy bean. Fermenting soy is often done by allowing raw soybeans to grow mold, adding water and salt, and allowing the soy to ferment.

Food Sensitivity/Intolerance—A non-allergic food hypersensitivity is a term used widely for varied physiological responses associated with a particular food or compound found in a range of foods. Food intolerance may be an autoimmune reaction to a food, beverage, food additive, or compound found in foods that produces symptoms in one or more body organs and systems. A food sensitivity requires the presence of immunoglobin G (IgG) antibodies against the food or substance. The result is that the body cannot completely process a food, resulting in partially digested proteins and sugars. This happens especially with processed foods like grains, milk, and sugars. An alternative to IgG testing is the ALCAT test, which exposes your white blood cells to over 350 different foods and chemicals, measuring how they react to a wide variety of things in your current diet and daily life.

Functional Medicine—A medical practice that addresses the underlying causes of disease using a systems-oriented approach and engaging both patient and practitioner in a therapeutic partnership. It is an evolution in the practice of medicine that better addresses the healthcare needs of the 21st century. By shifting the traditional, disease-centered focus of medical practice to a more patient-centered approach, functional medicine addresses the whole person, not just an isolated set of symptoms. Functional medicine practitioners spend time with their patients, listening to their histories and looking at the interactions among genetic, environmental, and lifestyle factors that can influence long-term health and complex, chronic disease. In this way, functional medicine supports the unique expression of health and vitality for each individual.

GAPS Diet (Gut and Psychology Syndrome Diet)—A modern development of the Specific Carbohydrate Diet, created by Dr. Natasha Campbell-McBride, which intends to heal digestive disorders and psychological issues. The premise is that there is a direct correlation between the state of intestinal flora and brain chemistry. By cleaning or healing the gut, according to Campbell-McBride, the patient will lose weight while treating a variety of medical conditions. The nutritional component of the GAPS diet has three phases: diet, supplementation, and detoxification and lifestyle changes. The diet plan offers a do-not-eat list that changes depending on the program phase. The purpose of the GAPS diet nutritional component is to heal the previous damage that foods have done to the gut.

Gastroesophageal Reflux Disease (GERD)/Acid Reflux—A chronic symptom of mucosal damage caused by stomach acid coming up from the stomach into the esophagus. GERD is usually caused by changes in the barrier between the stomach and the esophagus, including abnormal relaxation of the lower esophageal sphincter, which normally holds the top of the stomach closed, impaired expulsion of gastric reflux from the esophagus, or a hiatal hernia.

Gene Modifier—A gene that influences the expression of another gene. For example, one gene controls whether eye color is blue or brown, but other (modifier) genes can also influence the color by affecting the amount or distribution of pigment in the iris.

Genetic Mutation/Gene Mutation—A change or alteration in the DNA sequence. Mutations cause changes in the genetic code that can lead to disease. Mutations occur in two ways: one, they can be inherited by a parent, or two, they can be acquired during a person's lifetime when cells are exposed to environmental triggers such as ultraviolet radiation, pollution, and toxic chemicals. Specific mutations can prevent necessary chemical reactions in the body from occurring, and can inhibit the body's ability to digest foods, detox effectively, transport substances between cells, and utilize nutrients appropriately.

Genetically Modified Organism (GMO)—An organism with genetic material that has been altered using genetic-engineering techniques. Long-term effects of genetically modified foods are unknown.

Glutathione—Glutathione is produced in the human liver and plays a key role in intermediary metabolism, immune response, and health, though many of its mechanisms and much of its behavior await further medical understanding. It is also known as gamma-glutamylcysteineglycine and GHS. It is a small protein composed of three amino acids: cysteine, glutamic acid, and glyceine. Glutathione, in purified, extracted form, is a white powder that is soluble in water and in alcohol. It is found naturally in many fruits, vegetables, and meats. However, absorption rates of glutathione from food sources in the human gastrointestinal tract are low.

Gluten—A protein found in wheat, rye, barley, and sometimes oats. Gluten causes an inflammatory response in the small intestine, which damages the tissues and results in an impaired ability to absorb nutrients from foods. Many individuals with ADHD and ASD are highly sensitive to gluten, even though initial lab work may not reflect celiac disease. Researchers believe that a combination of genetic and environmental factors trigger the sensitivity. Environmental events that may provoke celiac disease in those with a genetic predisposition to the disorder include surgery or a viral infection.

Gluten-Free/Casein-Free Diet (GFCF)—A diet that strictly eliminates the dietary intake of the naturally occurring proteins gluten (found most often in wheat, barley, rye, and commercially available oats) and casein (found most often in milk and dairy products). Despite an absence of scientific evidence, there have been advocates for the use of this diet as a treatment for autism and related conditions.

Gut Flora—A complex of microorganism species that live in the digestive tracts of animals and comprise the largest reservoir of human flora. In this context, "gut" is synonymous with "intestines," and "flora" with "microbiota" and "microflora"; the word "microbiome" is also in use. Gut flora's primary benefit to the host is the gleaning of energy from the fermentation of undigested carbohydrates and the subsequent absorption of short chain fatty acids. Intestinal bacteria also play a role in synthesizing vitamin B and vitamin K, as well as metabolizing bile acids, sterols, and xenobiotics. The human body carries about 100 trillion microorganisms in its intestines.

Gut Permeability—A condition by which the intestinal wall breaks down and becomes overly porous due to inflammation. Food molecules enter the bloodstream instead of being absorbed by the intestines. Their nutrients—including vitamins, minerals, and amino acids—that should have been absorbed by the intestines, metabolized, and used in the body, instead are simply lost. This condition also alters the metabolism of proteins, carbohydrates, and lipids in the body.

Hepatic Stress—A condition that results when the liver is working overtime to excrete toxins. When the body is not detoxifying adequately enough, it leads to an increase of free radicals, which, in turn, leads to an excretion of reactive byproducts into bile, producing toxic bile capable of damaging bile ducts and refluxing into the pancreas. This toxic bile, rich in free radicals, further damages the small-bowel mucosa, exacerbating hyperpermeability. In addition, by attempting to eliminate toxic oxidation products, the liver then depletes its reserves of sulfur-containing amino acids, which would have assisted in the detoxifying process.

Hepatitis B (Hep B)—An infectious inflammatory illness of the liver caused by the hepatitis B virus (HBV) that affects humans. Originally known as "serum hepatitis," the disease has caused epidemics in parts of Africa and Asia, including China. About a third of the world population has been infected at one point in their lives, including 350 million who are chronic carriers. The virus is transmitted by exposure to infected blood or body fluids such as semen and vaginal fluids, while viral DNA has been detected in the saliva, tears, and urine of chronic carriers. Perinatal infection is a major route of infection in endemic (mainly developing) countries. Other risk factors for developing HBV infection include working in a healthcare setting, transfusions, dialysis, acupuncture, tattooing, sharing razors or toothbrushes with an infected person, travel in countries where it is endemic, and residence in an institution. However, hepatitis B viruses cannot be spread by holding hands, sharing eating utensils or drinking glasses, kissing, hugging, coughing, sneezing, or breastfeeding.

Hippotherapy—*see Equine Therapy.*

Histadelia—An inherited condition found primarily in males and characterized by too much histamine in the blood. These elevated blood levels of histamine are caused by a metabolic imbalance known as under-methylation.

This is an important biochemical process, which is responsible for the elimination of histamine, as well as the production of certain neurotransmitters, and, if low, creates a deficiency in serotonin, dopamine, and norepinephrine. Sufferers often exhibit psychological, behavioral, and cognitive symptoms, including depression, suicidal thoughts, blank mind episodes, phobias, OCD, insomnia, muscle pain, hyperactivity, and addictive tendencies. Other symptoms include rapid metabolism (hunger), asthma, excess saliva, running eyes, seasonal allergies, frequent cold symptoms, profuse sweating, pruritis and other skin conditions, and headaches.

Histamine—An organic nitrogen compound involved in local immune responses, as well as in regulating physiological function in the gut and acting as a neurotransmitter. Histamine triggers the inflammatory response. Histamine increases the permeability of the capillaries to white blood cells and some proteins to allow them to engage pathogens in the infected tissues.

Holistic—A belief that a whole system of conditions must be analyzed rather than simply its individual components. Holistic practitioners consider all factors when treating illness, taking into account all of a patient's physical, mental, and social conditions in the treatment of illness.

Homeopathy/Homeopathic Medicine—A system of medical practice that treats a disease by administrating minute doses of a remedy that would, in larger amounts, produce in healthy persons symptoms similar to those of the disease. This system of alternative medicine originated in 1796 by Samuel Hahnemann. This practice is not recognized by the scientific community because of the lack of scientific evidence of its efficacy, but a similar method is used in the administering of allergy shots by medically recognized allergists.

Hormone—A chemical substance produced in the body that has a specific regulatory effect on the activity of certain cells or a certain organ or organs. *Also see Neurotransmitter.*

Hygiene Hypothesis—A theory that children not exposed to bacteria and dirt and given too many antibacterial soaps develop weak immune systems and are prone to adult allergies, asthma, etc. The premise is that the immune system needs to be exposed to bacteria in order to strengthen itself.

Hypoglycemia—An abnormally diminished content of glucose in the blood, or "low blood sugar."

Insomnia—The inability to obtain sufficient sleep, especially when chronic; difficulty in falling or staying asleep; sleeplessness.

Integrative Medicine—A healing-oriented medicine that takes the whole person (body, mind, and spirit) into account, including all aspects of lifestyle. It emphasizes the therapeutic relationship and makes use of all appropriate therapies, both conventional and alternative. A philosophy that neither rejects conventional medicine nor accepts alternative therapies uncritically. Recognition that good medicine should be based in good science, be inquiry-driven, and be open to new paradigms. Use of natural, effective, less invasive interventions whenever possible. Promotes prevention of illness as well as the treatment of disease.

Ketogenic Diet—A special high-fat, low-carbohydrate diet that helps to control seizures in some people with epilepsy. It is prescribed by a physician and carefully monitored. The name *ketogenic* means that it produces ketones in the body (keto = ketone, genic = producing). Ketones are formed when the body uses fat for its source of energy instead of carbohydrates found in sugar, bread, or pasta. Ketones are one of the more likely mechanisms of action of the diet, with higher ketone levels often leading to improved seizure control. However, there are many other theories for why the diet may work. This diet could produce some side effects, so careful monitoring is important.

Kidney—One of a pair of organs located in the right and left sides of the abdomen. The kidneys remove waste products from the blood and produce urine. As blood flows through the kidneys, the kidneys filter waste products, chemicals, and unneeded water from the blood. Urine collects in the middle of each kidney in an area called the renal pelvis. It then drains from the kidney through a long tube, the ureter, to the bladder, where it is stored until elimination. The kidneys also make substances that help control blood pressure and regulate the formation of red blood cells.

Lactose—The sugar found in milk and, to a lesser extent, milk-derived dairy products. Lactose intolerance, or hypolactasia, is the inability to digest lactose. It is not a disorder as such, but a genetically-determined characteristic.

Leaky Gut Syndrome—*see Gut Permeability.*

Learning Disability—A group of disorders characterized by inadequate development of specific academic, language, and speech skills. Types of learning disabilities include reading disability (dyslexia), mathematics disability (dyscalculia), and writing disability (dysgraphia). In order to be classified as learning disabled, an individual must meet certain criteria as determined by a professional (psychologist, pediatrician, etc.). This disorder affects the brain's ability to receive and process information and makes it problematic for a person to learn as quickly or in the same way as someone who is not affected by a learning disability. People with a learning disability have trouble performing specific types of skills or completing tasks if left to figure things out by themselves or if taught in conventional ways.

Liver—The largest solid organ in the body, situated in the upper part of the abdomen on the right side. The liver has a multitude of important and complex functions, including to manufacture proteins, such as albumin (to help maintain the volume of blood), and blood-clotting factors; to synthesize, store, and process fats, including fatty acids (used for energy) and cholesterol; to metabolize and store carbohydrates (used as the source for the sugar in blood); to form and secrete bile that contains bile acids to aid in the intestinal absorption of fats and the fat-soluble vitamins A, D, E, and K; to eliminate, by metabolizing or secreting, the potentially harmful biochemical products produced by the body, such as bilirubin, from the breakdown of old red blood cells and ammonia from the breakdown of proteins; and to detoxify, by metabolizing and/or secreting, drugs, alcohol, and environmental toxins.

Malabsorption—A state arising from abnormality in absorption of food nutrients across the gastrointestinal (GI) tract. Impairment can be of single or multiple nutrients, depending on the abnormality. This may lead to malnutrition and a variety of anemias.

Melatonin—A hormone derived from serotonin and produced by the pineal gland that plays a role in sleep, aging, and reproduction in mammals. Vitamin B3, B6, B9, and the amino acid tryptophan trigger the production of serotonin, which then triggers the production of melatonin in the brain.

Massage—*see Therapeutic Massage.*

Metallothionein (mt)—A cysteine-rich, heat-stable, low-molecular-weight family of proteins that can bind heavy metals such as cadmium, copper, mercury, and zinc. Functions attributed to mt include detoxification, storage, and regulation of these metals.

Mineral—The building blocks of rocks, a substance that occurs naturally in nature. Minerals nurture our soil and feed our plants. Plant-derived minerals are the best dietary source of minerals and should be eaten regularly so that they are abundant in the body. The seven major minerals are calcium, phosphorus, potassium, sulfur, sodium, chloride, and magnesium. Important "trace" or minor minerals necessary for mammalian life include iron, cobalt, copper, zinc, molybdenum, iodine, and selenium. Over twenty dietary minerals are necessary for mammals. They have different benefits, and no mineral can be termed as more beneficial or less beneficial. All minerals are critical for proper functioning of the body. Most of the minerals aid in body metabolism, detoxification, water balance, and bone health.

MTHFR (Gene Mutation)—A gene mutation that inhibits the body's ability to transform vitamin B12 into vital folate enzymes. A healthy MTHFR gene converts vitamin B12 to folate (B9), an essential vitamin for brain, spine, and nerve health. Folate/folic acid also produces healthy red blood cells and aids in rapid cell division.

Muscle Testing—*see Applied Kinesiology.*

Nambudripad's Allergy Elimination Techniques (NAET)—An allergy elimination technique devised by Devi Nambudripad, a California-based chiropractor and acupuncturist, for the treatment of allergy-related illness. It has been used successfully in the treatment of allergy-related ADHD and autism. It is a noninvasive procedure that uses muscle testing (applied kinesiology) and acupressure to reverse the allergy or sensitivity. This technique does not require any blood draws, scratch tests, or shots. If the children are small, an adult becomes the energy conduit. Large numbers of autism spectrum children have been studied following aggressive allergy elimination treatment (NAET) and have displayed remarkable success.

Naturopath (ND)—A doctor who practices naturopathy. NDs have a PhD in naturopathic medicine. Some MDs also become NDs and are referred to as NMDs.

Naturopathy (Naturopathic Medicine)—A system of medicine based on the healing power of nature. Naturopathy is a holistic system, meaning that naturopathic doctors (NDs) or naturopathic medical doctors (NMDs) strive to find the cause of disease by understanding the body, mind, and spirit of the person. Most naturopathic doctors use a variety of therapies and techniques, such as nutrition, behavior change, herbal medicine, homeopathy, and acupuncture. There are two areas of focus in naturopathy: one is supporting the body's own healing abilities, and the other is empowering people to make lifestyle changes necessary for the best possible health. While naturopathic doctors treat both short bouts of illness and chronic conditions, their emphasis is on preventing disease and educating patients. Naturopathy favors a holistic approach with noninvasive treatment and encourages minimal use of surgery and drugs to achieve optimal health.

Neonatal Intensive Care Unit (NICU)—An intensive care unit specializing in the care of ill or premature newborn infants.

Neurofeedback—A computer-aided technique for training the brain to regulate itself without the use of medication or invasive procedures. It is an operant conditioning tool that simply retrains the brain to behave normally and to arouse when appropriate and calm down when appropriate. It is a noninvasive treatment that does not shock or manipulate the brain in any way, but produces a measurable physiological effect on the brain. Neurofeedback helps improve alertness, attention, emotional regulation, behavior, cognitive function, and mental flexibility. It was introduced in the 1960s, and although it has not met scientific standards for efficacy, it is believed by many to be very effective in conjunction with biomedical treatment and traditional psychotherapy.

Neurotherapy—*see Neurofeedback.*

Neurotoxin—Any substance that causes damage to nerves or nerve tissue, such as arsenic and lead.

Neurotransmitters—Several chemical messengers that transmit nerve impulses across a synapse between nerve cells or from nerve cells to muscles and glands. Neurotransmitters play a major role in everyday life and functioning. Scientists do not yet know exactly how many neurotransmitters exist, but more than one hundred chemical messengers have been identified.

Norepinephrine—A hormone/neurotransmitter, secreted by the adrenal gland and similar to epinephrine, that is the principal neurotransmitter of sympathetic nerve endings supplying the major organs and skin. Norepinephrine controls heart rate and blood pressure and contributes to sleep, arousal, and emotions. Too much can create feelings of anxiety, while too little can create depression and numbness.

Nutrient—A substance that provides nourishment—e.g., the minerals that a plant takes from the soil or the constituents in food that keep a human body healthy and help it to live and grow. Used in an organism's metabolism, which must be taken in from its environment. Nutrients are used to build and repair tissues, regulate body processes, and are converted into energy.

Nutritional Deficiency—An absence or insufficiency of essential vitamins, minerals, and other nutrients. Nutritional deficiencies can be caused when a person's nutrient intake consistently falls below the recommended requirement or by metabolic issues and leaky gut syndrome. Nutritional deficiencies can lead to developmental problems, "failure to thrive," growth delays, and illness and disease.

Obsessive Compulsive Disorder (OCD)—An anxiety disorder characterized by unreasonable thoughts and fears (obsessions) that lead a person to do repetitive behaviors (compulsions) to help relieve or manage the anxious, fearful, or worrysome feelings. Consciously, one often realizes that their thoughts are unreasonable and tries to stop them. This usually increases the distress, and the individual is driven to perform more compulsive acts.

Organic Foods—Foods that are produced using methods of organic farming that do not involve modern synthetic inputs such as synthetic pesticides and chemical fertilizers. Organic foods are also not processed using irradiation, industrial solvents, or chemical food additives. The organic farming movement arose in the 1940s. Organic food production is a heavily regulated industry. Organic certification is a process for producers of organic food and other organic agricultural products. In general, any business directly involved in food production can be certified, including seed suppliers, farmers, food processors, retailers, and restaurants.

Osteopathy—A form of alternative health care that emphasizes the interrelationship between structures and functions of the body, as well as the body's ability to heal itself. Osteopaths facilitate the healing process, principally by the practice of manual and manipulative therapy. The scope of practice of osteopathic practitioners varies by country. Osteopathic physicians in the U.S. are doctors and are most often integrative physicians trained in both Eastern and Western medicine practices. Note: Osteopaths trained outside the U.S. may not be physicians and are more limited in practice.

Pancreas—A gland situated near the stomach that secretes a digestive fluid into the intestine through one or more ducts and also secretes the hormone insulin.

PANDAS—A term used to describe children who have a rapid onset of OCD-type symptoms, and/or tic disorders that are thought to be due to an autoimmune response to a strep infection. It is believed that the body continues to produce antibodies to the strep bacteria, which mistakenly react in a part of the brain called the basal ganglia. The basil ganglia controls a body's movement and behavior, thus creating the symptoms.

Parasite (Intestinal)—An organism that lives on or in an organism of another species, known as the host, and obtains nourishment from the host. Many parasites live within our intestines and are virtually harmless. Others cause gastrointestinal problems, malnutrition, acute diarrhea, and constipation, and are an unsuspected cause of many illnesses. Two types of parasites include tapeworms and roundworms. They attach themselves to the lining of the small intestines, causing internal bleeding and the loss of essential nutrients. They may not produce obvious symptoms and may cause the slow loss of iron in the body of the host. The second type are protozoa, tiny one-celled organisms that can be the cause of acute or chronic diarrhea or even constipation, fatigue, joint pain, dizziness, or hives.

Pervasive Developmental Disorder (PDD)—A group of conditions that involve delays in the development of many basic skills. Most notable among them are problems with fine and gross motor skills and the inability to socialize with others or communicate due to speech delays. Children with these conditions often are confused in their thinking and generally have problems understanding the world around them. Because these conditions are typically identified in children around three years of age (a critical period in a child's development), they are called developmental disorders. The condition actually starts far earlier than age three, but parents often do not notice a problem until the child is a toddler who is still not walking, talking, or developing in similar ways as other children of the same age.

Note: The American Psychiatric Association (APA) announced the publication in May 2013 of their new diagnostic manual, which removed Pervasive Developmental Disorder—Not Otherwise Specified as an independently listed condition (as well as Asperger's) and instead replaced it with a sole diagnosis of Autistic Spectrum Disorder (ASD).

Prebiotic—Nondigestible dietary fiber that triggers the growth of healthy gut bacteria. The most common type of prebiotic is the soluble fiber inulin. Best sources include asparagus, chicory, garlic, leek, onion, and artichoke.

Probiotic—A preparation (as a dietary supplement) containing live bacteria (such as lactobacilli) that benefit humans and animals—e.g., by restoring the balance of microflora in the digestive tract.

Psoriasis—An autoimmune disease that produces a noncontagious, reddish, scaly rash often located over the surfaces of the elbows, knees, scalp, and around or in the ears, navel, genitals, or buttocks. Chronic plaque psoriasis affects many people around the world. About ten to fifteen percent of patients with psoriasis develop joint inflammation (inflammatory arthritis).

Psychiatrist—A physician (MD) who specializes in the diagnosis and treatment of mental illness. A psychiatrist must receive additional training and serve a supervised residency in his or her specialty. He or she may also have additional training in a psychiatric specialty, such as child psychiatry or neuropsychiatry. Psychiatrists often prescribe medication.

Psychologist—A doctorate-level clinician specializing in diagnosing and treating diseases of the brain, emotional disturbances, and behavioral problems. A doctoral degree is usually required for independent practice as a psychologist. Psychologists with a PhD or Doctor of Psychology (PsyD) qualify for a wide range of teaching, research, clinical, and counseling positions in universities, healthcare services, elementary and secondary schools, private industry, and government agencies. Psychologists with a doctoral degree often work in clinical positions or in private practices, but they also sometimes teach, complete educational assessments, conduct research, or carry out administrative responsibilities. In a clinical setting, a psychologist uses talk therapy and other noninvasive modalities to treat clients. A psychologist will often refer to a psychiatrist or other medical doctor if medication is warranted. Psychologists cannot prescribe medication.

Psychotherapist—A masters degree–level clinician who engages clients in "talk therapy" or in other noninvasive modalities using a variety of therapeutic theoretical approaches in order to improve quality of life, satisfaction in relationships, functioning in society, performance in work or play, and general psychological health and well-being. Psychotherapists have diverse educational and training backgrounds. A master's degree as well as a state license is required for independent practice. Some disciplines include Licensed Marriage and Family Therapists (LMFT), Licensed Professional Counselors (LPC), and Licensed Clinical Social Workers (LCSW). Psychotherapists cannot prescribe medication.

Pyrrole Disorder—An abnormality in biochemistry resulting in the overproduction of urinary pyrrole called OHHPL (hydroxyhemoppyrrolin-2-one), which leaches zinc and essential B3 and B6 vitamins from the body. It was first discovered in the late 1950s by a team of Canadian researchers led by Abram Hoffer, MD, when they identified a novel compound in the urine of patients with schizophrenia. In the 1960s, Dr. Hoffer and colleagues published clinical outcomes of schizophrenic and other mentally ill patients with high urinary pyrrole levels, showing that treatment with a high dose of vitamin B3 normalized the levels and treated clinical symptoms. In the 1970s, Carl Pfeiffer, MD, showed similar results with high levels of vitamin B6 and zinc, the current treatment of choice.

Reflexology—A system of massage used to relieve tension and treat illness, based on the theory that there are reflex points on the feet, hands, and head linked to every part of the body.

Reiki—A healing technique based on the principle that the therapist can channel energy into the patient by way of touch to activate the natural healing processes of the patient's body and restore physical and emotional well-being.

Rotation Diet—A plan that requires eating different foods throughout the day in a four-day period to decrease the likelihood of developing new allergies or sensitivities. People with mild food intolerances may find that if they follow the rotation diet, they can eventually tolerate certain foods better.

Seizure—A sudden disruption of the brain's normal electrical activity, accompanied by altered consciousness and/or other neurological and behavioral manifestations. Epilepsy is a condition characterized by recurrent seizures that may include repetitive muscle jerking called convulsions.

Sensory Processing Disorder—A condition in which the brain has trouble receiving and responding to information that comes in through the senses. The condition used to be called sensory integration dysfunction. Some people with sensory processing disorder are oversensitive to things in their environment. Common sounds may be painful or overwhelming. The light touch of a shirt may chafe the skin. Individuals with sensory processing disorder may lack coordination, are unable to tell where their limbs are in space, and have difficulty engaging in conversation and play. Sensory processing problems are usually identified in children but can also be present in adults. These problems are commonly seen in those with developmental disorders like autism.

Serotonin—A chemical derived from the amino acid tryptophan and widely distributed in the tissues of the body. It acts as a neurotransmitter, constricts blood vessels at injury sites, and controls mood, appetite, and sleep cycles. Too little serotonin can cause depression, sadness, social withdrawal, and impaired attention span.

The Specific Carbohydrate Diet—A nutritional regimen, created by Dr. Sidney V. Haas and popularized by biochemist and author Elaine Gottschall, which restricts the use of complex carbohydrates (disaccharides and polysaccharides) and eliminates refined sugar, all grains, and starch from the diet. It is promoted as a way of reducing the symptoms of irritable bowel syndrome (IBS), Crohn's disease, ulcerative colitis, celiac disease, and autism. Gottschall believed that, due to damage to the microvili in the body, these microvili lack the ability to break down specific types of carbohydrates (i.e., disaccharides and polysaccharides), resulting in dysbiosis (the overgrowth of harmful bacterial flora). This condition is known as dysbiosis, which causes the production of mucus and other symptoms. The diet aims to starve off the bacteria by removing its source of nutrients from the digestive system. In a 1924 study in the *American Journal of Diseases of Children*, Haas reported, "In cases which the diet can be controlled for a sufficiently long time, recovery ensues in every instance and without nutritional relapse."[1] In 2011, researchers at the University of Massachusetts Medical Center published the results of a pilot study that investigated the use of an SCD-like diet in treating inflammatory bowel disease (IBD). One hundred percent of patients treated with the new diet showed significant improvement in their symptoms.[2] Additionally, the majority of subjects were able to reduce their reliance on medications to treat their IBD.[3]

Therapeutic Massage—To use a broad definition, the manipulation of superficial layers of muscle and connective tissue to enhance their function and promote relaxation and well-being. There are more than eighty recognized massage techniques, from Ayurvedic to Swedish.

Thrush—*see Candida.*

Tourette's Syndrome—An inherited neuropsychiatric disorder with onset in childhood, characterized by multiple physical (motor) tics and at least one vocal (phonic) tic. These tics characteristically wax and wane, can be suppressed temporarily, and are preceded by a premonitory urge. Tourette's is defined as part of a spectrum of tic disorders, which includes provisional, transient, and persistent (chronic) tics. Tourette's is not always correctly identified because most cases are mild, and the severity of the tics decreases for most children as they pass through adolescence. Between 0.4% and 3.8% of children ages five to eighteen may have Tourette's, while the prevalence of other tic disorders in school-age children is higher, with the more common tics of eye blinking, coughing, throat clearing, sniffing, and facial movements. Extreme Tourette's in adulthood is a rarity, and Tourette's does not adversely affect intelligence or life expectancy. Genetic and environmental factors play a role in the etiology of Tourette's, and many alternative physicians know how to treat the condition without medication. Comorbid conditions (co-occurring diagnoses other than Tourette's) such as attention-deficit hyperactivity disorder (ADHD) and obsessive-compulsive disorder (OCD) are present in many patients seen in tertiary specialty clinics.

Vision Therapy—Also known as vision training, it is used to improve vision skills such as eye movement control, eye coordination, and teamwork. It involves a series of procedures carried out in both home and office settings, usually under professional supervision by a behavioral optometrist. Vision therapy can be prescribed when a comprehensive eye examination indicates that it is an appropriate treatment option for the patient. The specific program of therapy is based on the results of standardized tests, the needs of the patient, and the patient's signs and symptoms. Programs typically involve eye exercises and the use of lenses, prisms, filters, occluders, specialized instruments, and/or computer programs. The course of therapy may last weeks to several years, with intermittent monitoring by the eye doctor.

Vitamin—Any of a group of organic compounds that are essential for normal growth and nutrition. Derived from food, the body requires adequate intake in the diet because the body cannot make vitamins on its own.

Yeast—*see Candida.*

Endnotes

Chapter 2

1 Susan Ridge and Nicole Samra, "Information Paper on Hypoglycemia," *Hypoglycemic Health Association*, www.hypoglycemia.asn.au/2012/information-paper-on-hypoglycemia/ (March 13, 2012).

Chapter 4

1 American Speech-Language-Hearing Association (ASHA) Ad Hoc Committee, "Childhood Apraxia of Speech, www.asha.org/policy/TR2007–00278/#sec1.1.2 (accessed May, 2007).

Chapter 5

1 Stephen J. Blumberg, PhD, Matthew D. Bramlett, PhD, et al., "Changes in Prevalence of Parent-reported Autism Spectrum Disorder in School-aged U.S. Children: 2007 to 2011–2012," *National Health Statistics Reports*, no. 65 (20 Mar. 2013). www.cdc.gov/nchs/data/nhsr/nhsr065.pdf (accessed 10 Jun. 2013).

2 P. Gail Williams, Lonnie L. Sears and Annmarie Allard (May 2004) "Sleep problems in children with autism," *Journal of Sleep Research* 13, no.3 (2004), 265–268.

3 Douglas Woods, Raymond Miltenberger, *Tic Disorders, Trichotillomania, and Other Repetitive Behavior Disorders: Behavioral Approaches to Analysis and Treatment* (New York: Springer 2006), 89; Dusan Kolar, Amanda Keller, Maria Golfinopoulos, Lucy Cumyn, Cassidy Syer, and Lily Hechtman, "Treatment of adults with attention deficit/hyperactivity disorder," *Neuropsychiatry Disease and Treatment* 4, no. 2 (2008), 389–403.

4 Ibid.

5 *ADDitude Magazine* Editors, "Oppositional Defiant Disorder: What parents need to know about ODD—including symptoms and treatment information," *ADDitude*, www.additudemag.com/adhd-web/article/4646.html (accessed 27 Sept. 2013).

6 Tantam, D. and Prestwood, S. (1999). *A Mind of One's Own: A Guide to the Special Difficulties and Needs of the More Able Person with Autism or Asperger's Syndrome*. 3rd ed. London: National Autistic Society.

Chapter 6

1 Kenneth Bock, M.D., *Healing the New Childhood Epidemics: Autism, ADHD, Asthma, and Allergies: The Groundbreaking Program for the 4-A Disorders* (New York: Ballantine Books, 2008).

2 DC Lagace, JK Yee, CA Bolaños, AJ Eisch, "Juvenile administration of methylphenidate attenuates adult hippocampal neurogenesis," *Biology Psychiatry* 60, no. 10 (2006), 1121–1130.

3 P. J. Santosh, G. Baird, N. Pityaratstian, E. Tavare, and P. Gringras, "Impact of comorbid autism spectrum disorders on stimulant response in children with attention deficit hyperactivity disorder: a retrospective and prospective effectiveness study," *Child: Health Care and Development* 32, no. 5 (2006), 575–583.

4 Slavica K. Katusic, M.D., Robert C. Colligan, Ph.D., Amy L. Weaver, M.S., Robert G. Voigt, M.D., and William J. Barbaresi, M.D., "Stimulant Medication Treatment of Target Behaviors of Children with Autism: A population based study," *Journal of Developmental and Behavioral Pediatrics* 29, no. 2 (2008), 75–81.

5 U.S. Drug Enforcement Administration, "Drug Fact Sheets: Methylphenidate—Ritalin," www.justice.gov/dea/druginfo/concern_meth.shtml

6 Kenneth Bock, M.D., *Healing the New Childhood Epidemics: Autism, ADHD, Asthma, and Allergies: The Groundbreaking Program for the 4-A Disorders* (New York: Ballantine Books, 2008).

7 CCHR, "School shooters/school related violence committed by those under the influence of psychiatric drugs," *CCHR International,* www.cchrint.org/school-shooters/ (accessed 1 Feb, 2013).

8 U.S. National Library of Medicine, "Drug Fact Sheets: Methylphenidate," National Institute of Health; *Medline Plus* www.nlm.nih.gov/medlineplus/druginfo/meds/a682188.html

9 HC Kimko, JT Cross, DR Abernethy, "Pharmacokinetics and clinical effectiveness of methylphenidate." *Clinical Pharmacokinetics* 37 no. 6, (1999), 457–70.

10 Randal G. Ross, M.D, "Psychotic and Manic-like Symptoms during Stimulant Treatment of Attention Deficit Hyperactivity Disorder," *American Journal of Psychiatry* 163, no. 7 (2006), 1149–1152.

11 U.S. National Library of Medicine, "Drug Fact Sheets: Methylphenidate," National Institute of Health; Medline Plus www.nlm.nih.gov/medlineplus/druginfo/meds/a682188.html

12 RG Ross, "Psychotic and manic-like symptoms during stimulant treatment of attention deficit hyperactivity disorder," *American Journal Psychiatry* 163, no. 7 (2006), 1149–1152; CA Soutullo, DelBello MP, Ochsner JE et al. "Severity of bipolarity in hospitalized manic adolescents with history of stimulant or antidepressant treatment," *Journal Affective Disorders* 70, no. 3 (2002) 323–327.

13 M. Lerner, T. Wigal, "Long-term safety of stimulant medications used to treat children with ADHD," *Pediatric Annual* 37, no. 1 (2008), 37–45.

14 M. Kraemer, J. Uekermann, J. Wiltfang, B. Kis, "Methylphenidate-induced psychosis in adult attention-deficit/hyperactivity disorder: report of 3 new cases and review of the literature." *Clinical Neuropharmacology* 33, no. 4 (2010) 204–206.

15 RG Ross, "Psychotic and manic-like symptoms during stimulant treatment of attention deficit hyperactivity disorder," *American Journal of Psychiatry* 163, no. 7 (2006), 1149–1152.

Chapter 7

1 Claudia R. Morris, MD and Marilyn C. Agin, MD, "Syndrome of Allergy, Apraxia, and Malabsorption: Characterization of a Neurodevelopmental Phenotype That Responds to Omega 3 and Vitamin E Supplementation," *Alternative Therapies* Vol. 15, No. 4 (July/August 2009).

2 Kenneth Bock, M.D., *Healing the New Childhood Epidemics: Autism, ADHD, Asthma, and Allergies: The Groundbreaking Program for the 4-A Disorders* (New York: Ballantine Books, 2008).

3 James B. Adams, et al., "Toxicological Status of Children with Autism vs. Neurotypical Children and the Association with Autism Severity," *Biology Trace Elements Resource Springer Science & Business Media* (Aug. 2012), 1–10, www.rescuepost.com/files/adams-et-al-2012-tox-status-of-asd-children-blood-and-urine.pdf

4 Karen C Lindell, Martin Kohlmeier, and Steven H Zeisel, "Status of nutrition education in medical schools," *Journal of Clinical Nutrition* 83 (2006), 941S-944S.

5 Claudia R. Morris, MD and Marilyn C. Agin, MD, "Syndrome of Allergy, Apraxia, and Malabsorption: Characterization of a Neurodevelopmental Phenotype That Responds to Omega 3 and Vitamin E Supplementation," *Alternative Therapies* Vol. 15, No. 4 (July/August 2009).

Chapter 8

1 Moises Velasquez-Manoff, "An Immune Disorder at the Root of Autism," *New York Times,* 25 Aug. 2012, www.nytimes.com/2012/08/26/opinion/sunday/immune-disorders-and-autism .html?pagewanted=all&_r=0 (accessed 15 February. 2013).

2 Peadar N. Kirke, James L. Mills, Anne M. Molloy, et al., "Impact of the MTHFR C677T Polymorphism on Risk of Neural Tube Defects: Case-Control Study," *BMJ*, no. 328 (June 24, 2004), 1535–1536.

3 Bianca Garilli, ND, "MTHFR Mutation: A Missing Piece in the Chronic Disease Puzzle," *Holistic Primary Care* (18 Jun. 2012), http://holisticprimarycare.net/topics/topics-a-g/functional-medicine/1353-mthfr-mutation-a-missing-piece-in-the-chronic-disease-puzzle (accessed 10 Nov. 2012).

4 Xudong Liu, Fatima Solehdin, Ira L. Cohen, et al., "Population and Family-Based Studies Associate the MTHFR Gene with Idiopathic Autism in Simplex Families," *J. Autism Dev Disord.*, no. 41 (2011), 938–944.

5 Crott, J. et al., "Effects of dietary folate and aging on gene expression in the colonic mucosa of rats: implications for carcinogenesis," *Carcinogenesis* 22, no. 7 (2004), 1019–1025.

6 K. Malmberg, HLWargelius, P. Lichtenstein, L. Oreland, JO Larsson, "ADHD and Disruptive Behavior scores—associations with MAO-A and 5-HTT genes and with platelet MAO-B activity in adolescents, *BMC Psychiatry* 8, no. 28 (2008), 8–28.

7 G. Frazzetto, G DiLorenzo, V. Carola, et. al., "Early trauma and increased risk for physical aggression during adulthood: the moderating role of MAOA genotype," *PLoS ONE* 2, no. 5 (2007), e486

8 Medical Xpress "Researchers find genetic link to autism known as CHD8 mutation." Medical Xpress 3 – Press Release (Jul 2014), 1–2. http://medicalxpress.com/news/2014-07-genetic-link-autism-chd8-mutation.html

9 Faraneh Vargha-Khadem, David G. Gadian, Andrew Copp and Mortimer Mish "FOXP2 and the Neuroanatomy of Speech and Language" *Nature Reviews: Journal of Neuroscience* 6 (2005), 131–137.

10 Sebastian Haesler, Christelle Rochefort, Benjamin Georgi, Pawel Licznerski, Pavel Osten, and Constance Scharff, "Incomplete and Inaccurate Vocal Imitation after Knockdown of *FoxP2* in Songbird Basal Ganglia Nucleus Area X," PLOS *Biology Journal* 5, no. 12 (2007), www.ncbi.nlm.nih.gov/pmc/articles/PMC2100148/

11 Rabbi Eric R. Braverman, M.D, "Memories of Carl C. Pfeiffer, Ph.D., M.D. Physician, Scientist, Teacher and Philanthropist," *Journal of Orthomolecular Medicine* 4, No. 1, (1989), 5–7, www.ortho molecular.org/library/jom/1989/pdf/1989-v04n01-p005.pdf.

12 Donna Gates, The Little-Known Link between Blood Type and Autism (and Why It Matters to Everyone), *Body Ecology*, http://bodyecology.com/articles/link_ autism_blood_type.php (accessed 10 Sept. 2013); Donna Gates, *Body Ecology Diet: Recovering Your Health and Rebuilding Your Immunity* (California: Hay House, 2011).

13 Peter J. D'Adamo *Eat Right For Your Blood Type: The Individualized Diet Solution to Staying Healthy, Living Longer & Achieving Your Ideal Weight* (New York: Putnam Adult, 1997).

14 JB Adams, LJ Johansen, LD Powell, D. Quig, RA Rubin, "Gastrointestinal flora and gastrointestinal status in children with autism—comparisons to typical children and correlation with autism severity," *BMC Gastroenterology* 11, no. 22 (2011), 11–22.

15 William Shaw, PhD, *Biological Treatments for the Autism and PDD* (Kansas: Great Plains Laboratory, 2001),+ www.biologicaltreatments.com/book/ch6.asp

16 Nicholas A. Pawlowski, MD, "Your Baby's Health: All about Allergies," *The Mayo Clinic*, (Mar. 2003), http://customers.hbci.com/~wenonah/new/allergy.htm (accessed 10 Jan, 2013).

17 "Nutritional Disease: Food Allergies and Intolerances," *Encyclopedia Britannica*, www.britannica.com/EBchecked/topic/422916/nutritional-disease/247897/Food-allergies-and-intolerances

18 Richard Robinson, Jill Granger, and Teresa Odle, "Allergies," *Gale Encyclopedia of Medicine* 3 "Allergies," (2006).

19 Claudia R. Morris, MD and Marilyn C. Agin, MD, "Syndrome of Allergy, Apraxia, and Malabsorption: Characterization of a Neurodevelopmental Phenotype That Responds to Omega 3 and Vitamin E Supplementation," *Alternative Therapies* Vol. 15, No. 4 (July/August 2009).

20 Liz Szabo, "Autism tied to autoimmune disorders in immediate family," *USA Today*, 10 Aug. 2010, http://usatoday30.usatoday.com/news/health/2009–07–12-autism13_N.htm (accessed 22 Oct. 2012).

21 Krans, Brian, "Mom's Weak Thyroid Ups the Risk for Autism," *Healthline News*, 16 Aug. 2013, http://www.healthline.com/health-news/children-mothers-with-thyroid-problems-more-likely-to-have-autistic-kids-081613 (accessed 1 Aug. 2014).

22 Mervyn Susser, *Causal thinking in the health sciences: Concepts and strategies of epidemiology* (New York: Oxford, 1973); Osteopathic Medicine and Autism.

23 Mark Sisson, "Environmental Toxins and Gene Expression," (Dec. 2009), www.marksdailyapple.com/environmental-toxins-and-gene-expression/#axzz2gJKpNkIz.

24 W.J. Walsh, A. Usman, J. Tarpey, and T Kelly, *Metallothionein and Autism*, Second Edition, Pfeiffer Treatment Center, Naperville, IL (2002).

25 Ibid.

Chapter 9

1 Lindsey Biel, OTR/L, "Parenting Your Preemie with Sensory Issues," *Sensory Integration Focus Magazine*, (Autumn 2008), http://sensorysmarts.com/Preemie_SIF_Aut2008.pdf

2 H. Als, L. Gilkerson, F.H. Duffy Gilkerson, et al., "A three-center randomized control trial of individual's developmental care for very low-birth-weight preterm infants: Medical, neurodevelopmental parent and care giving effects," *J. Dev Behav Pediatr*, No. 24 (2003), 399–408.

3 Sue Hyland, "Primitive Reflexes: Moro," *Optimizing Neurological Development*, http://suehyland.co.uk/ond/primitive-reflexes/#moro

4 Patricia S. Lemer. *Outsmarting Autism*, World Association Publishers, Pittsburgh, PA: (June 2014).

5 Ray Medina, "How Infants Acquire Their Gut Flora," (9 Oct. 2012), http://syontix.com/how-infants-acquire-their-gut-flora/; "The infant intestinal microbiome: friend or foe?" Mshvildadze M., *Early Human Development* 86, no. 1 (2010), 67–71.

6 Beth Lambert and Victoria Kobliner, MS, RD, *A Compromised Generation—The Epidemic of Illness in America's Children* (USA: Sentient Publishing, 2010), 60–62.

7 Natasha Campbell-McBride, *Gut and Psychology Syndrome. Natural Treatment for Autism, ADHD/ADD, Dyslexia, Dyspraxia, Depression and Schizophrenia* (Cambridge, UK: Medinform, 2010).

8 Steven Lamm, MD, Boosting Your Immunity with Enzymes, *New York University School of Medicine* (24 Jan. 2013), www.doctoroz.com/videos/boosting-your-immunity-enzymes?page=2

9 Beth Lambert and Victoria Kobliner, MS, RD, *A Compromised Generation—The Epidemic of Illness in America's Children* (USA: Sentient Publishing, 2010), 32–34.

10 The Philadelphia's Children Hospital, "A Look at Each Vaccine: The Hepatitis B Vaccine," *Vaccine Education Center*, www.chop.edu/service/vaccine-education-center/a-look-at-each-vaccine/hepatitis-b-vaccine.html (accessed 27 Sept. 2013).

11 Childstats.gov, "Child Population: Number of Children (In Millions) Ages 0–17 In The United States By Age, 1950–2012 And Projected 2013–2050," *Forum on Child and Family Statistics*, www.childstats.gov/americaschildren/tables/pop1.asp (accessed 27 Sept. 27, 2013).

12 Burton A. Waisbren, Sr. M.D., "How Safe Is Universal Hepatitis B Vaccination?" Burton A. Waisbren, Sr., M.D., F.A.C.P.

13 Dr. Mercola, "Refuse This Routine Procedure—Or Expose Your Baby's Brain to Severe Danger," Mercola.com, 3 Nov. 2010, http://articles.mercola.com/sites/articles/archive/2010/11/03/hepatitis-b-vaccines-at-birth.aspx (accessed 10 Feb. 2013).

14 Chan F. "Limitations of Ultrasound," *Perinatal Society of Australia and New Zealand*, 1st Annual Congress. Freemantle, Australia, 1997.

15 Manual F. Casanova, M.D., "Is a Prenatal Ultrasound Safe?" *Blog at Wordpress*, http://fetalsonosafety.com/2013/05/23/autism-researcher-dr-manuel-f-casanova-and-ultrasound/ (accessed 3 Aug. 2012).

16 M.F. Casanova, M.D.," Potential teratogenic effects of ultrasound on corticogenesis: Implications for autism," *Medical Hypotheses* 75, No.1 (July 2010), 53–58.

17 Pasko Rakic, M.D., "Ultrasound Affects Embryonic Mouse Brain Development," *Yale School of Medicine*, (7 Aug. 2006), http://news.yale.edu/2006/08/07/ultrasound-affects-embryonic-mouse-brain-development (accessed 1 Oct. 2013).

18 Shawn Centers, DO, FACOP, "Osteopathy: A Philosophy and Methodology for the Effective Treatment of Children with Autism," Autism Science Digest: *The Journal of Autism One* 1 (Apr. 2011), 101–109, www.autismone.org/content/osteopathy-philosophy-and-methodology-effective-treatment-children-autism-shawn-k-centers-do (accessed 5 May 2013).

19 Robert Melillo, M.D., *Disconnected Kids* (New York: Penguin Group, 2009), 59–60.

20 Matthew L. Speltz, "Case-Control Study of Neurodevelopment in Deformational Plagiocephaly," *Pediatrics* (Mar. 2010); Frymann, Viola, "Relation of Disturbances of Craniosacral Mechanism to Symptomatology of the Newborn: Study of 1250 Infants," *Journal of the American Osteopathic Association*, 65 (June, 1966), 1059–1075; Sally Goddard, *Reflexes, Learning And Behavior: A Window into the Child's Mind: A Non-Invasive Approach to Solving Learning & Behavior Problems* (Oregon: Fern Ridge Press, 2005).

21 Moises Velasquez-Manoff, "An Immune Disorder at the Root of Autism." *New York Times* (25 Aug. 2012), www.nytimes.com/2012/08/26/opinion/sunday/immune-disorders-and-autism.html?pagewanted=all (accessed 25 Aug. 2012).

22 Moises Velasquez-Manoff, *An Epidemic of Absence: A New Way of Understanding Allergies and Autoimmune Diseases.* (New York: Scribner, 2012).

23 Kenneth Bock, M.D., *Healing the New Childhood Epidemics: Autism, ADHD, Asthma, and Allergies: The Groundbreaking Program for the 4-A Disorders* (New York: Ballantine Books, 2008), 92–93.

Chapter 10

1 Claudia R. Morris, MD and Marilyn C. Agin, MD, "Syndrome of Allergy, Apraxia, and Malabsorption: Characterization of a Neurodevelopmental Phenotype That Responds to Omega 3 and Vitamin E Supplementation," *Alternative Therapies* Vol. 15, No. 4 (July/August 2009).

2 S. Melanie Lee, Jennifer Li, Gloria Tran, Bana Jabri, Talal Chatila and Sarkis Mazmanian, "The Toll-Like Receptor 2 Pathway Establishes Colonization by a Commensal of the Human Microbiota," *Science* 20 vol. 332 no. 6032 (May 2011), 974–977.

3 Center for Disease Control and Prevention, "Possible Side Effects of Vaccines," www.cdc .gov/vaccines/vac-gen/side-effects.htm#hepb

4 Natasha Campbell-McBride, *Gut and Psychology Syndrome. Natural Treatment for Autism, ADHD/ADD, Dyslexia, Dyspraxia, Depression and Schizophrenia* (Cambridge, UK: Medinform, 2010).

5 JL Rodrigues, JM Serpeloni, BL Batista, S. Souza, F. Jr. Barbosa. "Identification and distribution of mercury species in rat tissue following administration of thimerosal or methyl mercury. *Archives of Toxicology* 84 (2010), 891–896.

6 David A. Geier, B.A., Mark R. Geier, M.D., Ph.D, "Early Downward Trends in Neurodevelopmental Disorders Following Removal of Thimerosal-Containing Vaccines," *Journal of American Physicians and Surgeons* 11, no. 1 (2006), 8–13.

7 Richard Nilson, "Polysorbate 80 Side Effects," *Live Strong*, 18 Sept. 2010, www.livestrong .com/article/262369-polysorbate-80-side-effects/

8 DA Geier, "An assessment of the impact of thimerosal on childhood neurodevelopmental disorders," *Pediatric Rehabilitation* 6, no. 2, (April-June 2003), 97–102.

9 Anita Manning, "Vaccine-autism link feared." *USA Today*, 16 Aug. 1999, http://onibasu.com/archives/am/10091.html

10 David Kirby, "Vaccine Court Awards Millions to Two Children with Autism," *Huffington Post*, 14 Jan. 2013, www.huffingtonpost.com/david-kirby/post2468343_b_2468343.html

11 Staff editor, "New Published Study Verifies Andrew Wakefield's Research on Autism—Again (MMR Vaccine Causes Autism)," *The Liberty Beacon* (21 Jun. 2013). www.thelibertybeacon.com/2013/06/21/new-published-study-verifies-andrew-wakefields-research-on-autism-again-mmr-vaccine-causes-autism/

12 My Health News Daily, "More schools get non-medical exemptions from vaccines," *Fox News* (Sept 21, 2012), www.foxnews.com/health/2012/09/21/more-schoolkids-get-non-medical-exemptions-from-vaccines/ (accessed 1 Oct. 2013).

13 Christine E. Schneemilch MD, Thomas Schilling MD, "Effects of general anaesthesia on inflammation," *Best Practice & Research Clinical Anaesthesiology* 18, no.3 (2004), 293–504.

14 Zhongcong Xie, M.D., Ph.D., et al., "Selective Anesthesia-induced Neuroinflammation in Developing Mouse Brain and Cognitive Impairment," *Journal of Anesthesiology* 18, no. 3. (2013), 502–515.

15 Alice Park, "Can Anesthesia Raise the Risk of ADHD? A new study finds that children who have multiple surgeries early on have a higher risk of learning disabilities later,"*Time Magazine*, 2 Feb. 2012, http://healthland.time.com/2012/02/02/can-anesthesia-raise-the-risk-of-adhd/

16 Denise Mann, "Anesthesia before Age 3 May Raise Risk of Learning Delays: Study Research found even one exposure is associated with language deficits by age 10," *U.S. News Report*, 20 Aug. 2012, http://health.usnews.com/health-news/news/articles/2012/08/20/anesthesia-before-age-3-may-raise-risk-of-learning-delays-study

17 " What is Applied Kinesiology?" ICAK-USA. Archived from the original on 30 November 2007, www.drlarrydirect.com/pages/What-is-Applied-Kinesiology%3F.html

18 Jacob Teitelbaum, MD; Devi S. Nambudripad, MD, PhD, DC, et al, "Improving communication skills with Allergy-related Autism Using Nambudripad's Allergy Elimination Techniques: A Pilot Study," *Journal of Integrative Medicine* 10, no. 5 (Oct/Nov. 2011), 36–43.

19 Devi S. Nambudripad, M.D., D.C., L.Ac., Ph.D., *Say Good-bye to Allergy-related Autism* (Illinois: Delta Publishing, 2006).

20 Glyconutrients References, "Scientific Validation," www.glyconutrientsreference.com/whatare glyconutrients/scientificvalidation.html

21 Crook, William G. M.D., *The Yeast Connection: A Medical Breakthrough* (New York: Vintage Books, 1986).

22 Akansha Jain, Shubham Jain, and Swati Rawat, "Emerging fungal infections among children: A review on its clinical manifestations, diagnosis, and prevention," *Journal of Pharmacy BioAllied Sciences* 2, no. 4 (2010), 314–320.

Chapter 11

1 Michael Gershon, M.D., *The Second Brain: A Groundbreaking New Understanding of Nervous Disorders of the Stomach and Intestine* (New York: HarperCollins, 1998).

2 Ibid.

3 Alan Swartz, "A.D.H.D Seen in 11% of U.S. Children as Diagnoses Rises," *New York Times*, 31 March, 2013, www.nytimes.com/2013/04/01/health/more-diagnoses-of-hyperactivity-causing concern.html?pagewanted=all&_r=0 (accessed 10 Sept. 2013).

4 Stephen J. Blumberg, PhD, Matthew D. Bramlett, PhD, et al., "Changes in Prevalence of Parent-reported Autism Spectrum Disorder in School-aged U.S. Children: 2007 to 2011–2012," *National Health Statistics Reports*, no. 65 (20 Mar. 2013). www.cdc.gov/nchs/data/nhsr/nhsr065.pdf (accessed 10 Jun. 2013).

Chapter 12

1 Julie Deardorff, "Doubts cast on food intolerance testing: Allergists and gastroenterologists question the use of expensive but sought-after analyses," *Chicago Tribune*, 11 Apr. 2012.

2 Annette Nay, PhD, "Untreated Food Allergies Cause MS," 2009, www.three-peaks.net/annette/allergies-death.htm (accessed Mar. 2013).

3 Robert J. Doman, M.D., "Food Sensitivities: The Hidden Problems," *Journal of the National Association for Child Development* 4, no. 2 (1984).

4 Beth Lambert and Victoria Kobliner, MS, RD, *A Compromised Generation—The Epidemic of Illness in America's Children* (USA: Sentient Publishing, 2010), 7–9.

5 Dr. Ben F. Feingold, M.D., *Why Your Child Is Hyperactive*, (New York: Random House, 1975).

6 Jenny McCarthy, *Louder Than Words: A Mother's Journey in Healing Autism* (New York: Penguin Group, 2008).

7 Hyla Cass, M.D., "Is Your Medication Robbing You of Nutrients Part 2: Getting Specific," *Huffington Post*, 9 Sept. 2010, www.huffingtonpost.com/hyla-cass-md/is-your-medication-robbin_1_b_691711.html (accessed 5 Feb. 2013).

8 Dr. Anurag Singh, "Gluten Intolerance: Is the Lack of probiotics and vitamin C to Blame?" *European Journal of Clinical Nutrition* Published online ahead of print, doi: 10.1038/ ejcn.2012.197

9 Jonathan Landsman, "What your doctor won't tell you about Vitamin D," *Natural Health 365*, 27 Jun. 2013, www.naturalhealth365.com/category/vitamin_d (accessed 30 Apr. 2013).

10 Claudia R. Morris, MD and Marilyn C. Agin, MD, "Syndrome of Allergy, Apraxia, and Malabsorption: Characterization of a Neurodevelopmental Phenotype That Responds to Omega 3 and Vitamin E Supplementation," *Alternative Therapies* Vol. 15, No. 4 (July/August 2009).

11 AJ Richardson, "Omega-3 fatty acids in ADHD and related neurodevelopmental disorders," *Internal Review of Psychiatry* 18, no. 2 (2006), 155–172.

12 Newsletter editor, "Studies confirm benefits of vitamin B6/magnesium therapy for autism, PDD, and ADHD," *Autism Research Review International* 20, no. 3 (2006), 5.

13 Hyla Cass, M.D., "Is Your Medication Robbing You of Nutrients Part 2: Getting Specific," *Huffington Post*, 9 Sept. 2010, www.huffingtonpost.com/hyla-cass-md/is-your-medication-robbin_1_b_691711.html (accessed 5 Feb. 2013).

14 Marty Hinz, Alvin Stein, Robert Neff, Robert Weinberg, and Thomas Uncini, "Treatment of attention deficit hyperactivity disorder with monoamine amino acid precursors and organic cation transporter assay interpretation," *Neuropsychiatric Disease and Treatment* 7 (2011), 31–38.

15 Michael R. Lyon, et al., "The Effects of L-Theanine on Objective Sleep Quality in Boys with Attention Deficit Hyperactivity Disorder (ADHD): a Randomized, Double-blind, Placebo-controlled Clinical Trial," *Alternative Medicine Review* 16, no. 4 (2011), 348–354.

16 NYU Langone Medical Center, "Carnitine: Therapeutic Uses," www.med.nyu.edu/content?ChunkIID=21450

17 L.J. Van Oudheusden, H.R. Scholte, "Efficacy of Carnitine in the treatment of children with attention-deficit hyperactivity disorder," *Prostaglandins, Leukotrienes and Essential Fatty Acids* 67, no. 1 (2002), 33–38.

18 "Dietary Reference Intakes for Energy, Carbohydrate, Fiber, Fat, Fatty Acids, Cholesterol, Protein,

and Amino Acids, *Acceptable Macronutrient Distribution Range (AMDR) reference and RDAs: Institute of Medicine (IOM)*, 5 Sept. 2002, www.iom.edu/reports/2002/dietary-reference-intakes-for-energy-carbohydrate-fiber-fat-fatty-acids-cholesterol-protein-and-amino-acids.aspx (accessed 2 Apr. 2013).

19 Cari Nierenberg and Louise Chang, M.D., "How Much Protein Do You Need," *WebMD*, 28 Feb. 2011, www.webmd.com/diet/healthy-kitchen-11/how-much-protein (accessed 2 Apr. 2013).

20 Cheryl Long and Tabitha Alterman, "Meet Real Free-Range Eggs," *Mother Earth News*, www.motherearthnews.com/real-food/tests-reveal-healthier-eggs.aspx#at xzz2gyRBriYP

Chapter 13

1 Claudia R. Morris, MD and Marilyn C. Agin, MD, "Syndrome of Allergy, Apraxia, and Malabsorption: Characterization of a Neurodevelopmental Phenotype That Responds to Omega 3 and Vitamin E Supplementation," *Alternative Therapies* Vol. 15, No. 4 (July/August 2009).

Chapter 14

1 Konstantin Monastyrsky, "Is Miralax the Next Vioxx? Getting mad or forgetful after taking a laxative? Well, according to the US Food and Drug Administration that's exactly what certain best-selling laxatives can do to you," www.gutsense.org/gutsense/the-role-of-miralax-laxative-in-autism-dementia-alzheimer.html (accessed 10 April. 2013).

2 Wim Caers, Glenn R. Gibson, Cyril W. C. Kendall, Kara D. Lewis, Yehuda Ringel, and Joanne L. Slavin, "Prebiotics and the Health Benefits of Fiber: Current Regulatory Status, Future Research, and Goals," *Journal of Nutrition* 142, no. 5 (2012), 962–974.

3 CNN iReport, "The 10 Health Benefits of Eating Turmeric," *CNN*, (28 Jul. 2013), http://ireport.cnn.com/docs/DOC-1012314 (accessed 5 Aug. 2013).

Chapter 15

1 Kelly Dorfman, MS, LND, *Cure Your Child with Food: The Hidden Connection Between Nutrition and Childhood Ailments* (New York: Workman Publishing, reprint 2013).

2 Joseph Mercola, M.D., "When You Heat Natural Plant Based Foods You Can Get Cancer Causing Acrylamide," 9 Jun. 2012, http://articles.mercola.com/sites/articles/archive/2012/06/09/when-you-heat-natural-plantbased-foods-you-can-get-acrylamide-and-cancer.aspx (accessed 3 Mar. 2013).

3 Jules Shepard and John Forberger, "What is Celiac Disease?" American Celiac Disease Alliance, http://1in133.org/info/#celiac.

4 David Perlmutter, MD, *Grain Brain: The Surprising Truth about Wheat, Carbs, and Sugar—Your Brain's Silent Killers* (USA: Little, Brown and Company, 2013).

5 Melissa Melton, "Why Are So Many Allergic to Wheat Now?" *Truth Stream Media*, http://truthstreammedia.com/why-are-so-many-allergic-to-wheat-now/ (2 May 2013).

6 KL Reichelt, AM Knivsberg, G. Lind, and M. Nødland, "Probable etiology and possible treatment of childhood autism," *Brain Dysfunction* 4 (1991), 308–319.

7 JB Adams, LJ Johansen, LD Powell, D. Quig, RA Rubin, "Gastrointestinal flora and gastrointestinal status in children with autism—comparisons to typical children and correlation with autism severity," *BMC Gastroenterology* 11, no. 22 (2011), 11–22.

8 Ann-Mari Knivsberg, Karl-L. Reichelt, Torleiv Høien, and Magne Nødland, "Effect of Dietary Intervention on Autistic Behavior," *Focus On Autism and Other Developmental Disabilities* 18, no. 4 (2003), 247–256.

9 Chia-Lin Hsu, MD, Delmar C.Y. Lin, MD, Chia-Lin Chen MD, PhD, Chin-Man Wang, Alice M.K. Wong, MD "The Effects of A Gluten and Casein-free Diet in Children with Autism: A Case Report," *Chang Gung Medical Journal* 32, No. 4 (2009), 459–465.

10 Frediani T, Zingoni AM, Ferruzzi F, Giardini O, Quintieri F, Barbato M, D'Eufemia P, Cardi E., "Food allergy and infantile autism," Department of Paediatrics, University of Rome La Sapienza, Italy, *Panminerva Medica* 37, no. 3 (1995), 137–41.

11 Dr. H.P. Maree, "Goat Milk and Its Use as a Hypo-Allergenic Infant Food," *Dairy Goat Journal* (1978), http://goatconnection.com/articles/publish/article_152.shtml (accessed 10 July, 2013).

12 Beth Lambert and Victoria Kobliner, MS, RD, *A Compromised Generation—The Epidemic of Illness in America's Children* (USA: Sentient Publishing, 2010).

13 Barbara L. Milton, "Fermented Soy Is Only Soy Food Fit for Human Consumption," *Natural News*, 3 Feb. 2009, www.naturalnews.com/025513_soy_food_soybeans.html (accessed 15, Jul. 2013).

14 Autism Spectrum Disorders Health Center, "Gluten Free/Casein Free Diets for Autism," *WebMD*, www.webmd.com/brain/autism/gluten-free-casein-free-diets-for-autism

15 Natasha Campbell-McBride, *Gut and Psychology Syndrome. Natural Treatment for Autism, ADHD/ ADD, Dyslexia, Dyspraxia, Depression and Schizophrenia* (2010), excerpted, www.gaps.me/?page_id=20. (accessed 12 Jan. 2013).

16 Mike Adams, "California-grown Lundberg rice shows near-zero metals' case closed on 'naturally occurring' excuse for lead in rice products," *NaturalNews.com* (14 Feb. 2014). (www.naturalnews .com/043903_lundberg_rice_heavy_metals_naturally_occurring.html (accessed Feb. 14, 2014).

Chapter 16

1 Neil Ward, "Assessment of chemical factors in relation to child hyperactivity," *Journal of Nutritional and Environmental Medicine* 7, (1997), 333–342.

2 Kelly Dorfman, MS, LND, "Eating at Whole Foods for Less Than $11 a Day," *Huffington Post*, 24 June 2013, www.huffingtonpost.com/kelly-dorfman/healthy-eating_b_3459288.html (accessed 14 Jul. 2013).

3 Arndt Manzel Jens Titze, Nir Yosef, Ralf A. Linker, Dominik N. Muller & David A. Hafler, "Sodium chloride drives autoimmune disease by the induction of pathogenic TH17 cells," *Nature International Weekly Journal of Science* 496 (2012), 518–522.

4 Ibid.

5 Asthma and Allergy Ltd., "Halotherapy: Dry saline aerosol inhalation," *Salt Cave*, www.saltcave .co.uk/Salt_Therapy.pdf

6 A.V.Chervinskaya, S.L. Konovalov, "Haloaerosol Therapy in the Rehabilitation of Asthma Patients," *Clinical Research Respiratory Center, St. Petersburg, Russia*—Annual meeting, Interastma, Palanga, Lithuania, May, 1999).

7 Denis Wilson, M.D., "This one soft drink ingredient may be slowing your thyroid," *Wilsons Temperature Syndrome*, 29 Dec. 2012, www.wilsonssyndrome.com/this-1-soft-drink-ingredient-might-be-slowing-your-metabolism/ (accessed 15 Jan. 2013).

8 Ibid.

9 Luke Yoquinto, "The Truth About Potassium Bromate," *Live Science*, 16 Mar. 2012, www.live-science.com/36206-truth-potassium-bromate-food-additive.html, (accessed 3 Mar. 2013).

10 Rachel Murphy, "How additives turn your little angel into the devil," *Daily Record*, 21 Oct. 1998.

11 Alfonso Efraín Campos-Sepúlveda, Et. al., "Neonatal Monosodium Glutamate Administration Increases Aminooxyacetic Acid (AOA) Susceptibility Effects In Adult Mice," *Proceedings of the Western Pharmacology Society* (2009) 72–74.

12 Science News Department, "Imaging children with ADHD: MRI technology reveals differences in neuro-signaling," *The American Medical Association Press Release* (December 4, 2003).

13 Swati S. More, Ashish P. Vartak, Robert Vince, "The Butter Flavorant, Diacetyl, Exacerbates beta-Amyloid Cytotoxicity," *Chemical Research in Toxicology* 25, *no. 10* (2012), 2083–2091.

14 Kristen of Food Renegade, "Decoding Labels: V8 Splash, Strawberry Kiwi, www.foodrenegade .com/decoding-labels-v8-splash-strawberry-kiwi/ (accessed 3 Jul. 2013).

15 El-Masry, Abdel-Rahman, McLendon, Schiffman, "Splenda alters gut microflora and increases intestinal p-glycoprotein and cytochrome p-450 in male rats," *Journal of Toxicology and Environmental Health* 71, no. 21 (2008), 1415–1429.

16 Nancy Appleton, PhD, "146 Reasons Sugar is Ruining Your Life," *Rheumatic.org*, http://rheumatic .org/sugar.htm (accessed 10 June 2013).

17 Dufault R, LeBlanc B, Schnoll R, Cornett C, Schweitzer L, Walling D, Hightower J, Patrick L, Lukiw WJ, "Mercury from chlor-alkali plants: Measured concentrations in food product sugar," *Environmental Health* 8 no. 2 (2009).

18 Weightlosstraps Online, "Does High Fructose Corn Syrup Cause Leaky Gut?" http://weight losstraps.com/64/does-high-fructose-corn-syrup-cause-leaky-gut/ (accessed 7, Sept. 2013).

19 Mark K. Shigenaga, PhD, "Overview: Diet, enteric bacterial invasion, and chronic inflammation," *Children's Hospital Oakland Research Institute* (2005).

20 Elaine Schmidt, "This is your brain on sugar: UCLA study shows high-fructose diet sabotages learning, memory," *UCLA Newsroom Press Release* (May 15, 2012).

21 Mark Hyman, M.D., "5 Reasons High Fructose Corn Syrup Will Kill you," *Huffington Post*, 13 May 2011, www.huffingtonpost.com/dr-mark-hyman/5-reasons-high-fructose-c_b_861913.html (accessed 19 Apr. 2013).

Chapter 17

1 Sayer Ji, "How GMO Farming and Food Is Making Our Gut Flora UNFRIENDLY," *Greenmedinfo*, 28 Mar. 2013, www.greenmedinfo.com/blog/how-gmo-farming-and-food-making-our-gut-flora-unfriendly (accessed 31 Mar. 2013).

2 Anthony Samsel and Stephanie Seneff, "Glyphosate's Suppression of Cytochrome P450 Enzymes and Amino Acid Biosynthesis by the Gut Microbiome: Pathways to Modern Diseases," *Entropy* 15, no. 4 (2013),1416–1463

Chapter 18

1 Nick Moskalev, PhD, "School shootings: How Can American Food Lead to American Blood," *Dye Diet*, 15 Dec. 2012, www.dyediet.com/2012/12/15/food-and-risk/school-shootings-how-american-food-leads-to-american-blood/ (accessed 23 Dec. 2012).

2 Ibid.

3 Mancy Oaklander, "New Fear about Food Dyes," *Prevention Magazine/Fox News*, 17 Jan. 2013, (accessed 20 Jan. 2013).

4 Storey HC et al., "A randomized controlled trial of the effect of school food and dining room modifications on classroom behavior in secondary school children," *European Journal of Clinical Nutrition* 65, no. 1 (2011), 32–38.

5 Belot M & James J., "Healthy school meals and educational outcomes," *Journal of Health Economics* 30, no. 3 (2011), 489–504.

6 C. Peter W. Bennett and Jonathan Brostoff, "The health of criminals related to behaviour, food, allergy and nutrition: a controlled study of 100 persistent young offenders," *Journal of Nutritional and Environmental Medicine* 7 (1997), 359–366.

7 C. Peter W. Bennett, Leonard M. McEwen, Helen C. McEwen, and Eunice L. Rose, "The Shipley

Project: treating food allergy to prevent criminal behaviour in community settings," *Journal of Nutritional and Environmental Medicine* 8 (1998), 77–83.

8 Ibid.

9 C. Bernard Gesch, CQSW, Sean M. Hammond, PhD, Sarah E. Hampson, PhD, Anita Eves, PhD, Martin J. Crowder, PhD, "Influence of supplementary vitamins, minerals and essential fatty acids on the antisocial behavior of young adult prisoners—Randomized, placebo-controlled trial," *The British Journal of Psychiatry* 181 (2002), 22–28.

10 University of Southern California, "Nutrition Key to Aggressive Behavior," *USC News Press Release* (November 16, 2004).

11 Neil Ward, "Assessment of chemical factors in relation to child hyperactivity," *Journal of Nutritional and Environmental Medicine* 7, (1997), 333–342.

12 C. Peter W. Bennett and Jonathan Brostoff, "The health of criminals related to behaviour, food, allergy and nutrition: a controlled study of 100 persistent young offenders," *Journal of Nutritional and Environmental Medicine* 7 (1997), 359–366; *Crime Times*, "Can Treating Food Allergies Prevent Anti-Social Behavior?" www.crimetimes.org/why.htm

Chapter 19

1 George J Georgiou, PhD, *Curing the Incurable with Holistic Medicine* (Florida: WHS Holdings, Ltd, 2009).

2 Amy S. Holmes, MD, "Metal Metabolism & Autism," *The Healing Center* (Mar. 5, 2002) www.healing-arts.org/children/metal-metabolism.htm.

3 W.J. Walsh, A. Usman, and J. Tarpey, "Disordered Metal Metabolism in a Large Autism Population," *Proceedings of the Amer. Psych. Assn.*; New Research: Abstract NR109, New Orleans, May, 2001.

4 Sameer Elsayed and Kunyan Zhang "Human Infection Caused by *Clostridium hathewayi*," *Emerging Infectious Diseases Journal* 10, no, 11 (2004), 1950–1952.

5 Natasha Campbell-McBride, *Gut and Psychology Syndrome. Natural Treatment for Autism, ADHD/ADD, Dyslexia, Dyspraxia, Depression and Schizophrenia* (2010), excerpted, www.gaps.me/?page_id=20. (accessed 12 Jan. 2013).

6 Sonya Doherty ND, "Yeast, Clostridia and Viruses," http://treatautism.ca/biomedical-treatment/digestion-and-inflammation/yeast-clostridia-and-viruses/; Sydney M. Finegold, et al., "Pyrosequencing study of fecal microflora of autistic and control children," *Anaerobe* 16, no, 4 (2010), 444–453.

7 Shaheen E Lakhan and Annette Kirchgessne, "Gut Inflammation in Chronic Fatigue Syndrome," *Nutrition and Metabolism* 7, no. 1 (2010), 1–10.

8 Dr. Robert Melillo, *Disconnected Kids* (New York: Penguin Group, 2009).

9 Kate Hoffman, Thomas F. Webster, Marc G. Weisskopf, Janice Weinberg, and Verónica M. Vieira1, "Exposure to Polyfluoroalkyl Chemicals and Attention Deficit/Hyperactivity Disorder in U.S. Children 12–15 Years of Age," *Environmental Health Perspectives* 118, no. 121 (2010), 1762–1767.

10 The National Institute of Environmental Health Sciences, "Perfluorinated Chemicals (PFCs)," (Report: Sept. 2012), www.niehs.nih.gov/health/materials/perflourinated_chemicals_508.pdf

11 Kate Hoffman, Thomas F. Webster, Marc G. Weisskopf, Janice Weinberg, and Verónica M. Vieira1, "Exposure to Polyfluoroalkyl Chemicals and Attention Deficit/Hyperactivity Disorder in U.S. Children 12–15 Years of Age," *Environmental Health Perspectives* 118, no. 121 (2010), 1762–1767.

12 Natural Defenses Resource Council "Our Children at Risk: The Five Worst Environmental Threats to Their Health: Pesticides," (1997), www.nrdc.org/health/kids/ocar/chap5.asp

13 Cho SC, Kim Y, Shin MS, Yoo HJ, Kim JW, Yang YH, Kim HW, Bhang SY, Hong YC, "Phthalates

exposure and attention-deficit/hyperactivity disorder in school-age children," *Biology Psychiatry* 15 no. 66 (2009), 958–963.

14 Hong YC, Kim JW, Park EJ, Shin MS, Kim BN, Yoo HJ, Cho IH, Bhang SY, Cho SC, "Biphenol A in relation to behavior and learning of school-age children," *Journal of Child Psychology Psychiatry* 54, no. 8 (2013), 890–899.

15 Lee DH, Jacobs DR and Porta M, "Association of serum concentrations of persistent organic pollutants with the prevalence of learning disability and attention deficit disorder," *Journal of Epidemiology Community Health* 61, no. 7 (2007), 591–596.

16 Carol Potera, "Mental Health: Molding a Link to Depression," *Environmental Health Perspective* 115, no. 11 (2007), A536.

17 MJ Mendell, "Indoor residential chemical emissions at risk factors for respiratory and allergic effects in children: a review," *Indoor Air* 17, no. 4 (2007), 259–277.

18 David Austin, "An epidemiological analysis of the 'autism as mercury poisoning' hypothesis," *International Journal of Risk and Safety in Medicine* 20 (2008), 135–142.

19 Ethen A. Huff, "How autism is linked to mercury toxicity—and what to do about it, *Natural News* www.naturalnews.com/039328_autism_mercury_toxicity_brain_pathology.html (3 Mar, 2013).

20 Julie Gabriel, *The Green Beauty Guide: Your Essential Resource to Organic and Natural Skin Care, Hair Care, Makeup, and Fragrances* (Deerfield Beach, FL: HCI Books, 2008).

21 A. Alberti, P. Pirrone, M Elia, *et al* "Sulphation deficit in 'low-functioning' autistic children—a pilot study," *Biological Psychiatry* 46, (1999), 420–424.

22 Zeyan Liew, MPH; Beate Ritz, MD, PhD; Cristina Rebordosa, MD, PhD, Pei-Chen Lee, PhD; Jørn Olsen, MD, PhD, "Acetaminophen Use During Pregnancy, Behavioral Problems, and Hyperkinetic Disorders," *JAMA Pediatrics* 168, no. 3 (2014) http://archpcdi .jamanetwork.com/article .aspx?articleid=1833486.

23 Antonio Y. Hardan, Lawrence K. Fung, Robin A. Libove, Tetyana V. Obukhanych, Surekha Nair, "A Randomized Controlled Pilot Trial of Oral N-Acetylcysteine in Children with Autism," *Biology Psychiatry* (2012) 956–961.

24 Jon E. Grant, JD, MD, MPH; Brian L. Odlaug, BA; Suck Won Kim, MD, "N-Acetylcysteine, a Glutamate Modulator, in the Treatment of Trichotillomania: A Double-blind, Placebo-Controlled Study," *Arch Gen Psychiatry* 66, no. 7 (Jul. 2009).

25 Westin A. Price, *Nutrition and Physical Degeneration* (California: Price Pottenger Nutrition, 8th ed. 2008).

Chapter 20

1 Georgia Davis, M.D., "Adrenal Fatigue for Children with Autism," *Autism One*, www.autism one.org/content/adrenal-fatigue-children-autism (accessed 27 Feb. 2013).

2 James Wilson, M.D., *Adrenal Fatigue: The 21st Century Stress Syndrome*. (California: Smart Publications, 2001.)

3 Ibid.

4 Dr. Christian Komor, "Protocols: Depression Self Care Recommendations," OCD Recovery Center www.ocdrecoverycenters.com/about/prot_depression.html; Australian Pumpkin Seed Company, "Pumpkin Seed Health Benefits," www.pumpkinseed.net.au/seedhealth benefits

5 Hoshiko, Sumi, Grether, Judith K.,et. al , "Are thyroid concentrations at birth associated with subsequent autism diagnosis," *Autism Research* 4, no. 6 (Aug. 2011).

6 Hesham M. Elgouhari, MD, "What is the utility of measuring the serum ammonia level in patients with altered mental status? *Cleveland Clinic Journal of Medicine* 76, no. 4 (2009), 252–254.

Chapter 21

1 Gehan A Mostafa and Leila Al-Ayadhi. "Reduced serum concentrations of 25-hydroxy Vitamin D in children with autism: Relation to autoimmunity," *Journal of Neuroinflammation* 9, (2012), 2.

2 Rhonda P. Patrick, PhD and Bruce N. Ames, PhD. "Vitamin D hormone regulates serotonin synthesis. Part 1: relevance for autism," *FASEB Journal* 28, (2014), 1–16.

3 Public Affairs Office, "New Study Linked DHA type of Omega-3 to better nervous system function: Deficiencies may factor into mental illness," *American Psychological Association Press Release,* (December 16, 2009).

4 S. Hirayama, K. Terasawa, R. Rabeler, T. Hirayama, T. Inoue, Y. Tatsumi,M. Purpura, R. Jäge "The effect of phosphatidylserine administration on memory and symptoms of attention-deficit hyperactivity disorder: a randomized, double-blind, placebo-controlled clinical trial," *Journal of Human Nutrition and Dietetics* Research Paper (2013), 1–8.

5 Scott Johnson, "Phosphatidylserine for ADHD," *Live Strong Foundation,* 5 Jul. 2011, www.live strong.com/article/485359-phosphatidylserine-for-adhd/#ixzz2PGB0G1UR (accessed 10 Mar. 2013.

6 Lawrence Wilson, M.D., "Autism: A Case History," *The Center for Development* (2008), http://dr lwilson.com/Articles/AUTISM%20BULLETIN%207–06.htm

7 Ibid.

8 F. Anwar, S, Latif, M. Ashraf and AH Gilani, "Moringa oleifera: a food plant with multiple medicinal uses," *Phytotherapy Research* 1 (2007), 17–25.

9 Anna L. Macready, Orla B. Kennedy, and Laurie T. Butler, "Flavonoids and cognitive function: a review of human randomized controlled trial studies and recommendations for future studies," *Genes Nutrition* 4, no. 4 (2009), 227–242.

Chapter 22

1 Jim Jealous D.O., "Conservations: healing and the natural world," *Alternative therapies in Health and Medicine* 3, no. 1 (1997), 68–75.

2 B. E. Arbuckle, "Cranial birth injuries," *Academy of Applied Osteopathy Yearbook 1945* 76 no. 1 (1945), 63.

3 R. Amin, "Osteopathic Medicine and Autism." March 13, 2006, http://studentdoctor.net/ blogs/omtguru/2006/03/osteopathic-medicine-and-autism.html

4 Blogger, March 13, 2006 (8:45 p.m.), "Osteopathic Medicine and Autism," http://omtommguru .blogspot.com/2006/03/osteopathic-medicine-and-autism.html (accessed 15 Oct. 2012).

5 Chugani, D.O., Musik et al, "Altered serotonin synthesis in the dentatothalamococrtical pathway in autistic boys," *Annals of Neurology* 42, no.10 (1997), 666–669.

6 DeLong, G.R., "Autism: new data suggesting new hypothesis: views and reviews," *Neurology* 52 (1999), 911–916; I. Rapin, "Autism in search of a home in the brain," *Neurology* 52 (1999), 902–904.

7 Frymann, V.M., R.E. Carney, et al, "Effect of Osteopathic Medical Management on Neurologic Development in Children," *Journal of the American Osteopathic Association* 92, no. 6 (1992), 729–744.

8 Erin L. Elster, D.C., "Upper Cervical Chiropractic Care for a Nine-Year Old Male with Tourette Syndrome, Attention Deficit Hyperactivity Disorder, Depression, Asthma, Insomnia, and Headaches: A Case Report," *Chiropractors Association,* 12 Jul. 2003, 1–11.

9 Hemat Allam, Nirvana Gamal Eldine, and Ghada Helmy, "Scalp Acupuncture Effect on Language Development in Children with Autism: A Pilot Study," *Journal of Alternative and Complementary Medicine* 14, no, 2 (2008), 109–114; DK, Cheuk, V Wong, WX Chen, "Acupuncture for autism spectrum disorders," *Department of Pediatrics and Adolescent Medicine, The University of Hong Kong Cochrane Database System Review* 9 (2011).

10 Xiang Chen, Xiao T. Wang, Zhen Zhang, Victor Kang, Barbie Zimmerman-Bier, "Acupuncture for the Treatment of Autism Spectrum Disorders," *Evidence Based Complementary Alternative Medicine*, www.ncbi.nlm.nih.gov/pmc/articles/PMC3235695/ (2011).

11 Devi S. Nambudripad, M.D., D.C., L.Ac., Ph.D., *Say Good-bye to Allergy-related Autism*, (Illinois: Delta Publishing, 2006).

12 Jacob Teitelbaum, MD; Devi S. Nambudripad, MD, PhD, DC, et al, "Improving communication skills with Allergy-related Autism Using Nambudripad's Allergy Elimination Techniques: A Pilot Study," *Journal of Integrative Medicine* 10, no. 5 (Oct/Nov. 2011), 36–43.

13 Brady Vincent and Dayne Bonzo, "Biomedical Analyses of a Holistic Peanut Allergy Treatment: NAET," *Medical Laboratory Sciences Weber State University, Utah* (2 Apr. 2011), 956–971.

14 Devi S. Nambudripad, M.D., D.C., L.Ac., Ph.D., *Say Good-bye to Allergy-related Autism* (Illinois: Delta Publishing, 2006), 180.

15 Natalie Sinn, Dr. Janet Bryan and Dr. Carlene Wilson, "Fish Oil Wins Over Children with ADHD," University of South Australia—*CSIRO Human Nutrition*, http://w3.unisa.edu.au/ researcher/ issue/2006january/story4.asp

16 Julie Behling-Hovdal, "Essential Oils for Brain Health" (August 13, 2012), www.essential survival.com.

17 Terry S. Friedmann, M.D., ABHM, "Attention Deficit and Hyperactivity Disorder (ADHD)," www.oilsofthegods.com/www.oilsofthegods.com/ADHD_RESEARCH.html

18 Carolyn L. Mein, *Releasing Emotional Patterns with Essential Oils* (California: Vision Ware Press, revised 2011).

19 Vani Hari, "Do You Know What's Really in Your Tea." *Food Babe*, 21 Aug. 2013.

Chapter 23

1 Gerry Leisman, Raed Mualem and Calixto Machado, "The integration of the neurosciences, child public health, and education practice: hemisphere-specific remediation strategies as a discipline partnered rehabilitation tool in ADD/ADHD," *Frontiers in Public Health* 1, no. 22 (2013).

2 Dr. Robert Melillo, *Disconnected Kids* (New York: Penguin Group, 2009), 7; Dr. Robert Melillo, *Autism: The Scientific Truth about Preventing, Diagnosing, and Treating Autism Spectrum Disorders—and What Parents Can Do Now* (New York: Penguin Group, 2013).

3 Rebecca Claire, Jan Martin and Tressie Taylor, *Fight Autism and Win: Biomedical Treatments That Work* (Illinois: JRT Publishing, 2012).

4 Sally Goddard, *Reflexes, Learning and Behavior: A Window into the Child's Mind: A Non-Invasive Approach to Solving Learning & Behavior Problems* (Oregon: Fern Ridge Press, 2005).

5 Daniel A Rossignol, Lanier W Rossignol, Scott Smith, Cindy Schneider, Sally Logerquist, Anju Usman, Jim Neubrander, Eric M Madren, Gregg Hintz, Barry Grushkin and Elizabeth A Mumper, "Hyperbaric treatment for children with autism: a multicenter, randomized, double-blind, controlled trial," *BMC Pediatrics* 9, no. 21 (2009); Collet, J.P., Vanasse, M., Marois, P., Amar, M., Goldberg, J., Lambert, J. et al. "Hyperbaric oxygen for children with cerebral palsy: A randomized multicentre trial." *The Lancet* 357, no. 9273 (2001), 582–586.

6 Monastra, VJ., Lynn, S., Linden, M., Lubar, JF., Gruzelier, J., LaVaque, TJ., "Electroencephalographic biofeedback in the treatment of attention-deficit/hyperactivity disorder," *Applied Psychophysiology and Biofeedback* 30, no. 2 (2005), 95–114.

7 A, Sajjad Haghshenasb, Reza Rostami,"Rehabilitation in Autism Spectrum Disorder (ASD): A Mixture of Neurofeedback Training and Auditory Integration Training (AIT)," *Procedia—Social and Behavioral Sciences* 30 (2011) 611–614.

8 Bahrami F, Movahedi A, Marandi SM, Abedi A, "Kata techniques training consistently decreases stereotypy in children with autism spectrum disorder," *Research in Developmental Disabilities* 33, no. 4 (2012), 1183–1193.

Chapter 24

1 Pål Surén, MD, MPH; Christine Roth, MSc; Michaeline Bresnahan, PhD; Margaretha Haugen, PhD; Mady Hornig, MD; Deborah Hirtz, MD; Kari Kveim Lie, MD; W. Ian Lipkin, MD; Per Magnus, MD, PhD; Ted Reichborn-Kjennerud, MD, PhD; Synnve Schjølberg, MSc; George Davey Smith, MD, DSc; Anne-Siri Øyen, PhD; Ezra Susser, MD, DrPH; Camilla Stoltenberg, MD, PhD, "Association Between Maternal Use of Medication Supplements and Risk of Autism Spectrum Disorders in Children," *Journal of the American Medical Association* 309, no.6 (2013), 570–577.

2 Christine Roth, MSc, ClinPsyD; Per Magnus, MD, PhD; Synnve Schjølberg, MSc, ClinPsyD; Camilla Stoltenberg, MD, PhD; Pål Surén, MD, MPH; Ian W. McKeague, PhD; George Davey Smith, MD, DSc; Ted Reichborn-Kjennerud, MD, PhD; Ezra Susser, MD, DrPH, "Folic Acid Supplements in Pregnancy and Severe Language Delay in Children," *Journal of the American Medical Association* 306, no.14 (2011), 1566–1573.

3 Allison Aubrey, "Are Organic Tomatoes Better?" (29 Mar, 2008) *NPR News*, www.npr.org/ templates/story/story.php?storyId=90914182

4 Leah Zerbe, "Pesticides in Food Linked to ADHD in Kids," *Rodale News*, www.rodale .com/ pesticides-and-food?page=0,0 (accessed 5 May, 2013).

5 Mike Adams, "'Organic' from China exposed: The shocking truth about 'organic' foods grown in the world's worst environmental cesspool," *NaturalNews.com* (21 Feb. 2013) www.naturalnews .com/039195_organic_foods_china_pollution_nightmare.html#ixzz2hQV9uTXg (accessed 21 Feb. 2013)

6 Michael K. Georgiff, "Nutrition and the developing brain: nutrient priorities and measurement," *American Journal of Clinical Nutrition* 85, no. 2 (2007), 6145–6205.

Chapter 25

1 Hy; Lu C, Barr DB, Pearson MA, Waller LA, "Dietary Intake and Its Contribution to Longitudinal Organophorus Pesticide in Urban/Suburban Children," *Environmental Health Perspectives* 116, no. 4, (April 2008).

2 Joanne K. Tobacman, "Review of Harmful Gastrointestinal Effects of Carrageenan in Animal Experiments." *College of Medicine, University of Iowa—Environmental Health Perspectives* 109, no. 10 (2001), 983–994.

Chapter 26

1 Kelly Dorfman, MS, LND, *Cure Your Child with Food: The Hidden Connection Between Nutrition and Childhood Ailments* (New York: Workman Publishing, reprint 2013).

2 Counsel on School Health, "The Crucial Role of Recess in School," *Journal of American Academy of Pediatrics* 131, no. 1 (2013), 183–188.

3 Dr. David L. Katz, M.D. MPH, FACPM, FACP, "Recess Not Ritalin," http://bigthink.com/ users/davidkatz (accessed 12 Sept. 2013).

4 Amika Singh, PhD; Léonie Uijtdewilligen, MSc; Jos W. R. Twisk, PhD; Willem van Mechelen, PhD, MD; Mai J. M. Chinapaw, PhD "Physical Activity and Performance at School: A Systematic Review of the Literature Including a Methodological Quality Assessment" *JAMA Pediatrics* 166, no. 1 (2012), 49–55.

5 Division of Sleep Medicine, "Importance of Sleep: 6 Reasons not to scrimp on sleep," *Harvard Medical Health Publications*, (Jan. 2006).

Chapter 29

1 Beth Lambert and Victoria Kobliner, MS, RD, *A Compromised Generation—The Epidemic of Illness in America's Children* (USA: Sentient Publishing, 2010), 24.

2 National Center for Immunization and Respiratory Diseases "State Vaccination Requirements," *CDC (Centers for Disease Control and Prevention)* Child and Adolescent Immunization Schedules www.cdc.gov/vaccines/vac-gen/laws/state-reqs.htm (accessed 12 Dec. 2012).

3 Markus Heinze, *VACCeptable Injuries: Increasing Childhood Diseases & Developmental Disorders* (CreateSpace Independent Publishing Platform, 2012).

4 Sherri J. Tenpenny, DO, *Saying No To Vaccines: A Resource Guide for All Ages* (Ohio: NMA Media Press, 2008).

5 Kate Birch, RS Hom (NA) and Cilla Whatcott, HD (RHom), *The Solution, Homeoprophylaxis: The Vaccine Alternative* (CreateSpace Independent Publishing Platform, 2012).

6 R. Webster Kehr, *The War Between Orthodox Medicine and Alternative Medicine* (eBook 2003), www.bibliotecapleyades.net/ciencia/ciencia_industrybigpharma42.htm (accessed 10 Nov. 2012).

7 Mike Adams, "Health Insurance Companies Invest Billions in Fast Food Chains." *NaturalNews*, www.naturalnews.com/028602_health_insurance_fast_food.html (accessed 10 June 2013).

Appendix A

1 Epilepsy Foundation: Colorado, "The Use of Medical Marijuana for the Treatment of Epilepsy," www.epilepsycolorado.org/index.php?s=10784&item=5985

2 UCIrvine News, "Boosting natural marijuana-like brain chemicals treats fragile X syndrome symptoms," University of California, Irvine, Press Release (September 25, 2012).

3 Patricia A. Murphy, *Treating Epilepsy Naturally: A Guide to Alternative and Adjunct Therapies* (New York: McGraw-Hill, 2001).

4 Esther Thelen, *A Dynamics Systems Approach to the Development of Cognition and Action* 4th ed. (Massachusetts: A Bradford Book/MIT Press, 1996, 4th ed.).

5 Danica Mamlet "Autism and Toilet Training," www.behavioradvisor.com/Autism&Toileting.html (accessed 19 Jan, 2013).

Glossary

1 Sidney V. Haas, "Value of the banana in the treatment of celiac disease," *American Journal of Diseases of Children* 28, no. 421 (1924), 421–437.

2 Barbara C. Olendzki, R.D., M.P.H., L.D.N., et al., "Pilot Testing a Novel Treatment for Inflammatory Bowel Disease," (UMASS Medical Center: Clinical and Translational Science Research Retreat, May. 2011) http://works.bepress.com/barbara_olendzki/46/ (accessed 14 May 2013).

3 Yunsheng Ma, MD, PhD, "A simple dietary message to improve dietary quality for metabolic syndrome," (UMASS Medical Center: Clinical Research Project, June, 2009—ongoing) www.umassmed.edu/Content.aspx?id=138546&linkidentifier=id&itemid=138546 (accessed 14 May 2013).

Index

About the Author

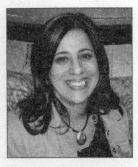

Jennifer Giustra-Kozek, LPC, NCC, has a master's degree in Community Counseling and a bachelor's degree in English/Criminal Justice from Western Connecticut State University. She is an accomplished licensed psychotherapist in private practice. She has more than fifteen years of clinical experience treating clients with an array of health disorders, including Asperger's, depression, anxiety, OCD, and ADHD.

Jennifer was a therapist at Silver Hill Hospital in New Canaan, Connecticut, treating victims and families after 9/11. In addition, she worked in the acute care and substance abuse unit of this hospital, treating adolescents as well as young adults. She began her private practice shortly thereafter, in 2002.

Once Jennifer began treating first responders and family members after the massacre at Sandy Hook Elementary School—perpetrated by a young man who was diagnosed with a mental illness associated with autism spectrum disorders—she knew she needed to get the message out that there were more natural and safe ways to treat these disorders.

Jennifer began consulting and blogging with thousands of moms through social media to teach them about alternative and natural solutions for treating autism spectrum disorders. Since the creation of her page on Facebook called "Healing ADHD & Asperger's Without Hurting," she has amassed a following of over 100,000 weekly visitors who turn to her for guidance and support, as they desperately search for help for their children.